CRC SERIES IN AGING

Editors-in-Chief

Richard C. Adelman, Ph.D.   George S. Roth, Ph.D.

VOLUMES AND VOLUME EDITORS

HANDBOOK OF BIOCHEMISTRY IN AGING
James Florini, Ph.D.
Department of Biology
Syracuse University
Syracuse, New York

HANDBOOK OF IMMUNOLOGY IN AGING
Marguerite M. B. Kay, M.D. and Takashi Makinodan, Ph.D.
Geriatric Research Education and Clinical Center
V.A. Wadsworth Medical Center
Los Angeles, California

SENESCENCE IN PLANTS
Kenneth V. Thimann, Ph.D.
The Thimann Laboratories
University of California
Santa Cruz, California

ALCOHOLISM AND AGING: ADVANCES IN RESEARCH
W. Gibson Wood, Ph.D.
Clinical Research Psychologist
Geriatric Research, Education, and Clinical
  Center
V.A. Medical Center
St. Louis, Missouri
Merrill F. Elias, Ph.D.
Professor of Psychology
University of Maine at Orono
Orono, Maine

TESTING THE THEORIES OF AGING
Richard C. Adelman, Ph.D.
Director
Institute of Gerontology
Professor of Biological Chemistry
University of Michigan
Ann Arbor, Michigan
George S. Roth, Ph.D.
Research Biochemist
Gerontology Research Center
National Institute on Aging
Baltimore City Hospitals
Baltimore, Maryland

HANDBOOK OF PHYSIOLOGY IN AGING
Edward J. Masoro, Ph.D.
Department of Physiology
University of Texas Health Science Center
San Antonio, Texas

IMMUNOLOGICAL TECHNIQUES APPLIED TO AGING RESEARCH
William H. Adler, M.D. and Albert A. Nordin, Ph.D.
Gerontology Research Center
National Institute on Aging
Baltimore City Hospitals
Baltimore, Maryland

CURRENT TRENDS IN MORPHOLOGICAL TECHNIQUES
John E. Johnson, Jr., Ph.D.
Gerontology Research Center
National Institute on Aging
Baltimore City Hospitals
Baltimore, Maryland

NUTRITIONAL APPROACHES TO AGING RESEARCH
Gairdner B. Moment, Ph.D.
Professor Emeritus of Biology
Goucher College
Guest Scientist
Gerontology Research Center
National Institute on Aging
Baltimore, Maryland

ENDOCRINE AND NEUROENDOCRINE MECHANISMS OF AGING
Richard C. Adelman, Ph.D.
Director
Institute of Gerontology
Professor of Biological Chemistry
University of Michigan
Ann Arbor, Michigan
George S. Roth, Ph.D.
Research Biochemist
Gerontology Research Center
National Institute on Aging
Baltimore City Hospitals
Baltimore, Maryland

Additional topics to be covered in this series include Cell Biology of Aging, Microbiology of Aging, Pharmacology of Aging, Evolution and Genetics, Animal Models for Aging Research, Detection of Altered Proteins, Insect Models, and Lower Invertebrate Models.

CRC Handbook on Pharmacology of Aging

Editors

Paula B. Goldberg, Ph.D.

Assistant Professor
Department of Pharmacology
The Medical College of Pennsylvania
Philadelphia, Pennsylvania

Jay Roberts, Ph.D.

Professor and Chairman
Department of Pharmacology
The Medical College of Pennsylvania
Philadelphia, Pennsylvania

CRC Series in Aging

Editors-in-Chief

Richard C. Adelman, Ph.D.

Director
Institute of Gerontology
Professor of Biological Chemistry
University of Michigan
Ann Arbor, Michigan

George S. Roth, Ph.D.

Research Chemist
Gerontology Research Center
National Institute on Aging
Baltimore City Hospitals
Baltimore, Maryland

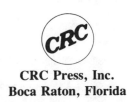

CRC Press, Inc.
Boca Raton, Florida

Library of Congress Cataloging in Publication Data (Revised)
Main entry under title:

Handbook on pharmacology of aging.

(CRC series in aging)
Bibliography: p.
Includes index.
1. Geriatric pharmacology. I. Goldberg, Paula B.
II. Roberts, Jay. III. Series. [DNLM: 1. Drug therapy—In old age—Handbook. 2. Aging—Drug effects—Handbooks. WT 100 H2335]
RC953.7.H36 1983   615.5'8'0880565   82-17829
ISBN-0-8493-3145-5

Direct all inquiries to CRC Press, Inc., 2000 Corporate Blvd., N.W., Boca Raton, Florida, 33431.

© 1983 by CRC Press, Inc.

International Standard Book Number 0-8493-3145-5

Library of Congress Card Number 82-17829
Printed in the United States

EDITORS-IN-CHIEF

Richard C. Adelman, Ph.D., is currently Director of the Institute of Gerontology at the University of Michigan, Ann Arbor, as well as Professor of Biological Chemistry in the Medical School. An active gerontologist for more than 10 years, he has achieved international prominence as a researcher, educator, and administrator. These accomplishments span a broad spectrum of activities ranging from the traditional disciplinary interests of the research biologist to the advocacy, implementation, and administration of multidisciplinary issues of public policy of concern to elderly people. He is the author and/or editor of more than 95 publications, including original research papers in refereed journals, review chapters, and books. His research efforts have been supported by grants from the National Institutes of Health for the past 13 consecutive years, and he continues to serve as an invited speaker at seminar programs, symposiums, and workshops all over the world. He is the recipient of the IntraScience Research Foundation Medalist Award, an annual research prize awarded by peer evaluation for major advances in newly emerging areas of the life sciences; and the recipient of an Established Investigatorship of the American Heart Association.

Dr. Adelman serves on the editorial boards of the *Journal of Gerontology, Mechanisms of Ageing and Development,* and *Gerontological Abstracts.* He chaired a subcommittee of the National Academy of Sciences Committee on Animal Models for Aging Research. As an active Fellow of the Gerontological Society, he was Chairman of the Biological Sciences section; a past Chairman of the Society Public Policy Committee; and is currently Chairman of the Research, Education and Practice Committee. He serves on National Advisory Committees which impact on diverse key issues dealing with the elderly, including a 4-year appointment as member of the NIH Study Section on Pathobiological Chemistry; the Executive Committee of the Health Resources Administration Project on publication of the recent edition of *Working with Older People — A Guide to Practice;* and a 4-year appointment on the Veterans Administration Advisory Council for Geriatrics and Gerontology.

George S. Roth, Ph.D., is a research chemist with the Gerontology Research Center of the National Institute on Aging in Baltimore, Md., where he has been affiliated since 1972. Dr. Roth received his B.S. in Biology from Villanova University in 1968 and his Ph.D. in Microbiology from Temple University School of Medicine in 1971. He received postdoctoral training in Biochemistry at the Fels Research Institute in Philadelphia, Pa. Dr. Roth has also been associated with the graduate schools of Georgetown University and George Washington University where he has sponsored two Ph.D. students.

He has published more than 70 papers in the area of aging and hormone/neurotransmitter action, and has lectured, organized meetings, and chaired sessions throughout the world on this subject.

Dr. Roth's other activities include fellowship in the Gerontological Society of America, where he has served in numerous capacities, including chairmanship of the 1979 midyear conference on "Functional Status and Aging." He is presently Chairman of the Biological Sciences Section and a Vice President of the Society. He has twice been selected as an exchange scientist by the National Academy of Sciences and in this capacity has established liaisons with gerontologists, endocrinologists, and biochemists in several Eastern European countries. Dr. Roth serves as an editor of *Neurobiology of Aging* and is a frequent reviewer for many other journals including *Mechanisms in Aging and Development, Life Sciences, The Journal of Gerontology, Science* and *Endocrinology.* He also serves as a grant reviewer for several funding agencies including the National Science Foundation. In 1981 Dr. Roth was awarded the Annual Research Award of the American Aging Association.

THE EDITORS

Paula Bursztyn Goldberg, Ph.D., is Assistant Professor of Pharmacology at the Medical College of Pennsylvania (MCP).

Dr. Goldberg received a B.S. degree in Pharmacy from the Columbia University College of Pharmacy (1962); a Ph.D. degree in Pharmacology from the Downstate Medical Center, State University of New York (1968); and postdoctoral training in muscle electrophysiology at the College of Physicians and Surgeons of Columbia University (1968) and at the Downstate Medical Center (1971 to 1972) and in pharmacogerontology at MCP (1972 to 1973).

Prior to completing her postdoctoral training, Dr. Goldberg assumed a Visiting Professorship at the School of Pharmacy of the University of Costa Rica (1969), where she developed a curriculum in pharmacology. Concurrent with her appointments at MCP, she has been Adjunct Clinical Instructor at the School of Pharmacy of Temple University (1975 to 1976), Adjunct Associate Professor in the Department of Biological Sciences of Drexel University (1976 to 1977), Consultant on matters relating to pharmacology and aging for the National Institute on Aging as well as other organizations, and a columnist for the publications, *"Geriatric Nursing."*

Dr. Goldberg is a member of several prestigious professional societies, among them the American Society for Pharmacology and Experimental Therapeutics, the Gerontological Society of America, American Federation for Clinical Research, Society for Experimental Biology and Medicine, New York Academy of Science, Physiological Society of Philadelphia, American Heart Association, and the honor societies, Sigma Xi and Rho Chi. In recognition of her contributions to research, curriculum development, and other activities in the area of aging, she has been elected a Fellow of the Gerontological Society of America. Prior distinction in the areas of pharmacy and pharmacology led to recognition through Rho Chi Awards, the J. C. Olshansky Gold Medal and the L. Leiterman Gold Medal from the Columbia University College of Pharmacy. Among her activities are included service on the Finance Committee of the Gerontological Society of America, Public Information Committee of the American Society for Pharmacology and Experimental Therapeutics, the Biomedical Research Committee of the Philadelphia Geriatric Center, and the Committee on Animal Models for Research on Aging of the Institute of Laboratory Animal Resources.

Dr. Goldberg's research interests center around pharmacogerontology and the cardiovascular system, relating especially to mechanisms of aging at the autonomic/cardiac neuroeffector junction and at the cardiac plasma membrane and receptor levels, as can be elucidated with the use of pharmacological probes. Her research in this area has been funded through the National Institute on Aging and through local chapters of the American Heart Association. Her expertise is recognized on the national and international scene so that she is a frequent contributor to scientific meetings, symposia, and review publications.

Jay Roberts, Ph.D., is Professor and Chairman of Pharmacology at the Medical College of Pennsylvania (MCP).

Dr. Roberts initiated his graduate studies in pharmacology at Cornell University Medical College in 1949. He received his Ph.D. in 1953. He taught pharmacology to medical and graduate students and developed his research programs in cardiovascular pharmacology at Cornell until he left to assume a Professorship of Pharmacology at the University of Pittsburgh School of Medicine. He continued his activities in cardiovascular and autonomic pharmacology and was selected to serve on the Pharmacology Study Section. He was appointed Professor and Chairman of Pharmacology at MCP in 1970. His interest in aging developed in the early 1970s and in recognition of his contribution to the field of aging, he was elected a Fellow of the Gerontological Society of America. He is also a Fellow of the College of Physicians of Philadelphia, of the American College of Cardiology, and of the American

College of Clinical Pharmacology. His interests in the effect of age on drug action has resulted in contributions to symposia on the biology of aging and numerous publications.

He has helped organize several symposia on various topics on aging and is a member of the organizing committee of the Philadelphia Symposium on Aging. He has served as a consultant to the National Institutes on Aging and was recently elected Chairman of the Geriatrics Division of the Committee of Revision to the U.S. Pharmacopeia Convention. He is a member of the most prestigious societies in his field of expertise and has served as President of the Cardiac Muscle Society.

He has served on many editorial boards of various pharmacology journals including *Journal of Pharmacology and Experimental Therapeutics, Journal of Cardiovascular Pharmacology*, and *Journal of Clinical Pharmacology*. He is also a member of the editorial board of the *Journal of Gerontology*. Dr. Roberts has published extensively in the field of cardiovascular and autonomic pharmacology and in the area of the effects of aging on drug action. His publication titles number over 170. His interests are wide and his contributions are highly regarded. He is recognized as an educator, teacher, and researcher.

CONTRIBUTORS

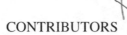

Steven I. Baskin, Pharm.D., Ph.D.
Team Leader
Cardiac Pathophysiology
U.S. Army Medical Research Institute of
  Chemical Defense
Aberdeen Proving Ground, Maryland

Barbara S. Beckman, Ph.D.
Assistant Professor
Department of Pharmacology
Tulane University
School of Medicine
New Orleans, Louisiana

C. Paul Bianchi, Ph.D.
Professor and Chairman
Department of Pharmacology
Jefferson Medical College
Thomas Jefferson University
Philadelphia, Pennsylvania

Kitt Booher
Research Assistant
Department of Pharmacology
Georgetown University
Schools of Medicine and Dentistry
Washington, D.C.

Peter Cervoni, Ph.D.
Head, Cardiovascular Biological Research
Medical Research Division
American Cyanamid Company
Pearl River, New York

Peter S. Chan, Ph.D.
Group Leader
Department of Cardiovascular Biological
  Research
Medical Research Division
American Cyanamid Company
Pearl River, New York

James W. Fisher, Ph.D.
Professor and Chairman
Department of Pharmacology
Tulane University
School of Medicine
New Orleans, Louisiana

Paula B. Goldberg, Ph.D.
Assistant Professor
Department of Pharmacology
The Medical College of Pennsylvania
Philadelphia, Pennsylvania

Allan H. Goldfarb, Ph.D.
Assistant Professor
Exercise Science Laboratory
University of Maryland
College Park, Maryland

Frederick J. Goldstein, Ph.D.
Professor
Department of Pharmacology and
  Toxicology
Philadelphia College of Pharmacy and
  Science
Philadelphia, Pennsylvania

Akira Horita, Ph.D.
Professor
Department of Pharmacology
                            and
Adjunct Professor
Department of Psychiatry andBehavioral
  Sciences
University of Washington Medical School
Seattle, Washington

Rosaline R. Joseph, M.D.
Director, Hematology/Oncology
Professor of Medicine
Medical College of Pennsylvania
Philadelphia, Pennsylvania

Donald Kaye, M.D.
Professor and Chairman
Department of Medicine
The Medical College of Pennsylvania
Philadelphia, Pennsylvania

**Nallanna Lakshminarayanaiah, Ph.D.,
  D.Sc.**
Professor
Department of Pharmacology
Jefferson Medical College
Thomas Jefferson University
Philadelphia, Pennsylvania

David Richey, Ph.D.
Scientific Director
New Compound Evaluation and Licensing
Smith Kline & French Laboratories
Philadelphia, Pennsylvania

Jay Roberts, Ph.D.
Professor and Chairman
Department of Pharmacology
The Medical College of Pennsylvania
Philadelphia, Pennsylvania

G. Victor Rossi, Ph.D.
Chairman
Department of Pharmacology and
　Toxicology
　　　　　　and
Associate Dean
Research and Graduate Studies
Philadelphia College of Pharmacy and
　Science
Philadelphia, Pennsylvania

Jerome Santoro, M.D.
Clinical Assistant Professor
Department of Medicine
Medical College of Pennsylvania
Philadelphia, Pennsylvania

Frank G. Standaert, M.D.
Professor and Chairman
Department of Pharmacology
Georgetown University
Schools of Medicine and Dentistry
Washington, D.C.

Richard C. Veith, M.D.
Clinical Investigator
Geriatric Research, Education, and Clini-
　cal Center
Seattle Veterans Administration Medical
　Center
　　　　　　and
Associate Professor
Department of Psychiatry and Behavioral
　Sciences
University of Washington
School of Medicine
Seattle, Washington

DEDICATION

To my wife, Marion, and my children, Hunt and Kathy, and to my departed mother and father, Evelyn and Harry, without whose encouragement, love and guidance, I would not be what I am.

Jay Roberts

To my children, Philip and the two Judys, and my parents, Henia and Hersz Bursztyn, for their generous love, support and patient understanding.

Paula Bursztyn Goldberg

TABLE OF CONTENTS

General Pharmacology

INTRODUCTION

Paula B. Goldberg

The pharmacological aspects of aging have only recently come to the foreground as an area requiring investigation and attention. Most likely this is due to the realization that as normal function declines with age, as homeostatic and adaptive capacities decline with age, and as the incidence of diseases increases with age, the elderly members in our society find themselves major consumers of drugs. As a result, they also find themselves in difficulties stemming from overmedication and drug misuse. Problems surrounding drug use or misuse by the elderly result from a sparse knowledge of the manner in which the elderly respond to drugs that may be different from the manner in which the very young and adults respond to drugs. Upon approaching drug compendia and learned texts of pharmacology, one immediately becomes impressed by the paucity of information regarding drug action and drug use in geriatric populations.

In general, when mechanisms of drug action are investigated, be it in laboratory animals or in man, usually it is done in only one age group or in as homogeneous an age group as possible. The same can be said for studies on drug toxicity and drug disposition. As pertains to studies in animals, age is not the usual basis for animal selection nor the characteristic reported in the literature. Rather, animals are selected on the basis of weight. Depending on the species used and the weight range selected, the ages of the individual animals may represent a very narrow or a very wide range. For example, in using rats as the animal model, the following considerations may apply. Sprague-Dawley rats, weighing between 200 and 300 g, because of their obesity, represent very young animals, that are relatively close in age. On the other hand, Fischer 344 rats or Wistar rats, which are much leaner, weighing between 200 and 300 g, represent adult animals whose ages may vary between perhaps 4 and 12 months. Using dogs as an animal model, without selecting for strain, the difficulties also become apparent. A 6 to 10 kg dog may be an old small strain or a very young large strain. Thus, experimentation in animals using weight as a criterion may mask significant results, or conversely, bring out significance where there might not be any. Furthermore, these considerations may apply to cases of divergent results obtained from different laboratories. But most important, studies on mechanisms of drug action, drug toxicity, and drug disposition do not take into consideration the age factor at all, so there is very little information on differences or similarities in relation to age.

With respect to drug trials in humans, the situation is also one of lack of information in older populations. Because of practical and ethical considerations, drugs are not commonly tested in old subjects or patients. The usual volunteer is a subject or patient between 18 and 40 years of age, and most likely male. Thus, drug information gathered in such an "average" population may be inappropriate for application in other, younger or older populations. It comes as no surprise then, that elderly patients encounter greater difficulty from drug use than younger adults.

Aside from the practical, clinical need for information, pharmacological aspects of aging are being delved into because of their utility in elucidating basic mechanisms of aging. This is accomplished through experimentation with drugs whose basic mechanism of action at the cellular and molecular level is relatively well understood. By studying the effects of such drugs in a model of aging over a wide range of ages, differences in drug action with age can help dissect the fundamental change that occurs in that model. For example, autonomic agonists and antagonists, acting at neuroeffector junctions, can be used to uncover age-related changes in the neural environment and in the postjunctional effectors; enzyme inhibitors and stimulants (e.g., digitalis glycosides, barbiturates) can help uncover age-related changes in different enzyme systems. Thus, pharmacogerontology can play a vital role in unraveling the riddles for aging, while providing a basis for rational therapy and a means for improving the quality of late life.

Because of this perceived growing interest in pharmacological aspects of aging, it was thought appropriate and useful to find out what the pharmacologically relevant data base consists of in this area. Accordingly, work on this volume was undertaken for the purpose of compiling a comprehensive, current, and reliable information source on pharmacology as it relates to aging. It was intended to serve those using aging data in research, in the clinics, for education, for service, and in other related areas.

It is felt that for the most part, the overall objective of this volume was achieved. This was due in great measure to the willingness of the many contributors to participate in this venture: to undertake the task of sifting through the literature and to transform the accumulated bits and pieces of information into a coherent review. However, as work began, it became increasingly clear that not all the original expectations for this volume could be met. This stemmed primarily from the nature of the literature in this area, upon which it is worthwhile to comment at this juncture for the purpose of sharing gained insights.

The first problem encountered was that of literature searching. Even with the help of computer data bases, precise vocabularies, and sophisticated reference librarians, this task was not straightforward. Primarily, the difficulty lies in the linguistics of the term "age". Terms such as "age", "age factors", and "aging" are used in the data bases to index literature on aging not only from birth to death, but also on aging of embryos, on aging during early postnatal development, on aging during maturation, and on aging in late life. A secondary difficulty in regard to searching the literature was that of the possibility of completely overlooking data relevant to aging. It cannot be estimated how much of the literature which contains incidental information on aging is missed because its main focus is on other topics and thus would not be indexed with aging literature at all.

Another disappointment relating to the literature, or rather to the state of the art, is simply the fact that not all areas or drug categories of interest to pharmacology have been researched in relation to aging, be it in humans or in laboratory animals. Although the intention had been to include material in every category of pharmacologic agents, some categories were omitted either because no literature was found or because that which had been found was too fragmentary for review. Thus, the areas covered represent those in which at least a moderate amount of work in relation to aging has been done.

Finally, an observation relating to the quality of aging studies in pharmacology is appropriate. For a study to be meaningful with respect to age factors, many other factors need to be controlled and characterized in the particular system used. For example, whether human or laboratory animal, it is important to describe such factors as gender, environment, nutritional status, breeding status, physiological state, pathological conditions, genetics, and others. All of these factors influence response to drugs, not only age. The literature, however, does not include such information for the most part. Furthermore, age itself is not clearly defined. Thus, weights of animals are sometimes indicated instead of age; or descriptive terms, such as young, adult, old, are used instead of actual ages. This made it difficult to interpret findings. With respect to this volume, because of a lack of uniformity in describing experimental conditions, it precluded tabulation of data in many instances.

The one most gratifying aspect of compiling this volume was the realization that for an area of pharmacology which in the past has received very little attention, a good deal of information is available which can already be put to practical use. This is especially true of what is known regarding changes with age in basic processes involved in drug disposition. It is also true of what is known regarding changes in effector organ responsiveness to certain drugs, especially cardiovascular and central nervous system drugs. However, it is also instructive to note the enormous gaps that exist in our knowledge of changes in drug action with respect to age. This is perhaps more important for it can serve to point towards future directions for research.

PHARMACOKINETICS AND DRUG DISPOSITION

David P. Richey

INTRODUCTION

There are two reasons why the study of pharmacokinetics in an elderly population merits attention. The first is the rather basic assumption that it is worthwhile to study pharmacokinetics in a variety of physiological states in order that we learn better how drugs are handled by the body. The second reason derives from the general recognition that aged patients experience a far greater incidence of adverse drug reactions than do their younger counterparts; it is natural to hope that a better understanding of the pharmacokinetics prevailing in an aged population will help explain the reason for this excess of adverse reactions and thereby provide us with a means to reduce them.

Pharmacologic effects — both the primary pharmacotherapeutic effect and the adverse drug effect — are related to the concentration of a drug at its end organ or site of action. There are examples demonstrating that the essential sensitivity of older subjects to a given drug concentration is altered in the elderly,[1,2] but more commonly and probably more importantly, there exist functional changes in the older subjects' drug handling mechanisms. There are pharmacokinetic data to illustrate this latter situation, which will be presented as this discussion proceeds.

PHYSIOLOGIC CHANGES IN THE ELDERLY

In addition to the overt and external changes that accompany aging, there are a number of other important changes in organ and tissue structure and function which occur and are relevant to the way the body handles drugs. It warrants mentioning also that these important changes are not simply exerted abruptly sometime in the 5th or 6th decade; instead, most of them begin in the 3rd or 4th decade and only reach functional significance at a more advanced age.

One notable physiologic change is the relative increase of body fat content in older people. In addition, there is a decrease in the amount of body water. The net effect of these two alterations is that relatively polar drugs and their metabolites are less well distributed throughout the body in older people; the obverse of this is that the highly lipid-soluble drugs tend to be better distributed and to reside longer in subjects with greater-than-average fatty tissue. Such age-related changes can be reflected in the apparent volume of distribution of a drug.

Another and one of the most important age-related physiologic changes that occurs is a decrease in cardiac output. With an onset in the 3rd decade, the cardiac output decrement is roughly 1%/year.[3] By age 60, the total cardiac output is reduced roughly 30%. Perfusion is not reduced by a uniform amount in all parts of the body, however.[4] Myocardial blood flow is reduced only very slightly and cerebral blood flow is down roughly 10 to 20%. The maintenance of good blood flow to these areas is accomplished at the expense of splanchnic blood flow, however, which decreases at the rate of roughly 1.5%/year as cardiac output decreases. This means that by age 60, renal blood flow has been reduced by 40 or 50%. As a result, a comparable reduction occurs in the glomerular filtration rate and in creatinine clearance; blood urea nitrogen is thereby increased 40 to 50%. Reduced blood flow in the intestine, liver, and kidneys is often manifested in altered handling of drugs by these tissues, namely in drug absorption, metabolism, and excretion.

Absorption

The absorption of drugs has not been studied as often or in as much detail as have other aspects of drug handling.[5] Since most drugs are absorbed by passive diffusion through the intestinal wall, they may be expected to behave differently than actively transported substances such as glucose or calcium, and a case has been made that reduced intestinal blood flow could indeed have an effect on the absorption of drugs.[6] Fortunately, such an effect would be expected to be greater for those compounds that are already most rapidly absorbed and, therefore, is probably not of much practical importance. An age-related decrease in gastric acid secretion has been suggested to mitigate against drug absorption but there is no evidence for this. The most reasonable view at the present time is that defects in drug absorption are not a clinically important aspect of drug therapy in the elderly.

Metabolism

Most drugs are not excreted in their original intact structure but are metabolized to more easily excreted, generally more polar, forms. The bulk of this metabolism occurs in the liver. Early studies in rats showed that mature animals lose their drug metabolizing capability with increasing age, and that this decrease results in increased serum levels of administered drugs and a corresponding increase in the intensity or duration of the effects of the drugs.[7,8] Although good evidence of an age-related decrease in liver activity is lacking for man, there is ample evidence of a greatly altered handling of many drugs known to be extensively metabolized in man prior to their excretion. Reduced hepatic activity in older patients may be manifested either in a reduced first pass effect (on newly absorbed drug entering via the portal vein) or in a lower extraction and metabolism of circulating drug. A number of review articles have described these reports and Table 1 presents these data.[9-11]

Excretion

In addition to many drug metabolites, a number of compounds are excreted unchanged through the kidneys. We have already mentioned the decreased renal activity due to reduced renal blood flow in older subjects. Most polar metabolites are cleared predominantly by simple glomerular filtration and cannot be reabsorbed in the renal tubule. A few compounds, such as the acidic metabolites of some antibiotics, are actively excreted at the tubule by specific transport systems. Naturally, decreased kidney function is often reflected in a decreased clearance of drugs or their metabolites. A knowledge of the functional state of the kidney is useful, therefore, in helping to estimate a patient's capacity to handle and excrete a given drug and for this purpose, creatinine clearance values are sometimes indicative of drug clearance. It bears mention, of course, that not every drug is cleared in a fashion parallel with creatinine.

Plasma Protein Binding

Drugs in the circulation are bound to varying degrees by plasma proteins. The nature of this binding is not clearly understood, but is presumed to be either of an ionic or hydrogen bonding type, since it is freely reversible. Although little detailed evidence is available, the current view is that the plasma albumin fraction is responsible for the majority of drug binding.

The physiologic effect of a drug is determined by that amount of drug free and not bound by plasma proteins; the percentage bound may vary widely. Phenylbutazone is approximately 98% bound whereas antipyrine is bound only negligibly, if at all. Since plasma albumin decreases an average of 10 to 20% between ages 30 and 70, the older patient often displays a decrease in the amount of a drug commonly bound to plasma proteins. Like decreased metabolism or decreased excretion, decreased binding of a drug results in a larger concentration of free drug in the older patient. This is of practical significance primarily for drugs that are highly bound.

Although there is a paucity of drug binding data, it is generally believed that a decrease in drug binding represents a decrease in the total number of sites available for that drug, but that the affinity constant for its binding is generally unaltered. Table 2 presents data published on drug binding in different age groups.

Table 1
AGE-RELATED PHARMACOKINETIC DATA

	Age[a] (year)	Peak plasma concentration (μg/mℓ)	V_d (ℓ/kg)	$t^{1/2}$ (hr)	Clearance rate (mℓ/min/kg)	Ref.
Antibiotics						
Penicillin G, i.v.	25			0.55		14
	77			1.0		
Procaine penicillin, i.m.	25			10		14
	77			18		
Sulfamethizole	24		0.345	1.75		15
	81		0.338	3.02		
Cephradine	24—33			0.53	5.04	16
	70—88			1.2	2.03	
Netilmicin, i.v.	54			2.3		17
	74			5.0		
Tetracycline	27			3.5		18
	75			4.5		
Dihydrostreptomycin	27			5.2		18
	75			8.4		
Mecillinam	<30	2.6		0.88		19
(pivmecillinam)	>65	2.3		3.97		
Kanamycin	20—50			1.78		20
	50—70			2.48		
	70—90			4.70		
Propicillin	20—30		0.43	0.57		21
	60—80		0.26	0.66		
Doxycycline, i.v.	20—28		0.73	11.9		22
	42—55		0.70	17.7		
Amoxicillin, i.v.	(Young)			1—1.5		23
	89			2.67		
Cefazolin, i.v.	24—33			1.57	1.11	16
	70—88			3.15	0.57	
Tranquilizers						
Diazepam	30		0.85	32		24
	65		1.4	70		
Chlordiazepoxide	25	0.86	0.42	10.1	0.61	25
	69	0.69	0.52	16.2	0.34	
Nitrazepam	21—38	0.039	2.4	28.9		13
Inactive	66—89	0.022	4.8	40.4		
	25		2.9	33.0		26
Healthy	75		2.7	32.5		
Oxazepam	25		0.64	5.1	1.54	27
	53		0.76	5.6	1.70	
Chlormethiazole	27	0.55		6.15	222	28
	70	2.90		6.34	35	
β-Blocking agents and cardiac drugs						
Propranolol	29	0.048		3.58		29
p.o.	80	0.110		3.61		
i.v.	29		3.0	2.53	13.2	29
	80		2.7	4.23	7.8	
Practolol	27			7.1		30
	80			8.6		
Metoprolol	23			3.5		31
	67			5.0		
Digoxin	27			51	1.11	32
	72			73	0.88	
	34—61		5.3	36.8	1.7	33
	72—91		4.1	69.6	0.8	
Quinidine, i.v.	23—34		2.39	7.25	4.04	34
	60—69		2.18	9.70	2.64	

Table 1 (continued)
AGE-RELATED PHARMACOKINETIC DATA

	Age[a] (year)	Peak plasma concentration (µg/mℓ)	V_d (ℓ/kg)	$t^{1/2}$ (hr)	Clearance rate (mℓ/min/kg)	Ref.
Lidocaine, i.v.	24		0.65	1.34	7.6	35
	65		1.13	2.33	8.1	
Analgesics						
Morphine, i.v.	26—32		3.2	2.9	14.7	36
	61—80		4.7	4.5	12.4	
Aspirin	20—40	35.0	0.08		0.40	37
	>65	40.5	0.11		0.28	
	21	129	3.8	2.38		38
	77	99	5.5	3.71		
Antipyrine	27		0.60	12.5		39
	79		0.56	16.8		
	26			12.0		40
	78			17.4		
i.v.	18—39			12.7		41
	40—59			f38 13.8		
	60—92			14.8		
Aminopyrine	25—30			3.85		42
	65—85			8.25		
Indomethacin	20—50			1.53		43
	71—83			1.73		
Paracetamol	24		1.03	1.82	6.36	15
(acetaminophen)	81		1.05	3.03	5.05	
	28		0.86	1.75	5.67	44
	77		0.77	2.17	4.23	
Acetanilide	<35			1.45		45
	>65			2.07		
	23		0.64	1.57	5.83	46
	81		0.59	1.75	5.50	
Miscellaneous						
Amylobarbital	20—40			22.8		47
	>65			86.6		
Phenobarbital	20—40			71		48
	50—60			77		
	>70			107		
Carbenoxolone	<40		0.1	16.3	0.078	49
	>65		0.1	22.9	0.055	
Phenylbutazone	26			81		50
	78			105		
	24	0.172		87		15
	81	0.165		110		
Isoniazid	<35			1.4		45
	>65	(Fast acetylators)		1.5		
	<35			3.7		
	>65	(Slow acetylators)		4.2		
Warfarin	31		0.19	37	0.063	2
	76		0.20	44	0.054	
Quinine	20—40	1.1	3.20		3.22	37
	>65	2.3	1.74		6.62	
Imipramine	<65			19.0		51
	>65			23.8		
Vitamin K, i.v.	Young	(No drugs)			3.29	52
	Elderly				3.51	
	Young	(On warfarin)			3.94	
	Elderly				7.80	

[a]   Age group or mean age.

Table 2
PLASMA PROTEIN BINDING

	Age[a] (year)	Plasma albumin (gm %)	Maximum plasma binding (%)	Clearance (mℓ/min/kg)	Ref.
Phenytoin	<50	4.0	82.4		53
	>50	3.4	83.6		
	<43			0.44	54
	>67			0.70	
i.v.	<45	4.1	(727 μmol/ℓ)		54
	>67	2.9	(595 μmol/ℓ)		
Phenylbutazone	27	4.2	96		55
	79	3.6	94		
Sulfadiazine	27	4.2	50		55
	79	3.6	45		
Salicylate	27	4.2	72		55
	79	3.6	73		
Warfarin	31		98.6		2
	76		98.5		
	<45	3.9	(561 μmol/ℓ)		56
	>65	3.0	(451 μmol/ℓ)		
Quinidine, i.v.	29		75	4.04	34
	66		72	2.64	
Chlormethiazole	27		45.4		57
	70	3.7	44.4		
Phenobarbituric acid	<50	4.1	41.8		53
	>50	3.4	41.9		
Penicillin G	<50	3.9	42.4		53
	>50	3.8	45.1		

[a] Age group or mean age.

PHARMACOKINETICS

A semilogarithmic plot of plasma drug concentration vs. time almost always has a terminal phase that is linear on such a graph. This is true whether the drug is administered orally or parenterally. The slope of this terminal (elimination) phase allows one to determine $t_{1/2}$, the biologic half-life of the drug and k_{el}, the elimination constant.

$$\text{slope} = \frac{k_{el}}{2.3} \qquad (1)$$

$$t_{1/2} = \frac{0.693}{k_{el}} \qquad (2)$$

The total "effect" of the drug can be represented by AUC, the area under the plasma concentration vs. time curve from time zero to infinity. Then, assuming that essentially all of the drug dose was absorbed, the effective distribution volume, V_d, of the drug can be calculated.

$$V_d = \frac{\text{dose}}{\text{AUC } k_{el}} \qquad (3)$$

An alternate means of calculating V_d is to extrapolate the linear (terminal elimination) phase back to time zero to determine a hypothetical zero time concentration, C_0. Then

$$V_d = \frac{dose}{C_0} \qquad (4)$$

Finally, the rate of drug clearance can be calculated:

$$Cl = \frac{0.693 V_d}{t_{1/2}} \qquad (5)$$

A more detailed treatment of pharmacokinetics, particularly with reference to aging was published in 1978.[12] Interested readers are referred to that publication for an extension of the above considerations.

Next, a few warning comments are in order. Most pharmacokinetic data published are a result of acute experiments utilizing a single dose; the differences observed in acute experiments may become even greater on chronic dosing. Furthermore, pharmacokinetic data obtained with older patients are almost invariably more heterogeneous than those obtained with younger patients, owing to the considerable variation in the rate and onset of the aging process in different individuals. In addition to this variation, there may exist significant differences in the physical activity level of older subjects; this alone may result in large differences in the rates of metabolism and excretion, as noted for nitrazepam.[13] Also, it is worth mentioning that the constants calculated are highly dependent on the model the particular investigator uses for fitting his data.

What is actually seen in clinical practice is the sum of the various drug handling capacities of the patient. Decreases in metabolic capability may be exacerbated by reduced renal function; on the other hand, changes in the apparent volume of drug distribution may either exacerbate or nullify reduced renal function. The interplay between these elements can be difficult to determine. We hope that by reference to the overall mass of data available and presented in Table 2, it may be possible for the clinician to have a clearer expectation of the pharmacokinetic situation prevailing in his patient for a given kind of drug.

REFERENCES*

1. **Reidenberg, M. M., Levy, M., Warner, H., Coutinho, C. B., Schwartz, M. A., Yu, G., and Cheripko, J.,** Relationship between diazepam dose, plasma level, age and central nervous system depression, *Clin. Pharmacol. Ther.,* 23, 371, 1978.
2. **Shepherd, A. M., Hewick, D. S., Moreland, T. A., and Stevenson, I. H.,** Age as a determinant of sensitivity to warfarin, *Br. J. Clin. Pharmacol.,* 4, 315, 1977.
3. **Brandfonbrenner, M., Landowne, M., and Shock, N. W.,** Changes in cardiac output with age, *Circulation,* 12, 557, 1955.
4. **Bender, A. D.,** The effect of increasing age on the distribution of peripheral blood flow in man, *J. Am. Geriatr. Soc.,* 13, 192, 1965.
5. **Bender, A. D.,** Effect of age on intestinal absorption: implications for drug absorption in the elderly, *J. Am. Geriatr. Soc.,* 16, 1131, 1968.

---

* Manuscript was submitted in early 1979, since that time more recent material is available.

6. **Richey, D. P. and Bender, A. D.,** Effects of human aging on drug absorption and metabolism, in *Physiology and Pathology of Human Aging,* Goldman, R. and Rockstein, M., Eds., Academic Press, New York, 1975, 59.
7. **Kato, R., Vassanelli, P., Frontino, G., and Chiesara, E.,** Variation in the activity of liver microsomal drug-metabolizing enzymes in rats in relation to the age, *Biochem. Pharmacol.,* 13, 1037, 1964.
8. **Kuhlmann, K., Oduah, M., and Coper, H.,** Uber die wirkung von barbituraten bei ratten verschiedenen alters, *Naunyn Schmiedebergs Arch. Pharmakol.,* 265, 310, 1970.
9. **Richey, D. P. and Bender, D.,** Pharmacokinetic consequences of aging, in *Annual Reviews of Pharmacology and Toxicology,* Vol. 17, Elliott, H. W., George, R., and Okun, R., Eds., Annual Reviews, Palo Alto, Calif., 1977, 49.
10. **Triggs, E. J. and Nation, R. L.,** Pharmacokinetics in the aged: a review, *J. Pharmacokinet. Biopharm.,* 3, 387, 1975.
11. **Crooks, J., O'Malley, K., and Stevenson, I. H.,** Pharmacokinetics in the elderly, *Clin. Pharmacokinet.,* 1, 280, 1976.
12. **Levy, G.,** Pharmacokinetic assessment of the effect of age on the disposition and pharmacologic activity of drugs, *Adv. Exp. Med. Biol.,* 97, 47, 1978.
13. **Iisalo, E., Kangas, L., and Ruika, I.,** Pharmacokinetics of nitrazepam in young volunteers and aged patients, *Br. J. Clin. Pharmacol.,* 4, 646 P, 1977.
14. **Leikola, E. and Vartia, K. O.,** On penicillin levels in young and geriatric subjects, *J. Gerontol.,* 12, 48, 1957.
15. **Triggs, E. J., Nation, R. L., Long, A., and Ashley, J. J.,** Pharmacokinetics in the elderly, *Eur. J. Clin. Pharmacol.,* 8, 55, 1975.
16. **Simon, V., Malerczyk, V., Tenschert, B., and Mohlenbeck, F.,** Geriatric pharmacology of cefazolin, cephradine, and sulfisomidine, *Arzneim. Forsch.,* 26, 1378, 1976.
17. **Welling, P. G., Baumeuller, A., Lau, C. C., and Madsen, P. O.,** Netilmicin pharmacokinetics after single intravenous doses to elderly male patients, *Antimicrob. Agents Chemother.,* 12, 328, 1977.
18. **Vartia, K. O. and Leikola, E.,** Serum levels of antibiotics in young and old subjects following administration of dihydrostreptomycin and tetracycline, *J. Gerontol.,* 15, 392, 1960.
19. **Ball, A. P., Viswan, A. K., Mitchard, M., and Wise, R.,** Plasma concentrations and excretion of mecillinam after oral administration of pivmecillinam in elderly patients, *J. Antimicrob. Chemother.,* 4, 241, 1978.
20. **Kristensen, M., Hansen, J. M., Kampmann, J., Lumholtz, B., and Siersback-Nielsen, K.,** Drug elimination and renal function, *J. Clin. Pharmacol.,* 14, 307, 1974.
21. **Simon, C., Malerczyk, V., Muller, U., and Muller, G.,** Zur pharmakokinetik von propicillin bei geriatrischen patienten im vergleich zu jungeren erwachsenen, *Dtsch. Med. Wochenschr.,* 97, 1999, 1972.
22. **Simon, C., Malerczyk, V., Engelke, H., Preuss, I., Grahmann, H., and Schmidt, K.,** Die pharmakokinetik von doxycyclin bei niereninsuffizienz und geriatrischen patienten im vergleich zu jungeren erwachsenen, *Schweiz. Med. Wochenschr.,* 105, 1615, 1975.
23. **Ball, A. P., Barford, T., Gilbert, J., Johnson, T., and Mitchard, M.,** Prolonged serum elimination half-life of amoxycillin in the elderly, *J. Antimicrob. Chemother.,* 4, 385, 1978.
24. **Klotz, U., Avant, G. R., Hoyumpa, A., Schenker, S., and Wilkinson, G. R.,** The effects of age and liver disease on the disposition and elimination of diazepam in adult man, *J. Clin. Invest.,* 55, 347, 1975.
25. **Shader, R. I., Greenblatt, D. J., Harmatz, J. J., Franke, K., and Koch-Wesser, J.,** Absorption and disposition of chlordiazepoxide in young and elderly male volunteers, *J. Clin. Pharmacol.,* 17, 709, 1977.
26. **Castelden, C. M., George, C. F., Marcer, D., and Hallett, C.,** Increased sensitivity to nitrazepam in old age, *Br. Med. J.,* 1, 10, 1977.
27. **Shull, H. J., Wilkinson, G. R., Johnson, R., and Schenker, S.,** Normal disposition of oxazepam in acute viral hepatitis and cirrhosis, *Ann. Int. Med.,* 84, 420, 1976.
28. **Nation, R. L., Vine, J., Triggs, E. J., and Learoyd, B.,** Plasma level of chlormethiazole and two metabolites after oral administration to young and aged human subjects, *Eur. J. Clin. Pharmacol.,* 12, 137, 1977.
29. **Castleden, C. M. and George, C. F.,** The effect of ageing on the hepatic clearance of propranolol, *Br. J. Clin. Pharmacol.,* 7, 49, 1979.
30. **Castleden, C. M., Kaye, C. M., and Parsons, R. L.,** The effect of age on plasma levels of propranolol and practolol in man, *Br. J. Clin. Pharmacol.,* 2, 303, 1975.
31. **Kendall, M. J., Brown, D., and Yates, R. A.,** Plasma metoprolol concentrations in young, old, and hypertensive subjects, *Br. J. Clin. Pharmacol.,* 4, 497, 1977.
32. **Ewy, G. A., Kapadia, G. G., Yao, L., Lullin, M., and Marcus, F. I.,** Digoxin metabolism in the elderly, *Circulation,* 39, 449, 1969.
33. **Cusack, B., Horgan, J., Kelly, J., Lavan, J., Noel, J., and O'Malley, K.,** Pharmacokinetics of digoxin in the elderly, *Br. J. Clin. Pharmacol.,* 6, 439 P, 1978.

34. **Ochs, H. R., Greenblatt, D. J., Woo, E., Franke, K., and Smith, T. W.,** Reduced clearance of quinidine in elderly humans, *Clin. Res.,* 24, 513 A, 1977.
35. **Nation, R. L., Triggs, E. J., and Selig, M.,** Lignocaine kinetics in cardiac patients and aged subjects, *Br. J. Clin. Pharmacol.,* 4, 439, 1977.
36. **Stanski, D., Greenblatt, D. J., and Lowenstein, E.,** Kinetics of intravenous and intramuscular morphine, *Clin. Pharmacol. Ther.,* 24, 52, 1978.
37. **Salem, S. A. and Stevenson, I. H.,** Absorption kinetics of aspirin and quinine in elderly subjects, *Br. J. Clin. Pharmacol.,* 4, 397 P, 1977.
38. **Cuny, G., Royer, R. J., Mur, J. M., Serot, J. M., Faure, G., Netter, P., Maillard, A., and Penin, F.,** Pharmacokinetics of salicylates in elderly, *Gerontology,* 25, 49, 1979.
39. **Liddell, D. E., Williams, F. M., and Briant, R. H.,** Phenazone (antipyrine) metabolism and distribution in young and elderly adults, *Clin. Exp. Pharmacol. Physiol.,* 2, 481, 1975.
40. **O'Malley, K., Crooks, J., Duke, E., and Stevenson, I. H.,** Effect of age and sex on human drug metabolism, *Br. Med. J.,* 3, 607, 1971.
41. **Vestal, R. E., Norris, A. H., Tobin, J. D., Cohen, B. H., Shock, N. W., and Andres, R.,** Antipyrine metabolism in man: influence of age, alcohol, caffeine, and smoking, *Clin. Pharmacol. Ther.,* 18, 425, 1975.
42. **Jori, A., Di Salle, E., and Quadri, A.,** Rate of aminopyrine disappearance from plasma in young and aged humans, *Pharmacology,* 8, 273, 1972.
43. **Traeger, A., Junze, M., Stein, G., and Ankermann, H.,** Zur pharmakokinetik von indomethazin bei alten menschen, *Z. Alternsforsch.,* 27, 151, 1973.
44. **Briant, R. H., Dorrington, R. E., Cleal, J., and Williams, F. M.,** The rate of acetaminophen metabolism in the elderly and the young, *J. Am. Geriat. Soc.,* 24, 359, 1976.
45. **Farah, F., Taylor, W., Rawlins, M., and James, O.,** Hepatic drug acetylation and oxidation: effects of aging in man, *Br. Med. J.,* 2, 155, 1977.
46. **Playfer, J. P., Baty, J., Lamb, J., Powell, C., and Price-Evans, D. A.,** Age-related differences in the disposition of acetanilide, *Br. J. Clin. Pharm.,* 6, 529, 1978.
47. **Ritschel, W.,** Age-dependent disposition of amylobarbital: analog computer evaluation, *J. Am. Geriatr. Soc.,* 26, 540, 1978.
48. **Traeger, A., Kiesewetter, R., and Kunze, M.,** Zur pharmakokinetic von phenobarbital bei erwachsenen und greisen, *Dtsch. Gesundheitswes.,* 29, 1040, 1974.
49. **Hayes, M. J., Sprackling, M., and Langman, M. J. S.,** Changes in the plasma clearance and protein binding of carbenoxolone with age and their possible relationship with adverse drug effects, *Gut,* 18, 1054, 1977.
50. **O'Malley, K., Crooks, J., Duke, E., and Stevenson, I. H.,** Effect of age and sex on human drug metabolism, *Br. Med. J.,* 3, 607, 1971.
51. **Nies, A., Robinson, D. S., Friedman, M. J., Green, R., Cooper, T. B., Ravaris, C. L., and Ives, J. O.,** Relationship between age and tricyclic antidepressant plasma levels, *Am. J. Psychiatry,* 134, 790, 1977.
52. **Shepherd, A. M. M., Wilson, N., and Stevenson, I. H.,** Vitamin K pharmacokinetics: response in young and elderly patients, *Clin. Pharmacol. Ther.,* 21, 117, 1977.
53. **Bender, A. D., Post, A., Meier, J. P., Higson, J. E., and Reichard, G.,** Plasma protein binding of drugs as a function of age in adult human subjects, *J. Pharm. Sci.,* 64, 1711, 1975.
54. **Hayes, M. J., Langman, M. J. S., and Short, A. H.,** Changes in drug metabolism with increasing age. II. Phenytoin clearance and protein binding, *Br. J. Clin. Pharmacol.,* 2, 73, 1975.
55. **Wallace, S., Whiting, B., and Runcie, J.,** Factors affecting drug binding in plasma of elderly patients, *Br. J. Clin. Pharmacol.,* 3, 327, 1976.
56. **Hayes, M. J., Langman, M. J. S., and Short, A. H.,** Changes in drug metabolism with increasing age. I. Warfarin binding and plasma proteins, *Br. J. Clin. Pharmacol.,* 2, 69, 1975.
57. **Nation, R. L., Learoyd, B., Barber, J., and Triggs, E. J.,** The pharmacokinetics of chlormethiazole following intravenous administration in the aged, *Eur. J. Clin. Pharmacol.,* 10, 407, 1976.

Cardiovascular Pharmacology

THE DIGITALIS GLYCOSIDES

Peter Cervoni and Peter S. Chan

INTRODUCTION

The digitalis glycosides play an important role in the treatment of atrial fibrillation of supraventricular origin with a rapid ventricular rate and in congestive heart failure (right and left ventricular failure). The glycosides are particularly useful in the aged when one considers the following statistics: Pedoe,[1] reporting on a 1975 survey of 400,000 prescriptions, indicated that 6% of the patients over age 65 were taking digoxin. If one considers that about 11% of modern U.S. society is over the age of 65,[2] then nearly 1 1/2 million Americans are taking digoxin. Corroborating this, it was estimated that in 1978 there were 23 million people in the U.S. over the age of 65,[3] and it has been noted that approximately 5% of elderly people at home are on some form of digitalis therapy.[4]

The digitalis glycosides have a relatively low therapeutic index.[5-8] Toxicity with the digitalis glycosides occurs at about 60% of the lethal dose,[6,7] and has been observed in about 20 to 30% of the individuals taking the drug,[7-10] although the range is slightly lower in hospitalized patients.[7,9] There are numerous reports in the literature that elderly patients are more prone to the toxic manifestations of digitalis therapy than are younger patients;[11-28] also that children can tolerate comparatively high doses of the digitalis glycosides without toxic manifestations.[29-31]

Age-related changes in susceptibility to the actions of the digitalis glycosides can result from changes in the responsiveness of the myocardium or from changes in the pharmaco-kinetic factors that regulate the concentration of the glycoside in the myocardium. Age-related changes in sensitivity or responsiveness to the glycosides are easily studied in hearts from aged animals, using in vitro techniques. However, in vivo it is difficult to dissociate changes in tissue responsiveness from changes in the way the elderly patient or aged animal handles the drug. The elderly patient often presents us with special problems such as impaired renal and liver function, electrolyte disturbances, pulmonary heart disease, or myocardial infarction, to name a few. We will attempt to review the data which provide some explanation for the alteration in the sensitivity of elderly patients to the digitalis glycosides.

Effects of aging on the cardiovascular system have been reviewed previously by Goldberg and Roberts,[32] and are also indicated in separate chapters in this Handbook. The alterations may be due to age per se or may be the result of co-existing pathology.[33] Roberts and Goldberg recently summarized some of the requirements for animal health care necessary for the successful conduct of pharmacological research in aging animals.[34] This approach may allow investigators to resolve the question of whether changes in cardiovascular reactivity to drugs are age-related or are due to other factors. Similarly, Gillette has reviewed some of the pharmacokinetic data required, and the possible consequences resulting from inadequate data.[35]

THERAPEUTIC VS. TOXIC ACTIONS

Several reviews have been published recently on the possible mechanisms of inotropic action of digitalis glycosides.[36,37] It has been postulated that the receptor for the inotropic action of the digitalis glycosides is the sodium and potassium-coupled adenosine triphos-phatase ($Na^+ + K^+$-ATPase) that is in the cardiac cell membrane.[38-43] Inhibition of $Na^+ + K^+$-ATPase by the glycosides leads to an accumulation of intracellular Na^+. It is further postulated that as Na^+ accumulates intracellularly, there is activation of a sodium-calcium

(Ca^{++}) coupled system which reestablishes steady-state Na^+ exchange at a higher intracellular Na^+ level. Thus, Ca^{++} influx is increased and developed tension with each action potential is increased.[45] Ca^{++} release from intracellular compartments has also been postulated to contribute to the digitalis glycoside inotropic action.[46] The inhibition of Na^+ + K^+-ATPase as a mechanism for digitalis action has been challenged by Okita et al.[47] who demonstrated in rabbit Langendorff preparations that significant Na^+ + K^+-ATPase activity exists after "washout" of the ouabain inotropic response. Similarly, Ten Eick et al.,[48] using rabbit papillary muscle and dog ventricular trabeculae, demonstrated that the inotropic effect of strophanthidin-3-bromoacetate could be dissociated temporally from both the electrophysiological and Na^+ + K^+-ATPase inhibitory activities.

Gerstenblith et al.,[49,50] using isolated cardiac trabeculae carnae of aged Wistar rats, studied the effects of paired pacing and the relation between ouabain-induced inotropy and Na^+ + K^+-ATPase inhibition. They found that age had no effect on tension development or on the maximal rate of tension development in response to paired pacing. The inotropic response to ouabain was less in preparations from senescent rats than from young adult rats. However, there was no age-dependent difference in ouabain-induced Na^+ + K^+-ATPase inhibition. The data suggest that the age-related diminution of response to ouabain results from an alteration in some step other than enzyme inhibition.

In contrast, Baskin et al.[51] reported that the activity of Na^+ + K^+-ATPase of brain, spinal cord, heart, and kidney of aged Fischer 344 rats was 50% less than in younger rats (toxicity to ouabain was inversely related to enzyme activity). Ouabain also inhibited the Na^+ + K^+-ATPase to a greater extent in older than in young rats. Wollenberger et al.[52] demonstrated that age (up to 5 to 6.5 years) did not alter the sensitivity of the guinea pig myocardium to ouabain. Aravarris[53] studied the effects of acetyldigoxin in elderly patients (60 to 86 years of age) with congestive heart failure. Using reduction of heart rate and elimination of congestion as the therapeutic endpoints, he found that the doses of acetyldigoxin were equal in elderly and young patients. The conclusion was that it is not necessary to reduce digitalis doses for the elderly. Chamberlain et al.,[54] studying elderly patients with atrial fibrillation (but with good renal function), noted that their sensitivity to digoxin was the same as in younger patients since therapeutic plasma levels of digoxin (levels producing similar decreases in ventricular rate) were the same in both groups. Age-related increases in sensitivity to ouabain, as measured by changes in intracellular action potential configuration of cardiac Purkinje fibers from dogs have been reported.[55] In these studies it was found that ouabain had a greater effect on Purkinje fiber action potentials from adult dogs than from young dogs. Ouabain uptake was greater in preparations from younger animals. The potential changes reported may represent toxic manifestations of ouabain rather than therapeutic actions, since the concentration of ouabain in the perfusion medium was relatively high ($2 \times 10^{-7}M$). The lethal dose of ouabain in guinea pigs has been shown to decrease by about 25% from birth to maturity (5.5 to 7.5 months), although no further change in the lethal dose occurred up to 5.5 to 6.5 years of age.[52] Kelliher and Roberts reported that adult rabbits (older than 12 weeks) were more sensitive to the arrhythmogenic effects of ouabain than were young rabbits.[56] Chen and Robbins also reported that the ouabain lethal dose was lower in 3- to 5-year-old albino rabbits than in younger animals.[57] Although heart weights decreased with age in this study, the aged animals were still more sensitive to ouabain when compared on the basis of units of heart weight. The digitalis glycosides also have been reported to cause more myocardial lesions in older cats than in younger ones.[58] The proposed mechanisms for the cardiotoxicity of the digitalis glycosides involve release of catecholamines from cardiac sympathetic nerves[56,59,60] and from the adrenal medulla[61] which sensitize the heart to the action of the glycosides, indirect actions on the central nervous system to increase sympathetic stimulation to the heart,[62] or direct cardiotoxic actions.[63,64] Most likely, the glycosides act on multiple sites in the "sympatho-adrenal" axis to produce cardiac arrhythmias.[65,66] In the rat, which is less sensitive to the lethal effects of the cardiac glycosides than other species, digitoxin and proscillaridin were reported to be 200 to 1000 times more toxic in young animals than in adult animals depending on the route of administration.[67,68] Since there were methodological problems in arriving at the lethal dose in the younger animals, these values may be only rough estimates.[67]

ABSORPTION

Some of the age-dependent changes that occur within the gastrointestinal (GI) tract have been reviewed by Bender[69] and Goldberg and Roberts[32] and are summarized by Dr. Richey in this handbook. To recapituate briefly, the pH and volume of basal and stimulated secretions decrease with age;[70,71] intestinal motility,[71] sphincter activity,[72] intestinal blood flow,[73] and the number of absorbing cells[72,74,75] also decrease with age. These changes could alter the absorptive capacity of the GI tract. In addition, special transport mechanisms have been found to be modified with age, decreasing the absorption of substances such as calcium, thiamine, galactose, and 3-methylglucose.[74,76,77]

Approximately 60 to 85% of an orally administered dose of digoxin is absorbed from the GI tract of normal individuals.[78,79] Patients with malabsorption syndrome[80] and elderly patients[26,81,82] appear to absorb less digoxin. However, Marcus has shown that if the dissolution of the digoxin tablets is greater than 65% in 1 hr [Federal Drug Administration (FDA) minimally accepted bioavailable digoxin tablet], then the absorption of digoxin is normal in individuals with malabsorption of fat and D-xylose.[28] Greenblatt et al.[83] demonstrated that absorption of preparations that were better than 70% bioavailable was comparable to an intravenous dose of digoxin. Caird[84] and Taylor et al.[4] noted that the absorption of digoxin in elderly patients was within normal limits.

DISTRIBUTION

Once a drug is absorbed, it is distributed through various body fluids and tissues. The distribution is dependent upon the chemical characteristics of the drug and upon body composition. For example, highly lipid-soluble drugs would tend to accumulate in obese subjects; thus appropriate adjustments in dose would have to be made. Age-related changes in body composition have been reviewed by Goldberg and Roberts.[32] In the elderly, body fat as a proportion of body weight increases about 35% while lean body mass as a percent of body weight decreases about 15%. This had led investigators to propose that body weight and size be taken into account in determining digitalis glycoside dosage.[19,85-88] Plasma volume decreases about 10% and total body water decreases about 15% with age. The decrease in total body water is reflected by a decrease in intracellular fluid but not extracellular fluid. Glantz et al.[89] demonstrated that young dogs had almost twice the ouabain volume of distribution per kilogram of body weight as adults. The young dogs were also shown to have almost twice the plasma volume and intracellular fluid space. In the young, more ouabain must be given to get the same plasma concentration as in the adults, because the mass of ouabain in rapid equilibrium with the plasma is diluted in a larger volume of distribution.

Approximately 75% of the digoxin in the bloodstream is not protein bound and is pharmacologically active.[90,91] There does not appear to be any change with age in protein binding of either ouabain or the glycosides.[89]

METABOLISM

After administration of an oral dose of digoxin, peak serum levels have been observed at 45 min to 2 hr.[4,79] Since about 90% of an orally administered dose of digoxin is excreted unchanged and only about 10% is excreted as metabolites,[19,92] it is unlikely that alterations in metabolism of digoxin, if they occur in old age, could alter blood levels sufficiently to account for changes in sensitivity to the drug. Peters et al.[93] studying digoxin metabolism in 100 patients, by the electron-capture gas-chromatographic method for analysis of metabolites, noted that 12.4% of the lipid-extractable cardenolenide in the 24-hr urine sample contained a reduced lactone ring, although the range was 2.2 to 52%. The level of metabolite was unaltered by age, sex, or dose, but increased as a function of duration of therapy.

EXCRETION

The excretion of digoxin in man is primarily through the kidneys, by glomerular filtration, regardless of the route of administration.[78,79] Approximately 60 to 90% of a single dose is excreted over 7 days.[79] Age-dependent changes in kidney function have been reviewed by Goldberg and Roberts[32] and Epstein[94] (also see chapter by Dr. Richey). Kidney function has been shown to decrease with age.[88-93,95-101] Renal blood flow,[100] renal plasma flow,[96,101] and glomerular filtration rate decrease with age.[96,101] Thus, elderly patients with moderate to severe impairment of renal function show a relatively high incidence of toxicity with the glycosides.[11,15,19,22,28,76,79,86-88,102-111] Altered renal function is probably the factor most responsible for altered drug levels in an aging population.[77] Bloom et al.[112] showed that in patients with normal renal function, 70% of the administered dose of digoxin appeared in the urine and 18% in the stools over 7 days. In patients with impaired renal function, only 15% appeared in urine and 6 to 36% appeared in the stools. Okada et al.[113] studied two groups of patients with mild congestive heart failure or atrial fibrillation. One group had normal renal function. They noted that there was a linear relationship between creatinine clearance and digoxin clearance following oral doses of digoxin in both groups of patients. However, since total body clearance was lower in patients with renal failure, steeper slopes were noted for the line relating steady-state digoxin concentrations to digoxin dose. Ewy et al.[19] report that, following intravenous administration of digoxin, higher levels of circulating glycosides were noted in elderly than in younger patients. Similar findings were reported by Marcus et al.[114] In addition they noted that nephrectomized dogs had higher levels of digoxin in plasma and in heart.[114] From the above, it is apparent that since kidney function is decreased in the elderly, the peak plasma concentrations and half-lives of the digitalis glycosides are higher than in younger individuals. Elderly patients with impaired renal function require smaller doses to achieve adequate blood levels.[11,12,54,88,104,109,115,116]

BLOOD AND TISSUE LEVELS VS. THERAPEUTIC AND TOXIC EFFECTS

In general, there is a positive correlation between digoxin plasma levels and digoxin dose.[91,113] Although Holt et al.[117] noted that there was a better correlation when daily dose was expressed in terms of total body weight, Dimant and Merrit[118] noted that in elderly patients there was no correlation between dose and plasma levels of digoxin.

There are conflicting reports on the correlation between myocardial levels of digoxin and plasma levels of digoxin. Marcus et al.[114] showed that myocardial digoxin levels in dogs correlated well with blood levels. Lichey et al.[119] measured plasma and myocardial digoxin levels in patients who had undergone cardiac surgery. A significant correlation existed between digoxin concentrations in plasma and papillary muscle. In atrial muscle, the correlation was poorer. This difference was attributed to the greater histological changes noted in atrial muscle than in papillary muscle. Biddle et al.[120] studied the relationship of tissue digoxin levels to serum digoxin levels through post-mortem examination of patients, mostly old ones who had been taking digoxin. They found that tissue digoxin levels were generally greater the higher the serum level, but the tissue-to-serum ratios were lower in the group judged toxic than in the group judged nontoxic.

There are also conflicting reports on the correlation of toxicity and digoxin blood levels. A positive correlation has been reported in some cases.[22,106,121] In other instances, cardiac toxicity in the elderly has been reported to occur several hours after serum digoxin levels fell from peak values.[4] While digoxin blood levels are generally higher in aged patients with toxic symptoms,[19,22,121,122] there does not appear to be a direct correlation, since both low and high digoxin blood levels have been shown to be associated with either therapeutic or toxic effects of the drug.[19,21,54,117,122-125] Several investigators have proposed that the variation in serum digoxin levels associated with toxicity may be due to differences in serum K^+ levels. Patients with symptoms of digoxin toxicity and serum levels that were generally considered nontoxic were also hypokalemic.[19,21,124,127-130] Other investigators have indicated that serum K^+ levels were not reliable prognosticators of toxicity.[22,117,131,132] It has also been proposed that the lack of correlation between serum digoxin levels and the therapeutic or toxic effects of digoxin may be due to other factors, such as severe underlying cardiac, thyroid, or pulmonary disease.[21,22,121,133]

ADVERSE REACTIONS

Adverse reactions to the cardiac glycosides include anorexia, vomiting, diarrhea, dizziness, headaches, visual disturbances, and cardiac arrhythmias.[6,15,18,78,79,106,134,135] In the elderly, anorexia may be more commonplace than nausea or vomiting and clouded or hazy vision more common than color vision.[5,136] Cardiac arrhythmias may occur without other toxic manifestations.[5,18,79,136,137] Allergic reactions, such as urticaria, skin eruptions, fever, and edema have been reported.[106,136] Other less common adverse reactions are fatigue and dysphagia.[135,139] Sudden deaths due to the digitalis glycosides in patients with elevated blood calcium levels have also been known to occur.[140-142]

REFERENCES

1. **Pedoe, H. D. T.**, Digoxin prescribing in general practice, *Lancet,* 2, 931, 1978.
2. **Kohn, R. R.**, Diseases and aging, *Fed. Proc., Fed. Am. Soc. Exp. Biol.,* 37, 2831, 1978.
3. **Butler, R. N.**, Aging: a challenge to medicine, *Conn. Med.,* 42, 529, 1978.
4. **Taylor, B. B., Kennedy, R. D., and Caird, F. I.**, Digoxin studies in the elderly, *Age, Ageing,* 3, 79, 1974.
5. **Bender, A. D.**, Pharmacologic aspects of aging: a survey of the effect of increasing age on drug activity in adults, *J. Am. Geriatr. Soc.,* 12, 114, 1964.
6. **Mason, D. T. and Braunwald, E.**, Digitalis and related preparations, in *Cardiovascular Diseases,* Brest, A. M. and Moyer, J. H., Eds., F.A. Davis, Philadelphia, 1968, 383.
7. **Chou, T. C.**, Digitalis-induced arrhythmias, *Mod. Treat.,* 7, 96, 1970.
8. **Lowenthal, D. T.**, Tissue sensitivity to drugs in disease states, *Med. Clin. North Am.,* 58, 1111, 1974.
9. **Mason, D. T., Zelis, R., Lee, G., Hughes, J. L., Spann, J. F., and Amsterdam, E. A.**, Current concepts and treatment of digitalis toxicity, *Am. J. Cardiol.,* 27, 546, 1971.
10. **Hurwitz, N. and Wade, O. L.**, Intensive hospital monitoring of adverse reactions to drugs, *Br. Med. J.,* 1, 531, 1969.
11. **Raisbeck, M. J.**, The use of digitalis in the aged, *Geriatrics,* 7, 12, 1952.
12. **Master, A. M.**, Practical consideration of digitalis administration, *N.Y. State J. Med.,* 55, 619, 1955.
13. **Crouch, R. B., Herrmann, G. R., and Hejtmanik, M. R.**, Digitalis intoxication, *Tex. J. Med.,* 52, 714, 1956.
14. **Wilson, G. M.**, Therapeutics in the elderly, in *Modern Trends in Geriatrics,* Hobson, W. and Hoeber, P. B., Eds., Harper Brothers, New York, 1957, 272.
15. **Fine, W.**, The effect of drugs on old people, *Med. Press (London),* 242, 4, 1955.
16. **Dreifus, L. S., McKnight, E. H., Katz, M., and Likoff, W.**, Digitalis intolerance, *Geriatrics,* 18, 494, 1963.
17. **Schott, A.**, Observations on digitalis intoxication. A plea, *Postgrad. Med. J.,* 40, 628, 1964.

18. **Herrmann, G. R.,** Digitoxicity in the aged, Recognition frequency and management, *Geriatrics,* 21, 109, 1966.
19. **Ewy, G. A., Kapadia, G. G., Yao, L., Lullin, M., and Marcus, F. I.,** Digoxin metabolism in the elderly, *Circulation,* 39, 449, 1969.
20. **Dall, J. C. L.,** Maintenance digoxin in elderly patients, *Br. Med. J.,* 2, 705, 1970.
21. **Smith, T. W. and Haber, E.,** Digitalis intoxication: the relationship of clinical presentation to serum digoxin concentration, *J. Clin. Invest.,* 49, 2377, 1970.
22. **Beller, G., Smith, T. W., Abelman, W. H., Haber, E., and Hood, W. B., Jr.,** Digitalis intoxication: a prospective clinical study with serum level correlations, *N. Engl. J. Med.,* 284, 989, 1971.
23. **Evered, D. C. and Chapman, C.,** Plasma digoxin concentrations and digoxin toxicity in hospital patients, *Br. Heart J.,* 33, 540, 1971.
24. **Thomas, J. H.,** The use and abuse of digitalis in the elderly, *Gerontol. Clin.,* 13, 285, 1971.
25. **Lee, P. V.,** Drug therapy: avoiding the pitfalls, *Med. World News, Geriatr. Issue,* 27, 1972.
26. **Armitage, D. P.,** Effects of digoxin (Letter to the Editor), *N. Engl. J. Med.,* 288, 1356, 1973.
27. **Kirsten, E., Rodstein, M., and Iuster, Z.,** Digoxin in the aged, *Geriatrics,* 28, 95, 1973.
28. **Marcus, F. I.,** Current status of therapy with digoxin, in *Current Problems in Cardiology,* Year Book Medical Publishers, Chicago, 1978, 1.
29. **Neill, C. A.,** The use of digitalis in infants and children, *Prog. Cardiovasc. Dis.,* 7, 399, 1965.
30. **Goldman, R. H.,** The use of serum digoxin levels in clinical practice, *J. Am. Med. Assoc.,* 229, 331, 1974.
31. **Giardina, A. C. V., Ehlers, K. H., Morrison, J. B., and Engle, M. A.,** Serum digitoxin concentrations in infants and children, *Circulation,* 51, 713, 1975.
32. **Goldberg, P. B. and Roberts, J.,** Influence of age on the pharmacology and physiology of the cardiovascular system, in *Special Review of Experimental Aging Research, Progress in Biology,* Elias, M. F., Eleftheriou, B. F., and Elias, P. K., Eds., Experimental Aging Research, Bar Harbor, 1976, 71.
33. **Lakatta, E. G.,** Alterations in the cardiovascular system that occur in advanced age, *Fed. Proc., Fed. Am. Soc. Exp. Biol.,* 38, 163, 1979.
34. **Roberts, J. and Goldberg, P. B.,** Changes in responsiveness of the heart during aging, *Fed. Proc., Fed. Am. Soc. Exp. Biol.,* 38, 1927, 1979.
35. **Gillette, J. R.,** Biotransformation of drugs during aging, *Fed. Proc., Fed. Am. Soc. Exp. Biol.,* 38, 1900, 1979.
36. **Schwartz, A., Lindenmayer, G. E., and Allen, J. C.,** The sodium-potassium adenosine triphosphatase: pharmacological, physiological and biochemical aspects, *Pharmacol. Rev.,* 27, 3, 1975.
37. **Lee, K. S. and Klauss, W.,** The subcellular basis for the mechanism of the inotropic action of the cardiac glycosides, *Pharmacol. Rev.,* 23, 193, 1971.
38. **Whittam, R.,** The asymmetrical stimulation of a membrane adenosine-triphosphatase in relation to active cation transport, *Biochem. J.,* 84, 110, 1962.
39. **Caldwell, P. C.,** The phosphorus metabolism of squid axons and its relationships to the active transport of sodium, *J. Physiol. (London),* 152, 545, 1960.
40. **Hokin, L. E., Dahl, J. L., Deupree, J. D., Dixon, J. F., Hackney, J. F., and Perdue, J. F.,** Studies on the characterization of the sodium-potassium transport adenosine triphosphate X. Purification of the enzyme from the rectal gland of *squalus acanthias, J. Biol. Chem.,* 248, 2593, 1973.
41. **Hoffman, J. F.,** The red cell membrane and the transport of sodium and potassium, *Am. J. Med.,* 41, 666, 1966.
42. **Lane, L. K., Copenhaver, J. H., Lindenmayer, G. E., and Schwartz, A.,** Purification and characterization of an ³H-ouabain binding to the transport adenosine triphosphatase from outer medulla of canine kidney, *J. Biol. Chem.,* 248, 7197, 1973.
43. **Kyte, J.,** The reactions of sodium and potassium ion-activated adenosine triphosphatase with specific antibodies. Implications for the mechanism of active transport, *J. Biol. Chem.,* 249, 3652, 1974.
44. **Langer, G. A. and Serena, S. D.,** Glycoside effects on ion exchange in perfused mammalian heart, *Ann. N.Y. Acad. Sci.,* 242, 689, 1974.
45. **Repke, K.,** Effect of digitalis on membrane adenosine triphosphatase of cardiac muscle, in *Proc. 2nd Int. Pharmacol. Meet., Prague,* Vol. 4, Drugs and Enzymes, Brodie, B. and Gillette, J. R., Eds., Pergamon Press, New York, 1965, 65.
46. **Lee, K. S., Hong, S. A., and Kang, D. H.,** Effect of cardiac glycosides on interaction of calcium with mitochondria, *J. Pharmacol. Exp. Ther.,* 172, 180, 1970.
47. **Okita, G. T., Richardson, F., and Roth-Schecter, B. F.,** Dissociation of the positive inotropic action of digitalis from inhibition of sodium-and-potassium-activated adenosine triphosphate, *J. Pharmacol. Exp. Ther.,* 185, 1, 1973.
48. **Ten Eick, R. E., Bassett, A. L., and Okita, G. T.,** Dissociation of electrophysiological and inotropic actions of strophanthidin-3-bromoacetate. Possible role of adenosine triphosphatase in the maintenance of the myocardial transmembrane Na^+ and K^+ gradients, *J. Pharmacol. Exp. Ther.,* 185, 12, 1973.

49. **Gerstenblith, G., Lakatta, E. G., Spurgeon, H., Shock, N. W., and Weisfeldt, M. L.,** Diminished ouabain sensitivity in the aged myocardium, *Fed. Proc., Fed. Am. Soc. Exp. Biol.,* 34, 365, 1975.

50. **Gerstenblith, G., Spurgeon, H. A., Froelich, J. P., Weisfeldt, M. L., and Lakatta, E. G.,** Diminished inotropic responsiveness to ouabain in aged myocardium, *Circ. Res.,* 44, 517, 1979.

51. **Baskin, S. I., Roberts, J., and DeSousa, B. N.,** Na$^+$ + K$^+$ ATPase and age-dependent digitalis toxicity, *Pharmacologist,* 19, 132, 1977.

52. **Wollenberger, A., Jehl, J., and Karsh, M. L.,** The influence of age on the sensitivity of the guinea pig and its myocardium to ouabain, *J. Pharmacol. Exp. Ther.,* 108, 52, 1952.

53. **Aravarris, C.,** The use of acetyldigoxin in the aged with congestive heart failure, *Geriatrics,* 24, 75, 1969.

54. **Chamberlain, D. A., White, R. J., Howard, M. R., and Smith, T. W.,** Plasma digoxin concentrations in patients with atrial fibrillation, *Br. Med. J.,* 3, 429, 1970.

55. **Rosen, M. R., Hordoff, A. J., Hodess, A. B., Verosky, M., and Vulliemoz, Y.,** Ouabain-induced changes in electrophysiological properties in neonatal, young, and adult canine Purkinje fiber, *J. Pharmacol. Exp. Ther.,* 194, 255, 1976.

56. **Kelliher, G. J. and Roberts, J.,** Effect of age on the cardiotoxic actions of digitalis, *J. Pharmacol. Exp. Ther.,* 197, 10, 1976.

57. **Chen, K. K. and Robbins, E. B.,** Influence of age of rabbits on the toxicity of ouabain, *J. Am. Pharm. Assoc.,* 33, 61, 1944.

58. **Dearing, W. H., Barnes, A. R., and Essex, W. E.,** Experiments with calculated therapeutic and toxic doses of digitalis: effects on the myocardial cell structure, *Am. Heart J.,* 25, 648, 1943.

59. **Donaldson, J., Minnich, J. L., and Barbeau, A.,** Ouabain-induced seizures in rats: regional and subcellular localization of ^{3}H-ouabain associated with Na$^+$-K$^+$-ATPase in brain, *Can. J. Biochem.,* 50, 888, 1972.

60. **Weaver, L. C., Akera, T., and Brody, T. M.,** Digoxin toxicity: primary sites of action on the sympathetic nervous system, *J. Pharmacol. Exp. Ther.,* 197, 1, 1976.

61. **Kelliher, G. J. and Roberts, J.,** A study of the antiarrhythmic action of certain beta blocking agents, *Am. Heart J.,* 87, 458, 1974.

62. **Gillis, R. A., Raines, A., Sohn, Y. J., Levitt, B., and Standaert, F. E.,** Neuroexcitatory effects of digitalis and their role in the development of cardiac arrhythmias, *J. Pharmacol. Exp. Ther.,* 183, 154, 1972.

63. **Spann, J. F., Jr., Sonnenblick, E. H., Cooper, T., Chidsey, C. A., Willman, V. L., and Braunwald, E.,** The intrinsic contractile state of heart muscle and its response to digitalis: two properties independent of cardiac norepinephrine stores, in *Factors Influencing Myocardial Contractility,* Tanz, R. D., Kavaler, F., and Roberts, J., Eds., Academic Press, New York, 1967, 579.

64. **Mason, D. T., Spann, J. F., Jr., and Zelis, R.,** New developments in the understanding of the cardiac glycosides, *Prog. Cardiovasc. Dis.,* 11, 443, 1969.

65. **Roberts, J. and Kelliher, G. J.,** The mechanisms of digitalis at the subcellular level, *Semin. Drug. Treat.,* 2, 203, 1972.

66. **Roberts, J., Kelliher, G. J., and Lathers, C. M.,** Mini-review: role of adrenergic influences in digitalis-induced ventricular arrhythmia, *Life Sci.,* 18, 665, 1976.

67. **Goldenthal, E. I.,** A compilation of LD50 values in newborn and adult animals, *Toxicol. Appl. Pharmacol.,* 18, 185, 1971.

68. **Scott, W. J., Beliles, R. P., and Silverman, H. I.,** The comparative acute toxicity of two cardiac glycosides in adult and newborn rats, *Toxicol. Appl. Pharmacol.,* 20, 599, 1971.

69. **Bender, A. D.,** Effect of age on intestinal absorption: implication for drug absorption in the elderly, *Geriatrics,* 16, 1331, 1968.

70. **Baron, J. H.,** Studies of basal peak acid output with an augmented histamine test, *Gut,* 4, 136, 1963.

71. **Prescott, L. F.,** Gastrointestinal absorption of drugs, *Med. Clin. North Am.,* 58, 907, 1974.

72. **Geokas, M. C. and Haverback, B. J.,** The aging gastrointestinal tract, *Am. J. Surg.,* 117, 881, 1969.

73. **Bender, A. D.,** The effect of increasing age on the distribution of peripheral blood flow in man, *J. Am. Geriatr. Soc.,* 13, 192, 1965.

74. **Bender, A. D.,** A pharmacodynamic basis for changes in drug activity with aging in the adult, *Exp. Gerontol.,* 1, 237, 1965.

75. **Cornes, J. S.,** Number, size, distribution of Peyer's patches in human small intestine. II. The effect of age on Peyer's patches, *Gut,* 6, 230, 1965.

76. **Bender, A. D.,** Pharmacodynamic principles of drug therapy in the aged, *J. Am. Geriatr. Soc.,* 22, 296, 1974.

77. **Richey, D. P. and Bender, A. D.,** Pharmacokinetic consequences of aging, *Ann. Rev. Pharmacol. Toxicol.,* 17, 49, 1977.

78. **Moe, G. K. and Farah, A. E.,** Digitalis and allied cardiac glycosides, in *Pharmacological Basis of Therapeutics,* Goodman, L. S. and Gilman, A., Eds., MacMillan, New York, 1965, 653.

79. **Doherty, J. E. and Kane, J. J.,** Clinical pharmacology and therapeutic use of digitalis glycosides, in *Cardiovascular Drugs,* Vol. 4, Antiarrhythmic, Antihypertensive and Lipid Lowering Drugs, Adis Press, Sydney, Australia, 1977, 135.

80. **Goldfinger, S. E., Heizer, W. D., and Smith, T. W.,** Absorption of digoxin in patients with malabsorption, in *Symposium on Digitalis,* Storstein, O., Ed., Glydendal Norsk Forlag, Oslo, Norway, 1973, 224.

81. **Huffman, D. H. and Azarnoff, D. L.,** Absorption of orally given digoxin preparations, *J. Am. Med. Assoc.,* 222, 957, 1972.

82. **Roe, P. F. and Abbot, A. L.,** Studies in serum digoxin, *Age Ageing,* 3, 106, 1974.

83. **Greenblatt, D. J., Duhme, D. W., Koch-Weser, J., and Smith, T. W.,** Equivalent bioavailability from digoxin elixir and rapid dissolution tablets, *J. Am. Med. Assoc.,* 229, 1774, 1974.

84. **Caird, F. I.,** Metabolism of digoxin in relation to therapy in the elderly, *Gerontol. Clin.,* 16, 68, 1972.

85. **Jeliffe, R. W.,** Administration of digoxin, *Dis. Chest.,* 56, 56, 1969.

86. **Marcus, F. I., Burkhalter, L., Cuccia, C., Pavlovich, J., and Kapadia, G. G.,** Administration of tritiated digoxin with and without a loading dose, *Circulation,* 34, 865, 1966.

87. **Ewy, G. A. and Marcus, F. I.,** Digitalis therapy in the aged, *Am. Fam. Physician,* 1, 81, 1970.

88. **Smith, T. W.,** Letter to the Editor: effects of digoxin, *N. Engl. J. Med.,* 288, 1356, 1973.

89. **Glantz, S. A., Kernoff, R., and Goldman, R. H.,** Age-related changes in ouabain pharmacology: ouabain exhibits a different volume of distribution in adult and young dogs, *Circ. Res.,* 39, 407, 1976.

90. **Lüllman, H. and van Zweiten, P. A.,** The kinetic behavior of cardiac glycosides *in vivo,* measured by isotope techniques, *J. Pharm. Pharmacol.,* 21, 1, 1969.

91. **Evered, D. C., Chapman, C., and Hayter, C. J.,** Measurement of plasma digoxin concentration by radioimmunoassay, *Br. Med. J.,* 3, 427, 1970.

92. **Marcus, F. I., Kapadia, G. J., and Kapadia, G. G.,** Metabolism of digoxin in normal subjects, *J. Pharmacol. Exp. Ther.,* 145, 203, 1964.

93. **Peters, U., Falk, L. C., and Kalman, S. M.,** Digoxin metabolism in patients, *Arch. Int. Med.,* 138, 1074, 1978.

94. **Epstein, M.,** Effects of aging on the kidney, *Fed. Proc., Fed. Am. Soc. Exp. Biol.,* 38, 168, 1979.

95. **Shock, N. W.,** Some physiological aspects of aging in man, *Bull. N.Y. Acad. Med.,* 32, 268, 1956.

96. **Wesson, L. G., Jr.,** Renal hemodynamics in physiological states, in *Physiology of the Human Kidney,* Wesson, L. G., Jr., Ed., Grune & Stratton, New York, 1969, 96.

97. **Shock, N. W.,** Physiological aspects of aging, *J. Am. Diet. Assoc.,* 56, 491, 1970.

98. **Lindeman, R. D.,** Age changes in renal function, in *The Physiology and Pathology of Human Aging,* Goldman, R. and Rockstein, M., Eds., Academic Press, New York, 1975, 9.

99. **Lewis, W. H., Jr. and Alving, A. S.,** Changes with age in renal function in adult men. I. Clearance of urea. II. Amount of urea nitrogen in blood. III. Concentrating ability of the kidneys, *Am. J. Physiol.,* 123, 500, 1938.

100. **Hollenberg, N. K., Adams, D. F., Solomon, H. S., Rashid, A., Abrams, L., and Merrill, J. P.,** Senescence and the renal vasculature in normal man, *Circ. Res.,* 34, 309, 1974.

101. **Davies, D. F. and Shock, N. W.,** Age changes in glomerular filtration rate, effective renal plasma flow and tubular excretory capacity in adult males, *J. Clin. Invest.,* 29, 496, 1950.

102. **Doherty, J. E., Perkins, W. H., and Wilson, M. C.,** Studies with tritiated digoxin in renal failure, *Am. J. Med.,* 37, 536, 1964.

103. **Bender, A. D.,** Geriatric Pharmacology. Age and its influence on drug action in adults, *Drug. Inform. Bull.,* 3, 153, 1969.

104. **Bayliss, E. M., Hall, M. S., Lewis, G., and Marks, V.,** Effects of renal function on plasma digoxin levels in elderly ambulant patients in domiciliary practice, *Br. Med. J.,* 1, 338, 1972.

105. **Doherty, J. E.,** The influence of renal function on digoxin metabolism, in *Symposium on Digitalis,* Storstein, O., Ed., Glydendal Norsk Forlag, Oslo, Norway, 1973, 168.

106. **Smith, T. W.,** Drug Therapy. Digitalis glycosides (second of two parts), *N. Engl. J. Med.,* 288, 942, 1973.

107. **Steiness, E.,** Renal excretion of digoxin, in *Symposium on Digitalis,* Storstein, O., Ed., Glydendal Norsk Forlag, Oslo, Norway, 1973, 178.

108. **Schapel, G. J., McGrath, B. P., Edwards, K. D. G., Hawkins, M. R., and Mitchell, A. S.,** Therapeutic serum digoxin concentration: relation to age, weights, sex and serum creatinine level, *Aust. N.Z. J. Med.,* 3, 606, 1973.

109. **Smith, T. W.,** Radioimmunoassay for serum digitoxin concentration: methodology and clinical experience, *J. Pharmacol. Exp. Ther.,* 175, 352, 1970.

110. **Rasmussen, K., Jervell, J., Storstein, L., and Gjerdrum, K.,** Digitoxin kinetics in patients with impaired renal function, *Clin. Pharm. Ther.,* 15, 6, 1972.

111. **Storstein, L.,** Influence of renal function on the pharmacokinetics of digitoxin, in *Symposium on Digitalis,* Storstein, O., Ed., Glydendal Norsk Forlag, Oslo, Norway, 1973, 158.

112. **Bloom, P. M., Nelp, W. B., and Tuell, S. H.,** Relationship of excretion of tritiated digoxin to renal function, *Am. J. Med. Sci.,* 251, 133, 1966.
113. **Okada, R. D., Hager, W. D., Graves, P. E., Mayersohn, M., Perrier, D. G., and Marcus, F. I.,** Relationship between plasma concentration and dose of digoxin in patients with and without renal impairment, *Circulation,* 58, 1196, 1978.
114. **Marcus, F. I., Peterson, A., Salel, A., Scully, J., and Kapadia, G. G.,** Metabolism of tritiated digoxin in renal insufficiency in dogs and man, *J. Pharmacol. Exp. Ther.,* 152, 372, 1966.
115. **Dall, J. L. C.,** Digitalis intoxication in elderly patients, *Lancet,* 1, 194, 1965.
116. **Doherty, J. E.,** The clinical pharmacology of digitalis glycosides, *Am. J. Med. Sci.,* 255, 382, 1968.
117. **Holt, D. W., Williamson, J. D., and Volans, G. N.,** Digoxin measurements in general practice, *Br. J. Pharmacol.,* 4, 321, 1977.
118. **Dimant, J. and Merrit, W.,** Serum digoxin levels in elderly nursing home patients: appraisal of routine periodic measurements, *J. Am. Geriatr. Soc.,* 26, 378, 1978.
119. **Lichey, J., Havestatt, C., Weinmann, J., Hasford, J., and Rietbrock, N.,** Human myocardium and plasma digoxin concentration in patients on long term digoxin therapy, *Int. J. Clin. Pharmacol.,* 16, 460, 1978.
120. **Biddle, J., Weintraub, M., and Lasagna, L.,** Relationship of serum and myocardial digoxin concentration to electrocardiographic estimation of digoxin intoxication, *J. Clin. Pharmacol.,* 18, 10, 1978.
121. **Christiansen, N. J. B., Kolendorf, K., Siersbaek-Nielsen, K., and Hansen, J.,** Serum digoxin values following a dosage regimen based on body weight, sex, age and renal function, *Acta Med. Scand.,* 194, 257, 1973.
122. **Smith, T. W. and Haber, E.,** The clinical value of serum digitalis glycoside concentration in the evaluation of drug toxicity, *Ann. N.Y. Acad. Sci.,* 179, 322, 1971.
123. **Waldorf, J. and Burch, J.,** Serum digoxin and empiric methods in identification of digitoxicity, *Clin. Pharmacol. Ther.,* 23, 19, 1978.
124. **Aronson, J. K., Grahame-Smith, D. G., and Wigley, F. M.,** Monitoring digoxin therapy. The use of plasma digoxin concentration measurements in the diagnosis of digoxin therapy, *Q.J. Med. New Ser.,* 57, 111, 1978.
125. **Penchas, S. and Zajicek, G.,** Plasma digoxin levels and the interbeat interval signal in atrial fibrillation, *Z. Kardiol.,* 67, 104, 1978.
126. **Bhalla, R. K., Basu, A. K., and Bhatia, M. L.,** Serum digoxin levels in adults with and without digoxin toxicity (a ^{86}Rb uptake inhibition study), *Ind. Heart J.,* 30, 208, 1978.
127. **Lown, B., Weller, J. M., Wyatt, N., Hoigne, R., and Merrill, J. P.,** Effects of alterations of body potassium on digitalis toxicity, *J. Clin. Invest.,* 31, 648, 1952.
128. **Davidson, S. and Surawicz, B.,** Ectopic beats and atrioventricular disturbances in patients with hypopotassemia, *Arch. Int. Med.,* 120, 280, 1967.
129. **Jørgensen, A. W. and Sorensen, O. H.,** Digitalis intoxication, *Acta Med. Scand.,* 188, 179, 1970.
130. **Shapiro, W.,** Correlative studies of serum digitalis levels and the arrhythmias of digitalis intoxication, *Am. J. Cardiol.,* 41, 852, 1978.
131. **Gotsman, M. S. and Schrire, V.,** Toxicity — a frequent complaint of digitalis therapy, *S. Afr. Med. J.,* 40, 590, 1966.
132. **Chung, E. K.,** The current status of digitalis treatment, *Mod. Treat.,* 8, 643, 1941.
133. **Smith, T. W.,** Digitalis toxicity. Epidemiology and clinical use of serum concentration measurements, *Am. J. Med.,* 58, 470, 1975.
134. **Chung, L. Y. and Thomas, J.,** Arrhythmias caused by digitalis toxicity, *Geriatrics,* 20, 1006, 1965.
135. **Lely, A. H. and Van Enter, C. H. J.,** Large-scale digitoxin intoxication, *Br. Med. J.,* 3, 337, 1970.
136. **Friend, D.,** Drug therapy and the geriatric patient, *Clin. Pharmacol. Ther.,* 2, 832, 1961.
137. **Soffer, A. L.,** The importance of atrio-ventricular dissociation in the diagnosis of digitalis intoxication, *Dis. Chest,* 41, 422, 1962.
138. **Kelton, J. G. and Scullin, D. C.,** Digitalis toxicity manifested by dysphagia, Letter to the Editor, *J. Am. Med. Assoc.,* 239, 613, 1978.
139. **Riccitelli, M. L. and Hirschfeld, H.,** Digitalis allergy: a study of 1720 skin tests on 430 patients, *J. Am. Geriatr. Soc.,* 9, 277, 1961.
140. **Schrager, M. W.,** Digitalis intoxication, *Arch. Int. Med.,* 100, 881, 1957.
141. **Somlyo, A. P.,** The toxicology of digitalis, *Am. J. Cardiol.,* 5, 523, 1960.
142. **Resnick, N.,** Digitalis: a double edged sword, *Med. Sci.,* 4, 31, 1964.

ANTIARRHYTHMIC DRUGS

Peter Cervoni and Peter S. Chan

INTRODUCTION

Recently, two excellent reviews on the mechanisms of arrhythmias and the pharmacology of the antiarrhythmic agents have been published.[1,2] In this section, several antiarrhythmic agents will be discussed in relation to the effects of aging on drug action and only brief summaries of the electrophysiologic actions of these agents will be presented.

LIDOCAINE

Lidocaine is generally considered to be the drug of choice in the treatment of ventricular arrhythmias[3-7] and those arrhythmias originating from digitalis glycosides.[8] While it is generally considered to be ineffective in the treatment of supraventricular arrhythmias, it is not without effect on atrial fibrillation.[9,10] However, the drug should be used with caution in patients with atrial fibrillation or in those treated with pacemakers.[11-14] The effects of lidocaine on the electrophysiologic properties of cardiac muscle and conducting tissues have been investigated.[15] Briefly, action-potential duration and effective refractory period are shortened, but the effective refractory period in relation to action-potential duration is increased, especially in ventricular muscle. Phase 4 diastolic depolarization and spontaneous firing of Purkinje fibers are decreased without decreasing diastolic depolarization. Membrane responsiveness is unchanged except at high concentrations, where it is decreased. Phase 0 depolarization of the action potential and conduction velocity are either unchanged or increased slightly.

Age-related changes in the electrophysiologic effects of lidocaine in Fisher 344 rat hearts have been extensively investigated by Goldberg et al.[16-19] Using isolated atrial preparations from animals 1 to 28 months of age, it was noted that membrane resting potential did not change with age. Action potential amplitude and Phase 0 depolarization (dV/dt) was decreased equally at all ages. The decrease in action potential amplitude by lidocaine was less as age increased from 1 to 24 months, but at 28 months, the decrease in overshoot was greater. Action potential duration at 95% repolarization and plateau duration increased more at 6 to 28 months than it did earlier, at 1 to 3 months. In perfused Langendorff preparations from the same species, in which atrioventricular block was surgically induced so that atrial and ventricular pacemaker activity could be studied, these investigators were able to show that lidocaine depressed ventricular rates more than atrial rates. Lidocaine depression increased with age in atria but decreased in ventricles. Asystole in both tissues decreased with age. In man, age-related changes in sensitivity to lidocaine have not been elucidated. The drug has been used effectively to treat arrhythmias following acute myocardial infarction in elderly patients[6,7] and has been shown to produce minimal effects on conduction in special conducting tissues in elderly patients.[20,21]

Various pharmacokinetic factors which have been shown to change with age alter responsiveness to lidocaine. Since only 35% of an oral dose of lidocaine is absorbed, and less than antiarrhythmic plasma levels are achieved, the drug is used intravenously.[22] Nation et al.[23] studied the kinetics of long-term infusions of lidocaine in aged subjects. Longer half-lives were noted in elderly than in normal young subjects. This was considered not to be due to a decrease in drug metabolizing enzyme, because no change in plasma clearance of lidocaine was observed. A possible explanation to account for the longer half-life is reduction in cardiac output, which has been shown to occur with increasing age,[24] and the concomitant reduction in hepatic blood flow. There is considerable supporting evidence in the literature that patients with chronic liver and heart diseases have elevated lidocaine levels after intravenous administration.[4,25-31] In patients with renal failure, the plasma clearance of lidocaine is normal.[26] However, more polar metabolites such as monoethylglycine xylide, xylidine, and 4-hydroxyxylidine, may accumulate and account for the toxicity of lidocaine.[23,32] Lidocaine binds to plasma protein, but only 6% remains in the bloodstream since the volume of distribution for the drug is very large.[23] This does not appear to be a factor in the aged.

Adverse reactions to lidocaine are grouped into central nervous system and cardiovascular types. Pfeiffer et al.[33] have indicated that adverse reactions occurred in 6.3% of the patients taking lidocaine and that they were more common in elderly patients. Factors predisposing to adverse effects from therapeutic dose levels are underlying diseases, including liver disease and low cardiac output states, both of which tend to reduce hepatic clearance of lidocaine. While idiosyncratic reactions to lidocaine are rare, there has been a recent report of profound depression of automaticity of the sinoatrial and atrioventricular nodes with cardiac asystole, in a 67-year-old patient, following a single 50-mg bolus of lidocaine.[34]

QUINIDINE

Quinidine has a long history of usefulness in the treatment and prevention of most atrial and ventricular arrhythmias. It has been shown to produce direct and indirect actions on the specialized tissues of the heart. The direct actions include:

1. A reduction in automaticity through an increase in resting membrane potential (less negative) and a slowing in the rate of Phase 4 repolarization of nodal tissue[35,36]
2. A slowing of conduction velocity in nodal, intra-atrial and His-Purkinje systems[35,37]
3. A prolongation of the effective refractory period in relation to action potential duration in Purkinje fibers and atrial muscle[38,39]
4. A decrease in excitability of atrial and ventricular muscle[36,38]
5. A decrease in membrane responsiveness[40]

The indirect action is an anticholinergic one, which increases sinoatrial rate and facilitates atrioventricular (AV) conduction. This action counteracts the direct actions of quinidine on sinoatrial rate and on conduction velocity and refractory period of the AV node.[2] While many electrophysiological changes in cardiac tissues have been demonstrated for quinidine, it appears that the mechanism for the antiarrhythmic action in man is related primarily to slowing of cardiac conduction.[37,41]

Earlier publications on the actions of quinidine in the elderly indicate that, while quinidine was effective in this patient population, it should be used with caution.[42,46] However, the supporting data are rather meager. The effects of quinidine on isolated cardiac tissues from young and aged animals have been studied.[47,48] Perfused Langendorff preparations from Fisher 344 rats were used, in which AV block was surgically induced, so that atrial and ventricular nodal activity could be studied simultaneously. Quinidine decreased ventricular rate more than atrial rate. The depressant effect of quinidine on nodal activity decreased with age, as did quinidine asystole.[47,48] Age-related changes in action potential amplitude, overshoot amplitude, plateau duration, and membrane responsiveness were demonstrated in isolated atrial preparations. However, the quinidine effects were not age related.[48] Recently, Nawrath and Eckel reported on the electrophysiological effects of quinidine on papillary muscles from 7 patients,[49] aged 7 to 60 years, who had undergone surgery. The underlying pathology was the same in young and elderly patients, viz., cardiac hypertrophy from chronic cardiac failure of II to III degree clinical severity. Quinidine, 10^{-5} to 10^{-4} M, decreased maximal upstroke velocity of the action potential, shortened the plateau phase of repolarization, and prolonged terminal repolarization. These actions were similar in all preparations and are similar to those reported for normal myocardium. Controlled studies in which the effects of quinidine are compared in young and elderly subjects are relatively few. However, studies in which the majority of the patients are elderly demonstrate that quinidine possesses similar antiarrhythmic properties to those reported for isolated and in vivo preparations.[37,42,50-52]

The effect of age on the pharmacokinetics of quinidine that may alter therapeutic and toxic levels are rather few in number. After oral administration, quinidine is generally considered to be promptly and completely absorbed.[1] The bioavailability of oral quinidine preparations is accounted for on the basis of first-pass hepatic metabolism.[51,53] Maximal effects occur within 1 to 3 hr.[53] Significant correlation of the prolongation of the QRS complex and the QTc interval with plasma levels of quinidine has been reported.[41] Recently, Meyerburg et al.[55] noted that cardiac arrest patients, who had adequate blood levels of quinidine, had no recurrent arrests for more than 12 months; while those in which cardiac arrest recurred invariably had unstable quinidine plasma levels. Thus, there appears to be good correlation between quinidine plasma levels and therapeutic effects. Quinidine is also used intravenously but with caution.[52,56-59] Peak plasma levels after intramuscular administration is about 45 to 90 min.[37] However, the use of quinidine by this route is limited because of erratic absorption and is often associated with tissue necrosis and pain at the site of injection.[53]

Quinidine is 60 to 80% bound to total plasma proteins[60] and to lipoproteins.[61] Binding is relatively insensitive to changes in any one serum protein, providing other proteins are in normal concentrations.[62] Hypo- or hyperlipoprotemia do not affect binding of quinidine.[56,62] Ochs et al.[63] reported that the percentage of unbound quinidine was similar in young and old healthy patients. Drayer et al. reported that quinidine binding to protein was not affected in patients with renal failure. Total protein binding is decreased in patients with alcoholic disease, suggesting that quinidine doses be reduced to one third of normal in such patients.[65]

Quinidine distributes rapidly extramuscularly.[56] In dogs, it has been shown to accumulate in kidney, lung, and liver in concentrations 20 to 40 times the steady-state plasma levels.[66]

Quinidine is metabolized primarily in the kidney to 3-hydroxyquinidine and 2'-oxoquinidine.[64] The metabolites have been shown to possess good antiarrhythmic activity in various animal models.[64] Patients with cirrhotic liver disease have longer plasma half-lives and greater volumes of distribution than normal subjects. Similarly, patients with congestive heart failure have higher quinidine blood levels,[58,67,68] which may be due to a reduction in the total body clearance of quinidine.

Only about 15 to 18% of the administered dose of quinidine is excreted unchanged by the kidneys. There are conflicting data regarding the effects of renal failure on the excretion rates and plasma levels of quinidine. Plasma levels have been reported to be increased in patients with renal failure.[64,67] However, Kessler et al.[69] reported that quinidine plasma levels and half-lives were similar in patients with and without reduced renal clearance. It is possible that the more polar metabolites which are excreted by the kidney may be cleared less well in patients with kidney disease than in those without kidney disease, and these metabolites contribute to the antiarrhythmic and toxic effects of quinidine.[64]

The reports on the toxicity of quinidine are also conflicting. Lown and Wolf[70] reported that 30% of the patients in their study who were receiving "ordinary" doses of quinidine, were forced to discontinue therapy because of untoward effects. Cohen et al.,[71] reviewing the Boston Collaborative Drug Surveillance Program, noted that 14% of the patients taking quinidine alone had adverse drug reactions such as: gastrointestinal distress, arrhythmias, fever, cinchonism, and dermatologic and hematologic abnormalities. About 1% of those patients exhibited syncope. Selzer and Wray[72] noted that 54 of 61 patients with quinidine syncope were also on digitalis, or digitalis had been discontinued so recently that its pharmacologic effects must have been present. A possible pharmacokinetic interpretation of this interaction between quinidine and digoxin is that quinidine may displace digoxin from its binding sites, and this may contribute to the increased cardiac effect of the two drugs.[73]

Adverse reactions to quinidine have been reported in patients who ingested quantities of antacids large enough to alkalinize the urine.[74] Dementia, agranulocytosis, leukopenia, and thrombocytopenia also have been reported in elderly patients taking quinidine.[75-78]

PROCAINAMIDE

Procainamide is another useful agent for the treatment and prevention of most atrial and ventricular arrhythmias.[1,2,54,79] The electrophysiological properties of procainamide appear to be the same as those described for quinidine.[1,2,54,79] Similarities in the electrophysiological properties of various antiarrhythmic agents led Vaughan Williams to propose a four-category classification system of antiarrhythmics.[80] Several other antiarrhythmic drug classification systems have evolved since then.[81-83]

Studies on the effects of procainamide in the young are lacking because indications for its use in this age group are rare.[84] Procainamide has been used successfully to treat various arrhythmias in adult and elderly patients.[50,79,85-93] However, since many elderly patients have functional impairment of various organs, the pharmacokinetics of procainamide in the elderly may be affected.

Procainamide is almost completely absorbed from the small intestines.[94-97] Oral and intramuscular absorption is erratic, incomplete, and unpredictable in early myocardial infarction, so the drug is usually given intravenously in this situation.[94] However, Lalka et al.[98] found that, in the immediate postinfarction period, the time to achieve steady-state plasma levels of procainamide after intravenous administration was the same as in normal patients, but that this steady-state level was higher. It appears that the patient with acute myocardial infarction has a lower total body clearance of procainamide than normal volunteers. Peak plasma levels appear in about 60 min.[54] Good correlation between therapeutic or toxic effects of procainamide and plasma concentrations of the drug have been reported by some investigators,[93,95,97,99,100] whereas others have found the correlation not as good as previously reported.[101,102] Approximately 15% of the procainamide at therapeutic plasma levels is bound to plasma protein.[94,103] It is unlikely that binding is a problem in the pharmacokinetics of procainamide.

Procainamide is bound to heart, kidney, liver, and lung tissues.[84] Schnitzer and Robertson found that the procainamide content of dog atria was about 1/100 the content of procainamide of the ventricles, 1 hr following an intravenous bolus injection.[104] These data provided support for the proposition that procainamide was more effective in ventricular arrhythmias than in atrial arrhythmias. However, Wenger et al.[105] found that although there was a statistically significant difference between the procainamide content of dog atria and ventricles, the atria contained only slightly less than the ventricles, so that tissue binding could not account for differences in action at the two sites. In the latter study, the procainamide dose was infused over 4 hr.[105]

The plasma half-life of procainamide in normal healthy volunteers is approximately 3 to 4 hr.[84,93,94,99] Approximately 50 to 60% of the administered dose is excreted in the urine unchanged.[84,94,106] Procainamide is acetylated in the liver to N-acetylprocainamide.[84,106,108] Detectable plasma levels of N-acetylprocainamide appear soon after oral administration, suggesting first-pass metabolism through the intestinal wall and/or liver.[84] Approximately 15% of an administered dose of procainamide is excreted in the urine, as N-acetylprocainamide, within 24 hr.[84-96] N-acetylprocainamide has antiarrhythmic and acute toxic properties similar to those of procainamide.[108-112] There appear to be two patient populations in which slow or rapid rates of procainamide acetylation have been identified.[84,103] It has been suggested recently that the procainamide acetylation status is best determined by measuring steady-state procainamide plasma levels and N-acetylprocainamide urinary excretion rates.[113]

Patients with impaired renal function (prerenal azotemia, uremia, and anephric) have significantly prolonged procainamide and *N*-acetylprocainamide plasma half-lives.[53,94,106,114-115] Dosage should be adjusted downward in these patients. Du Souich and Erill found that patients with chronic liver disease had a decrease in excretion of procainamide.[116] Since these patients had normal renal function, the apparent increase in the procainamide volume of distribution was attributed to an impairment in the oral absorption of the drug.

Adverse reactions to procainamide have recently been reviewed by Lawson and Jick.[117] The reaction categories include gastrointestinal, cardiovascular, central nervous system, and immunologic reactions. Gastrointestinal reactions include nausea, vomiting, or diarrhea.[2,117] Cardiovascular reactions include hypotension and conduction disturbances (ventricular ectopic beats, ventricular fibrillation, and asystole).[2,117] While central nervous system effects are rare, stimulation and psychosis have been reported.[118,119] Patients on long-term therapy with procainamide have been known to develop a lupus erythematosus-like syndrome,[120-123] characterized by symptoms such as fever and arthralgia. It has also been suggested that patients who are slow acetylator phenotypes may be prone to the development of this condition.[121] A circulating anticoagulant has also been identified in the lupus syndrome.[124] Other adverse reactions that have been reported recently are granulomatous hepatitis,[125] bone marrow granulomas and neutropenia,[126] and a hemolytic anemia, without lupus symptoms, in which the direct antiglobulin tests were consistently positive.[127]

PHENYTOIN (DIPHENYLHYDANTOIN)

Putnam and Merritt described the anticonvulsant actions of phenytoin in 1937.[128] In 1950, Harris and Kohernat reported on the use of phenytoin in experimental ventricular tachyarrhythmias in dogs, resulting from ligation of the left descending coronary artery.[129] The first successful use of phenytoin as an antiarrhythmic agent in man was described by Leonard in 1958.[130] Since that time, there have been numerous reports on the successful use of phenytoin in ventricular arrhythmias resulting from various causes, especially digitalis-induced arrhythmias.[131-141] However, several investigators have reported less than favorable results with phenytoin,[86,87,142] and its use has been limited because of the potential toxicity from intravenous or oral use.

The electrophysiologic actions of phenytoin resemble those of lidocaine.[1,2] Roberts and Goldberg[19] studied the electrophysiologic effect of phenytoin in isolated atria of Fischer 344 rats, ages 1 to 28 months. The concentration used was 10 mg/ℓ, which is reported to be the clinical therapeutic plasma level of the drug.[143] They reported that with increasing age, phenytoin increased the depression of the action potential overshoot and the rate of rise of the upstroke of the action potential (dV/dt). The increase in action potential duration and action potential plateau duration produced by phenytoin decreased with age. The phenytoin effect on action potential amplitude did not change with age. Reports on the effects of age on the actions of phenytoin are rare. Several earlier reports have indicated that infants and young children required larger doses of phenytoin than adults, per kilogram of body weight, in order to achieve therapeutic concentrations sufficient to control epilepsy.[144-146] However, Lambie and Caird recently have reported that even higher doses were needed in the elderly to obtain optimum serum concentrations for epilepsy control.[147]

Age-related changes in the pharmacokinetics of phenytoin have been reported. Oral absorption of phenytoin in man results in detectable blood levels in about 2 hr.[148] Peak plasma levels appear in about 8 hr,[148-150] and are maintained up to 12 hr.[148,149] However, to achieve steady-state plasma levels may take as long as 6 to 7 days without a loading dosage regimen.[143] Achlorhydria,[148] or alkalinization of the stomach contents with sodium bicarbonate solution,[151] does not alter oral absorption of phenytoin.

Furlanut et al.[152] reported that the correlation between dose and serum concentration for phenytoin was not good and that age did not affect the serum concentration to dose ratio.

Higher steady-state plasma levels were reported by Sherwin et al.[153] in the elderly. Dill et al.[149] reported that tissue levels of phenytoin correlated well with blood levels, but were two to three times higher. Kutt reported that blood and tissue phenytoin concentrations were related to the administered dose,[154] but the actual values depended more on rate of phenytoin metabolism. The concentration in red blood cells was reported to be equal to that found in plasma.[148] The plasma half-life of phenytoin in normal subjects is 18 to 24 hr.[148,149] Increased plasma clearance of phenytoin was observed in the elderly, but decreased absorption did not account for this effect.[155-156]

More than 90% of the phenytoin in blood is bound to serum albumin,[148,157] although it also binds to α-globulin and is known to compete with thyroxine for this binding site.[158] Phenytoin leaves the blood rapidly; a high percentage of it is excreted into the bile and is recirculated via the bile. Protein binding of phenytoin is decreased in patients with uremia; therefore, higher levels of unbound drug are reported in these subjects.[155,156,159-163] Shoeman and Azarnoff,[164] using an isoelectric focusing technique, noted that serum albumin was altered in uremia. In addition, they concluded that since the association constant was weak, phenytoin binding may have little or no clinical significance. Odar-Cederlöf and Borgå noted that treatment of uremic plasma with charcoal increased binding of phenytoin,[163] suggesting that an inhibitory factor was present in the blood or uremic patients and that it decreased phenytoin binding.

Phenytoin is metabolized almost completely in the liver.[165,166] Drugs that inhibit or induce liver microsomal metabolizing enzymes increase or decrease phenytoin is 5-(p-hydroxy-phenyl-5-phenyl-hydantoin). Lambie and Caird noted that the K_m (serum concentration at which metabolism was half-saturated) and V_{max} (maximum rate of metabolism) for phenytoin were the same for young and elderly subjects.[147] The observation that females have lower plasma levels of drugs which are metabolized by liver microsomal enzymes does not hold for phenytoin.[156,169,170]

Less than 5% of phenytoin administered per dose is excreted in the urine, unchanged. Hydroxylated phenytoin and its glucuronide metabolite are excreted via the kidneys by glomerular filtration and tubular secretion.[171] The relationships between renal function, protein binding, and plasma clearance of phenytoin were discussed above.

Adverse cardiovascular, central nervous system, and hematologic reactions to phenytoin have been reported. Cardiovascular reactions include arrhythmias,[172] sudden death,[173] and hypotension.[174] Recently the hypotensive effect of phenytoin was studied as a possible therapeutic regimen in hypertension.[175] While phenytoin produces an acute lowering of blood pressure, the effect is absent on chronic administration.[175] Central effects include nystagmus, ataxia, dysarthria, seizures, mental changes, and choreathetosis (abnormal involuntary movements).[176] Hematologic reactions include anemia, pancytopenia, reticulo-endothelial disorders, and a megaloblastic anemia.[2] Osteomalacia and erythema multiforma[178] have been also reported in elderly patients.[177,178]

PROPRANOLOL

The variety of arrhythmias in which propranolol has proven efficacy has been reviewed recently.[179] They range from atrial and ventricular arrhythmias arising from different causes, to catecholamine- and digitalis-induced arrhythmias.

The antiarrhythmic effects of propranolol result from the beta-adrenoceptor blocking properties of the drug[180] and its quinidine-like or membrane stabilizing properties.[181,182] The former action will antagonize the effects of sympathetic nerve stimulation and adrenergic or sympathomimetic drug action on the heart. The electrophysiologic effects of propranolol on the various parts of the heart are as follows: sinus node automaticity is decreased by depressing Phase 4 depolarization, resulting in slowing of sinus rate.[183,184] In atrial cells, the maximum rate of rise of the action potential and conduction velocity are decreased, while action potential duration and effective refractory period are unchanged.[182] In the atrioventricular node, conduction velocity is decreased and refractory period is increased.[182,184-186] In Purkinje fibers propranolol decreases automaticity, action potential duration, and effective refractory period.[187] The effective refractory period relative to action potential duration is increased.[187] The maximum rate of rise of the action potential and overshoot are decreased while the resting membrane potential is unchanged.[187] In ventricular muscle, propranolol does not change the ventricular fibrillation threshold.[188] The rate of depolarization of the ventricular action potential is decreased, but duration of conduction velocity is unchanged.[187] Propranolol prolongs the P-R interval, shortens the Q-T interval, but has no effect on the QRS complex of the electrocardiogram.[189,190]

The effect of age on tissue sensitivity to propranolol was studied by Roberts and Goldberg[19] in isolated atria of Fischer 344 rats, ages 1 to 28 months. Propranolol, at a concentration of 1 mg/ℓ decreased the maximum rate of rise of the action potential and increased action-potential duration, but age had no effect on these changes.[19] Conway[191] studied the effect of age on the cardiovascular responses to propranolol in man. Propranolol produced a greater fall in systolic blood pressure in elderly subjects than in young subjects. However, systolic blood pressure was higher in the elderly prior to propranolol treatment. Heart rate response to propranolol was the same in young and elderly subjects, but a greater fall in cardiac index was observed in the young than in the elderly (for further discussion, see chapter by Dr. Roberts).

The effects of age on the pharmacokinetics of propranolol are not well defined. Castleden et al.[192] reported that the mean peak plasma levels of propranolol in the elderly were about four times greater than those observed in children, suggesting that the propranolol dose be reduced in the elderly. Shand et al.[193] used two methods for calculating the propranolol dosage needed for studying blood levels in adults and children. When the oral dose was expressed on a milligram per kilogram basis, the propranolol plasma levels in children fell below the range of adult values.[193] If the oral dose was expressed on the basis of relative body surface area (milligram per square millimeter), then the plasma levels in children were in the higher range of adult values.[193]

The absorption of orally administered propranolol is 70 to 100% complete.[194,195] However, the variability in peak plasma levels after oral doses is five- to sevenfold, whereas the variability after intravenous dosing is about two- to two and one-half-fold.[193,195] Very little propranolol appears in blood after small oral doses, since the drug undergoes extensive hepatic binding.[194] The plasma half-life of propranolol after a single oral dose is about 3.2 hr and after a single intravenous dose, it is about 2.3 hr.[193] With chronic oral dosing, the plasma half-life is about 4.6 hr,[195,196] presumably because of saturation of hepatic binding sites. Under these conditions, the plasma concentration of propranolol is proportional to the dose.[195-197] About 93% of the administered dose is bound to plasma proteins.[196,198] Patients with Chron's disease, inflammatory arthritis, or renal failure exhibit increased protein binding.[199] Plasma protein binding is unchanged in patients with chronic hepatic disease or uncomplicated renal failure.[199]

The liver metabolizes almost all of the administered propranolol.[194,197,200,202] The major metabolite of propranolol is p-hydroxypropranolol, although at least six other metabolites have been identified.[202] Since the metabolites have pharmacologic and toxicologic properties that are similar to propranolol, their disposition is important.[203,204] Liver diseases such as alcoholic cirrhosis, chronic active hepatitis, and cryptogenic cirrhosis decrease plasma clearance of propranolol and increase the concentration of the free drug in the plasma.[205]

Less than 1% of the administered dose of propranolol is excreted unchanged in the urine,[202] and about 1 to 4% of the dose is excreted in the feces.[194] The metabolites of propranolol are excreted in the urine.[194] Peak blood and plasma concentrations of propranolol in patients with chronic renal failure are two to three times greater than in normal or dialyzed patients;[206] plasma half-life of propranolol is also increased. On the basis of these data, the authors recommended that, in patients with chronic renal failure, the propranolol dose be decreased and that the drug be used with caution.[206] However, Thompson et al.[207] noted that although the plasma half-life of radioactivity from a dose of radiolabeled propranolol was increased, the plasma half-life of propranolol and *p*-hydroxypropranolol was unchanged. They suggest that renal failure should not alter the clinically effective dose. Propranolol also is excreted in the milk of lactating mothers, but the amounts passed to the infant are considerably less than the usual therapeutic dose for infants.[208]

Adverse reactions to propranolol include nausea and diarrhea, fatigue, skin rash, mild visual disturbances, hypoglycemia, and development of congestive heart failure.[209] Greenblatt and Koch-Weser[210] reviewed the clinical toxicology of propranolol from the Boston Collaborative Drug Surveillance Program. About 9.9% of patients taking propranolol alone exhibit adverse reactions. Reactions other than those reported above were impaired cardiac perfusion and function, bradycardia and heart block, bronchospasm and pulmonary edema, and shock.[209] While adverse reactions were more common among the elderly, this was a trend that was not statistically significant.[210] Azotemic patients exhibited comparatively a greater incidence of reactions.[210] Long-term propranolol therapy has recently been shown to decrease glomerular filtration in normal subjects,[211] alopecia,[213] organic brain syndrome,[214] aggravated peripheral arterial insufficiency,[215] recurrent migraine,[216] and cheilostomatitis.[217] Sudden withdrawal of propranolol therapy has been reported to result in rebound angina and death.[218] One recent review does not support the concept of a rebound propranolol withdrawal reaction,[219] whereas another review suggests that the clinical setting may be a factor in this reaction.[220]

VERAPAMIL

Verapamil is a papaverine analogue that was first introduced as an antianginal agent but was subsequently found to possess antiarrhythmic activity.[221] The drug has proven efficacy in the treatment of supraventricular tachyarrhythmias, atrial flutter, and atrial fibrillation; it has limited usefulness in ventricular tachyarrhythmias.[222-231] Asystole has been known to occur in patients with sick sinus syndrome who present with atrial arrhythmias; verapamil should be used with caution in this group.[232,233]

Verapamil has a selective depressant action on the sinoatrial node and on conduction in the atrioventricular node.[234,235] In normal Purkinje fibers, verapamil has no effect on the resting membrane potential, action potential amplitude, nor on the upstroke of the depolarization phase of the action potential, but it abolishes the plateau of repolarization and increases the action potential duration at 100% of repolarization.[236] In Purkinje fibers that show a calcium-dependent slow response, verapamil suppresses rhythmic activity and depresses excitability.[236] In the His bundle, verapamil delays A-V conduction proximal to the bundle, without having any effect on atrial and intraventricular conduction.[237] The electrocardiographic effects of verapamil are manifested as a prolongation of the P-R interval, but there is no effect on the QRS, QT_c or R-R intervals.[228]

The influence of age on the electrophysiological effects of verapamil were studied by Goldberg et al.[17] and Roberts and Goldberg[19] in atria of Fischer 344 rats, ages 1 to 28 months. Decreases in action potential amplitude and overshoot became more pronounced with increasing age. Increases in action potential duration produced by verapamil became less pronounced with increasing age.

Verapamil has been used to treat paroxysmal supraventricular tachycardia in infants, ages 5 days to 18 months, but whether the drug was more or less efficacious in infants than in the elderly was not indicated.[231]

The pharmacokinetics of verapamil in man were studied recently by Schomerus et al.[238] Radiolabeled verapamil was administered orally and intravenously to 5 patients, ages 51 to 59, with normal kidney and liver function. About 92% of the oral dose was absorbed and peak concentrations appeared in 30 to 45 min. Approximately 88 to 92% of the drug was protein bound. Verapamil undergoes rapid inactivation during first-pass biotransformation in the liver. Thus, only 10 to 22% of the orally administered drug is bioavailable. The plasma half-life after intravenous administrations is 213 to 442 min. About 9 to 16% of the drug is excreted in the feces and 50% in the urine in 24 hr. About 80% of an intravenous dose is recovered from the urine and feces in 5 days.[238]

Verapamil has a relatively short history compared to the antiarrhythmic drugs discussed earlier. There are many studies lacking that could provide a better understanding of whether age-related changes in responses to verapamil are due to changes in tissue sensitivity or pharmacokinetic factors.

NEW ANTIARRHYTHMIC AGENTS

Several new antiarrhythmic agents have been introduced lately: amiodarone, aprindine, bretylium, disopyramide, mexiletine, potassium canrenoate, and tocainide. These agents have been reviewed,[1,2,239] but more studies are needed before their roles in antiarrhythmic therapy are established.

REFERENCES

1. **Mason, D. T., DeMaria, A. N., Amsterday, E. A., Vismara, L. A., Miller, R. R., Vera, Z., Lee, G., Zelis, R., and Massumi, R. A.,** Antiarrhythmic agents: mechanisms of action, clinical pharmacology and therapeutic considerations, in *Cardiovascular Drugs,* Vol. 1, Antiarrhythmic, Antihypertensive and Lipid Lowering Drugs, Avery, G. S., Series Ed., University Park Press, Baltimore, Md., 1977, 75.
2. **Lucchesi, B. R.,** Antiarrhythmic drugs, in *Cardiovascular Pharmacology,* Antonaccio, M., Ed., Raven Press, New York, 1977, 269.
3. **Frieden, J.,** Lidocaine as an antiarrhythmic agent, *Am. Heart J.,* 70, 713, 1965.
4. **Gianelly, R., Van der Groeben, J. O., Spivak, A. P., and Harrison, D. C.,** Effect of lidocaine on ventricular arrhythmias in patients with coronary artery disease, *N. Engl. J. Med.,* 277, 1215, 1967.
5. **Lown, B. and Wolf, M.,** Approaches to sudden death from coronary heart disease, *Circulation,* 44, 130, 1971.
6. **Löfmark, R. and Orinius, E.,** Restricted lignocaine in myocardial infarction, *Acta Med. Scand.,* 201, 89, 1977.
7. **Bergdahl, B., Karlsson, E., Magnusson, J. O., and Sonnhag, C.,** Lidocaine and the quaternary ammonium compound QX-572 in acute myocardial infarction. A comparative study, *Acta Med. Scand.,* 204, 311, 1978.
8. **Grossman, J. I., Lublow, L. A., Frieden, J., and Rubin, I. L.,** Lidocaine in cardiac arrhythmias, *Arch. Intern. Med.,* 121, 396, 1968.
9. **Danahy, D. T. and Aronow, W. S.,** Lidocaine-induced cardiac rate changes in atrial fibrillation and atrial flutter, *Am. Heart J.,* 95, 474, 1978.
10. **Dhingra, R. C., Deedwania, P. C., Lummings, J. M., Amat-Y-Leon, F., Wu, D., Denes, P., and Rosen, K. M.,** Electrophysiologic effects of lidocaine on sinus node and atrium in patients with and without sinoatrial dysfunction, *Circulation,* 57, 448, 1978.
11. **Nevins, M. A.,** Reevaluating the use of lidocaine, *Geriatrics,* 28, 48, 1973.
12. **Ryden, L. and Kosgren, M.,** The effect of lignocaine on the stimulation threshold and conduction disturbances in patients treated with pacemaker, *Cardiovasc. Res.,* 3, 415, 1969.
13. **Aravindakshan, V., Kuo, C.-S., and Gettes, L. S.,** Effect of lidocaine on escape rate in patients with complete atrioventricular block, a distal His bundle block, *Am. J. Cardiol.,* 40, 177, 1977.
14. **Sinatra, S. T. and Jeresaty, R. M.,** Enhanced atrioventricular conduction in atrial fibrillation after lidocaine administration, *J.A.M.A.,* 273, 1356, 1977.

15. **Bigger, J. T., Jr. and Mandel, W. J.,** Effect of lidocaine on the electrophysiological properties of ventricular muscle and Purkinje fibers, *J. Clin. Invest.,* 49, 63, 1970.

16. **Goldberg, P. B. and Roberts, J.,** Age effects on atrial and ventricular sensitivity to quinidine and lidocaine. II, *Gerontologist,* 15, 24, 1975.

17. **Goldberg, P. B., Stoner, S-A., and Roberts, J.,** Influence of age on activity of antiarrhythmic drugs in rat heart, *Adv. Exp. Med. Biol.,* 97, 309, 1978.

18. **Goldberg, P. B. and Roberts, J.,** Physiological and pharmacological changes of rat cardiac pacemakers with increasing age, *Adv. Exp. Med. Biol.,* 97, 315, 1978.

19. **Roberts, J. and Goldberg, P. B.,** Changes in responsiveness of the heart to drugs during aging, *Fed. Proc. Fed. Am. Soc. Exp. Biol.,* 38, 1927, 1979.

20. **Rosen, K. M., Lau, S. H., Weiss, M. B., and Damato, A. N.,** The effect of lidocaine on atrioventricular and intraventricular conduction in man, *Am. J. Cardiol.,* 25, 1, 1970.

21. **Bekheit, S., Murtagh, J. G., Morton, P., and Fletcher, E.,** Effect of lignocaine on conducting system of human heart, *Br. Heart J.,* 35, 305, 1973.

22. **Boyes, R. N., Scott, D. B., Jebson, P. J., Godman, M. J., and Julian, D. G.,** Pharmacokinetics of lidocaine in man, *Clin. Pharm. Ther.,* 12, 105, 1971.

23. **Nation, R. L., Triggs, E. J., and Selig, M.,** Lidocaine kinetics in cardiac patients and aged subjects, *Br. J. Clin. Pharm.,* 4, 439, 1977.

24. **Brandfonbrener, M., Landowne, M., and Schock, N. W.,** Changes in cardiac output with age, *Circulation,* 12, 557, 1955.

25. **Thompson, P. D., Rowland, M., and Melmon, K. L.,** The influence of heart failure, liver disease and renal failure on the disposition of lidocaine in man, *Am. Heart J.,* 82, 417, 1971.

26. **Thompson, P. D., Melmon, K. L., Richardson, J. A., Cohn, K., Steinbrunn, W., Cudihee, R., and Rowland, M.,** Lidocaine pharmacokinetics in advanced heart failure, liver disease, and renal failure in humans, *Ann. Intern. Med.,* 78, 499, 1973.

27. **Aps, C., Bell, J. A., Jenkins, B. S., Poole-Wilson, P. A., and Reynolds, F.,** Logical approach to lignocaine therapy, *Br. Med. J.,* 1, 13, 1976.

28. **Prescott, L. F., Adjepon-Yamoah, K. K., and Talbot, R. G.,** Impaired lignocaine metabolism in patients with myocardial infarction and cardiac failure, *Br. Med. J.,* 1, 939, 1976.

29. **Forrest, J. A. H., Finlayson, N. D. C., Adjepon-Yamoah, K. K., and Prescott, L. F.,** Antipyrine, paracetamol, and lignocaine elimination in chronic liver disease, *Br. Med. J.,* 1, 1384, 1977.

30. **Zito, R. A., Reid, P. R., and Longstreth, J. A.,** Variability of early lidocaine levels in man, *Am. Heart J.,* 94, 292, 1977.

31. **Zito, R. A. and Reid, P. R.,** Lidocaine kinetics predicted by indocyanine green clearance, *N. Engl. J. Med.,* 298, 1160, 1978.

32. **Beckett, A. J., Boyes, R. N., and Appleton, P. J.,** The metabolism and excretion of lignocaine in man, *J. Pharm. Pharmacol.,* 18(Suppl.), 76, 1966.

33. **Pfeiffer, H. J., Greenblatt, D. J., and Koch-Weser, J.,** Clinical use and toxicity of intravenous lidocaine. A report of the Boston Drug Surveillance Program, *Am. Heart J.,* 92, 168, 1976.

34. **Manyari-Ortega, D. E. and Brennan, F. J.,** Lidocaine-induced cardiac asystole, *Chest,* 74, 227, 1978.

35. **Hoffman, B. F.,** The action of quinidine and procaine amide on single fibers of dog ventricle and specialized conducting systems, *An. Acad. Bras. Cienc.,* 29, 365, 1958.

36. **West, T. C. and Amory, D. W.,** Single fiber recording of the effects of quinidine at atrial pacemaker sites in the isolated atrium of the rabbit, *J. Pharmacol. Exp. Therap.,* 130, 183, 1960.

37. **Josephson, M. E., Seides, S. F., Batsford, W. P., Weisfogel, G. M., Akhtar, M., Caracta, A. R., Lau, S. H., and Damato, A.,** The electrophysiological effects of intramuscular quinidine on the atrioventricular conducting system in man, *Am. Heart J.,* 87, 55, 1974.

38. **Wallace, A. G., Clive, R. E., and Sealy, W. C.,** Electrophysiologic effects of quinidine, *Circ. Res.,* 19, 960, 1966.

39. **Geddes, L. S. and Sandquest, V.,** Effect of quinidine on the differences between Purkinje and ventricular fibers, *Circulation,* 40, 88, 1969.

40. **Weidmann, S.,** Effects of calcium ions and local anesthetics on electrical properties of Purkinje fibers, *J. Physiol. (London),* 129, 568, 1955.

41. **Heissenbuttel, R. H. and Bigger, J. T., Jr.,** The effect of oral quinidine on intraventricular conduction in man: correlation of plasma quinidine with changes in QRS duration, *Am. Heart J.,* 80, 453, 1970.

42. **Weisman, S. A.,** Quinidine in geriatrics, *Geriatrics,* 4, 85, 1949.

43. **Yount, E. H., Rosenblum, M., and McMillan, R. L.,** Quinidine for chronic auricular flutter in the patients over 50, *Geriatrics,* 8, 19, 1953.

44. **Gotthold, E.,** Die chinidin-therapie des alterherzens, *Med. Monatsschr. (Stuttgart),* 15, 396, 1961.

45. **DeGraff, A. C.,** Drug therapy of cardiovascular disease, *Geriatrics,* 29, 51, 1974.

46. **Simon, A. P.,** Quinidine in elderly patients, *Am. Fam. Phys.,* 9, 127, 1974.

47. **Goldberg, P. B. and Roberts, J.,** Physiological and pharmacological changes of rat cardiac pacemakers with increasing age, *Adv. Exp. Med. Biol.,* 97, 315, 1978.
48. **Roberts, J. and Goldberg, P. B.,** Changes in responsiveness of the heart to drugs during aging, *Fed. Proc. Fed. Am. Soc. Exp. Biol.,* 38, 1927, 1979.
49. **Nawrath, H. and Eckel, L.,** Electrophysiological study of human ventricular heart muscle treated with quinidine: interaction with isoprenaline, *J. Cardiovasc. Pharmacol.,* 1, 415, 1979.
50. **Winkle, R. A., Gradman, A. H., and Fitzgerald, J. W.,** Antiarrhythmic drug effect assessed from ventricular arrhythmia assessment in the ambulatory electrocardiogram and treadmill test: comparison of propranolol, procainamide and quinidine, *Am. J. Cardiol.,* 42, 4731, 1978.
51. **Woo, E., Greenblatt, D. J., and Ochs, J. R.,** Short- and long-acting oral quinidine preparations. Clinical implications of pharmacokinetic differences, *Angiology,* 29, 243, 1978.
52. **Hirschfeld, D. S., Ueda, C. T., Rowland, M., and Scheinman, M. M.,** Clinical and electrophysiological effects of intravenous quinidine in man, *Br. Heart J.,* 39, 309, 1977.
53. **Harrison, D. C., Meffin, P. J., and Winkle, R. A.,** Clinical pharmacokinetics of antiarrhythmic drugs, *Progr. Cardiovasc. Dis.,* 20, 217, 1977.
54. **Moe, G. K. and Abildskov, J. A.,** Antiarrhythmic drugs, in *The Pharmacological Basis of Therapeutics,* Goodman, L. S. and Gilman, A., Eds., Macmillan, New York, 1975, 683.
55. **Meyerburg, R. J., Conde, C., Sheps, D. S., Appel, R. A., Kiem, L., Sung, R. J., and Castellanos, A.,** Antiarrhythmic drug therapy in survivors of pre-hospital cardiac arrest: comparison of effects of chronic ventricular arrhythmias and recurrent cardiac arrest, *Circulation,* 59, 855, 1979.
56. **Ueda, C. T., Hirschfeld, D. S., Scheinman, M. M., Rowland, M., Williamson, B. J., and Dzindzio, B. S.,** Disposition kinetics of quinidine, *Clin. Pharmacol. Ther.,* 19, 30, 1976.
57. **Greenblatt, D. J., Pfeiffer, H. J., Ochs, H. R., Franke, K., MacLaughlin, D. S., Smith, T. W., and Koch-Weser, J.,** Pharmacokinetic studies of quinidine in humans after intravenous, intramuscular and oral administration, *J. Pharmacol. Exp. Ther.,* 202, 365, 1977.
58. **Ueda, C. T. and Dzindzio, B. S.,** Quinidine kinetics in congestive heart failure, *Clin. Pharmacol. Ther.,* 23, 158, 1978.
59. **Woo, E. and Greenblatt, D. J.,** A reevaluation of intravenous quinidine, *Am. Heart J.,* 96, 829, 1978.
60. **Conn, H. J. and Luchi, R. J.,** Some quantitative aspects of binding by quinidine and related quinoline compounds by human serum albumin, *J. Clin. Invest.,* 40, 504, 1961.
61. **Nilsen, O. G.,** Serum albumin and lipoproteins as the quinidine binding molecules in normal sera, *Biochem. Pharmacol.,* 25, 1007, 1976.
62. **Kates, R. E., Sokoloski, T. D., and Comstock, T. J.,** Binding of quinidine to plasma proteins in normal subjects and in patients with hyperlipoproteinemias, *Clin. Pharmacol. Ther.,* 23, 30, 1978.
63. **Ochs, H. R., Greenblatt, D. J., Woo, E., and Smith, T. W.,** Reduced quinidine clearance in elderly persons, *Am. J. Cardiol.,* 42, 481, 1978.
64. **Drayer, D. E., Lowenthal, D. T., Restivo, K. M., Schwartz, A., Cooke, C. E., and Reidenberg, M. M.,** Steady state serum levels of quinidine and active metabolites in cardiac patients with varying degrees of renal function, *Clin. Pharmacol. Ther.,* 24, 31, 1978.
65. **Affrime, M. and Reidenberg, M. M.,** The protein binding of some drugs in plasma from patients with alcoholic liver disease, *Eur. J. Clin. Pharmacol.,* 8, 267, 1975.
66. **Hiatt, E. and Quinn, G.,** The distribution of quinine, quinidine, and cinchonine and cinchonidine in fluids and tissues of dogs, *J. Pharmacol. Exp. Therap.,* 83, 101, 1945.
67. **Conrad, K. A., Molk, B. L., and Chidsey, C. A.,** Pharmacokinetic studies of quinidine in patients with arrhythmias, *Circulation,* 55, 1, 1977.
68. **Ditlefsen, E. L.,** Quinidine concentration in blood and excretion in urine following parenteral administration as related to congestive heart failure, *Acta Med. Scand.,* 159, 105, 1957.
69. **Kessler, K. M., Lowenthal, D. T., Warner, H., Gibson, T., Briggs, W., and Reidenberg, M. M.,** Quinidine elimination in patients with congestive heart failure or poor renal function, *N. Engl. J. Med.,* 290, 706, 1974.
70. **Lown, B. and Wolf, M.,** Approaches to sudden death from coronary artery disease, *Circulation,* 44, 130, 1971.
71. **Cohen, I., Jick, H., and Cohen, I. S.,** Adverse reactions to quinidine in hospitalized patients: findings based on data from the Boston Collaborative Drug Surveillance Program, *Progr. Cardiovasc. Dis.,* 20, 151, 1977.
72. **Selzer, A. and Wray, H. W.,** Quinidine syncope: paroxysmal ventricular fibrillation occurring during treatment of chronic atrial arrhythmias, *Circulation,* 30, 17, 1964.
73. **Leahey, E. B., Jr., Reiffel, J. A., Drusin, R. E., Heissenbuttel, R. H., Lovejoy, W. P., and Bigger, J. T., Jr.,** Interaction between quinidine and digoxin, *J.A.M.A.,* 240, 533, 1978.
74. **Zinn, M. B.,** Quinidine intoxication from alkali ingestion, *Tex. Med.,* 66, 64, 1970.
75. **Gilbert, G. J.,** Quinidine dementia, *J.A.M.A.,* 237, 2093, 1977.
76. **Gilbert, G. J.,** Quinidine dementia (letter), *Am. J. Cardiol.,* 41, 791, 1978.

77. **Eisner, E. V., Carr, R. M., and MacKinney, A. R.,** Quinidine-induced agranulocytosis, *J.A.M.A.*, 238, 994, 1977.
78. **Castro, O. and Nash, I.,** Quinidine leukopenia and thrombocytopenia with a drug-dependent leukoagglutinin, *N. Engl. J. Med.*, 296, 572, 1977.
79. **Bigger, J. T., Jr. and Heissenbuttel, R. H.,** The use of procaine amide and lidocaine in the treatment of cardiac arrhythmias, *Progr. Cardiovasc. Dis.*, 11, 515, 1969.
80. **Vaughan Williams, E. M.,** Classification of antiarrhythmic drugs, in, *Symposium on Cardiac Arrhythmias (Elsinore, Denmark, 1970),* Sandø, E., Flensted-Jensen, E. and Olsen, K. H., Eds., Södertälje, Sweden, 1970, 449.
81. **Hoffman, B. F. and Bigger, J. T., Jr.,** Antiarrhythmic drugs, in *Drill's Pharmacology in Medicine*, 4th ed., DiPalma, J. R., Ed., McGraw-Hill, New York, 1971, 824.
82. **Singh, B. N. and Hauswirth, O.,** Comparative mechanisms of action of antiarrhythmic drugs, *Am. Heart J.*, 87, 367, 1974.
83. **Gettes, L. S.,** On the classification of antiarrhythmic drugs, *Mod. Conc. Cardiovasc. Dis.*, 58, 13, 1979.
84. **Karlsson, E.,** Clinical pharmacokinetics of procainamide, *Clin. Pharmacokinet.*, 3, 97, 1978.
85. **Giardina, E. V. and Bigger, J. T., Jr.,** Procainamide against reentrant ventricular arrhythmias. Lengthening R-V intervals of coupled ventricular premature depolarizations as an insight into the mechanism of action of procainamide, *Circulation*, 48, 959, 1973.
86. **Karlsson, E.,** Procainamide and phenytoin. Comparative study of their antiarrhythmic effects at apparent therapeutic plasma levels, *Br. Heart J.*, 37, 731, 1975.
87. **Karlsson, E., Kinman, A., and Sonnhag, C.,** Comparative evaluation of intravenous phenytoin, procainamide and practolol in the acute treatment of ventricular arrhythmias, *Eur. J. Clin. Pharmacol.*, 11, 1, 1977.
88. **Wellens, H. J. J., Bär, F. W. H. N., Lei, K. I., Düren, D. R., and Dohmen, H. J.,** Effect of procainamide, propranolol and verapamil on mechanism of tachycardia in patients with chronic recurrent ventricular tachycardia, *Am. J. Cardiol.*, 40, 579, 1970.
89. **Wu, D., Denes, P., Bauerfeind, R., Kehoe, R., Amat-Y-Leon, F., and Rosen, K. M.,** Effects of procainamide on atrioventricular reentrant paroxysmal tachycardia, *Circulation*, 57, 1171, 1978.
90. **Engel, T. R., Gonzalez, A. del C., Meister, S. G., and Frankel, W. S.,** Effect of procainamide on induced ventricular tachycardia, *Clin. Pharmacol. Ther.*, 24, 274, 1978.
91. **Reddy, C. P. and Lynch, M.,** Abolition and modification of reentry within the His-Purkinje system by procainamide in man, *Circulation*, 58, 1010, 1978.
92. **Wyse, D. G., McAnulty, J. H., and Rahimtoola, S. H.,** Influence of plasma drug level and the presence of conduction disease on the electrophysiologic effects of procainamide, *Am. J. Cardiol.*, 43, 619, 1979.
93. **Koch-Weser, J.,** Pharmacokinetics of procainamide in man, *Ann. N.Y. Acad. Sci.*, 179, 370, 1971.
94. **Koch-Weser, J. and Klein, S. W.,** Procainamide dose schedules, plasma concentrations and clinical effects, *J.A.M.A.*, 215, 1454, 1971.
95. **Weliky, I. and Neiss, E. S.,** Absorption of procainamide from the human intestine, *Clin. Pharmacol. Ther.*, 17, 248, 1975.
96. **Graffner, C., Johnnsson, G., and Sjogren, J.,** Pharmacokinetics of procainamide intravenously and orally as conventional and slow-release tablets, *Clin. Pharmacol. Ther.*, 17, 414, 1973.
97. **Giardina, E., Heissenbuttel, R., and Bigger, J. T., Jr.,** Correlation of plasma concentration with effect on arrhythmia, electrocardiogram and blood pressure, *Ann. Intern. Med.*, 78, 183, 1973.
98. **Lalka, D., Wyman, M. G., Goldreyer, B. N., Ludden, T. M., and Cannom, D. S.,** Procainamide accumulation kinetics in the immediate post myocardial infarction period, *J. Clin. Pharmacol.*, 18, 397, 1978.
99. **Koch-Weser, J.,** Serum procainamide levels as therapeutic guides, *Clin. Pharmacokinet.*, 2, 389, 1977.
100. **Scheinman, M. M., Weis, A. N., Shafton, E., Benowitz, N., and Rowland, M.,** Electrophysiologic effects of procainamide in patients with intraventricular conduction delay, *Circulation*, 49, 522, 1974.
101. **Wellens, H. J. J. and Durrer, D.,** Effect of procainamide, quinidine and ajmaline in the Wolff-Parkinson-White syndrome, *Circulation*, 50, 114, 1974.
102. **Mattiasson, I., Hanson, A., and Johansson, B. W.,** Massive doses of procainamide for ventricular tachyarrhythmias due to myocardial infarction, *Acta Med. Scand.*, 204, 27, 1978.
103. **Reidenberg, M. M., Drayer, D. E., Levy, M., and Warner, H.,** Polymorphic acetylation of procainamide in man, *Clin. Pharmacol. Ther.*, 17, 722, 1975.
104. **Schnitzer, R. N. and Robertson, P. A.,** Regional distribution of procainamide in the canine heart, *Clin. Res.*, 23, 8A, 1975.
105. **Wenger, T. L., Masterton, G. E., Abou-Dania, M. B., Bache, R. J., and Strauss, H. C.,** Myocardial procainamide concentration in canine atria and ventricles, *J. Cardiovasc. Pharmacol.*, 1, 155, 1979.
106. **Weilly, H. S. and Genton, E.,** Pharmacokinetics of procainamide, *Arch. Intern. Med.*, 130, 366, 1972.
107. **Dreyfuss, J., Bigger, J. T., Jr., Cohen, A. I., and Schreiber, E. C.,** Metabolism of procainamide in rhesus monkey and man, *Clin. Pharmacol. Ther.*, 13, 366, 1972.

108. **Drayer, E., Reidenberg, M. M., and Sevy, R. W.,** N-acetylprocainamide: an active metabolite of procainamide, *Proc. Soc. Exp. Biol. Med.,* 146, 358, 1974.
109. **Elson, J., Strong, J. M., and Lee, W.-K.,** Antiarrhythmic potency of N-acetylprocainamide, *Clin. Pharmacol. Ther.,* 17, 134, 1975.
110. **Drayer, D. E.,** Pharmacologically active metabolites, *Clin. Pharmacokinet.,* 1, 426, 1976.
111. **Atkinson, A. J., Lee, W.-K., Quinn, M. L., Kushner, W., Nevin, M. J., and Strong, J. M.,** Dose-ranging trial of N-acetylprocainamide in patients with premature ventricular contractions, *Clin. Pharmacol. Ther.,* 21, 575, 1977.
112. **Minchin, R. F., Ilett, K. F., and Paterson, J. W.,** Antiarrhythmic potency of procainamide and N-acetylprocainamide in rabbits, *Eur. J. Pharmacol.,* 47, 51, 1978.
113. **Lima, J. J. and Jusko, W. J.,** Determination of procainamide acetylator status, *Clin. Pharmacol. Ther.,* 23, 25, 1978.
114. **Gibson, T. P., Lowenthal, D. T., Nelson, H. A., and Briggs, W. A.,** Elimination of procainamide in end-stage renal failure, *Clin. Pharmacol. Ther.,* 17, 321, 1975.
115. **Drayer, D. E., Lowenthal, D. T., Woosley, R. L., Nies, A. S., Schwartz, A., and Reidenberg, M. M.,** Cumulation of N-acetylprocainamide, an active metabolite of procainamide in patients with impaired renal function, *Clin. Pharmacol. Ther.,* 22, 63, 1977.
116. **du Souich, P. and Erill, S.,** Metabolism of procainamide and p-aminobenzoic acid in patients with chronic liver disease, *Clin. Pharmacol. Ther.,* 22, 588, 1977.
117. **Lawson, D. H. and Jick, H.,** Adverse reactions to procainamide, *Br. J. Clin. Pharmacol.,* 4, 507, 1977.
118. **Kayden, H. J., Brodie, B. B., and Steele, J. M.,** Procaine amide, *Circulation,* 15, 118, 1957.
119. **McCrum, I. D. and Guidry, J. R.,** Procainamide-induced psychosis, *J.A.M.A.,* 240, 1265, 1978.
120. **Davies, D. M., Beedie, M. A., and Rawlins, M. D.,** Antinuclear antibodies during procainamide treatment and drug acetylation, *Br. Med. J.,* 3, 682, 1975.
121. **Heningsen, N. C., Cederberg, A., and Hanson, A.,** Effects of long-term treatment with procaine amide, *Acta Med. Scand.,* 198, 475, 1975.
122. **Kosowski, B. D., Taylor, J., and Lown, B.,** Long-term use of procainamide following acute myocardial infarction, *Circulation,* 42, 1204, 1973.
123. **Warner, W. A.,** Drug-induced lupus erythematosus, *Ariz. Med.,* 34, 172, 1977.
124. **Bell, W. R., Boss, G. R., and Wolfson, J. S.,** Circulating anticoagulant in the procainamide-induced lupus syndrome, *Arch. Intern. Med.,* 137, 1471, 1977.
125. **Rotmensch, H. H., Yust, I., Sieman-Igra, Y., Liron, M., Ilie, B., and Varinon, N.,** Granulomatous hepatitis: a hypersensitivity response to procainamide, *Ann. Intern. Med.,* 89, 646, 1978.
126. **Riker, J., Baker, J., and Swanson, M.,** Bone marrow granulomas and neutropenia associated with procainamide, report of a case, *Arch. Intern. Med.,* 138, 1731, 1978.
127. **Jones, G. W., George, T. L., and Bradley, R. D.,** Procainamide-induced hemolytic anemia, *Transfusion,* 18, 224, 1978.
128. **Putnam, T. J. and Merritt, H. H.,** Experimental determination of the anticonvulsant properties of phenyl derivatives, *Science,* 85, 525, 1937.
129. **Harris, A. S. and Kohernat, R. H.,** Effects of phenylhydantoin sodium and phenobarbital upon ectopic ventricular tachycardia in acute myocardial infarction, *Am. J. Physiol.,* 136, 505, 1950.
130. **Leonard, W. A., Jr.,** The use of diphenylhydantoin sodium in the treatment of ventricular tachycardia, *Arch. Intern. Med.,* 101, 714, 1958.
131. **Bernstein, H., Gold, H., Lang, T. W., Pappelbaum, S., Bazika, N., and Corday, E.,** Sodium diphenylhydantoin in the treatment of recurrent cardiac arrhythmias, *J.A.M.A.,* 191, 695, 1965.
132. **Conn, R. D.,** Diphenylhydantoin sodium in cardiac arrhythmias, *N. Engl. J. Med.,* 272, 277, 1965.
133. **Scherlag, B. J., Helfant, R. H., and Damato, A. N.,** The contrasting effects of diphenylhydantoin and procainamide on A-V conduction in the digitalis-intoxicated and the normal heart, *Am. Heart J.,* 75, 200, 1965.
134. **Helfant, R. H., Scherlag, B. J., and Damato, A. N.,** The electrophysiological properties of diphenylhydantoin sodium as compared to procainamide in the normal and digitalis-intoxicated heart, *Circulation,* 36, 108, 1967.
135. **Helfant, R. H., Scherlag, B. J., and Damato, A. N.,** Protection from digitalis toxicity with the prophylactic use of diphenylhydantoin sodium, *Circulation,* 36, 119, 1967.
136. **Mercer, E. N. and Osborne, J. A.,** The current status of diphenylhydantoin in heart disease, *Ann. Intern. Med.,* 67, 1084, 1967.
137. **Rosen, M., Lisak, R., and Rubin, I.,** Diphenylhydantoin in cardiac arrhythmias, *Am. J. Cardiol.,* 20, 674, 1967.
138. **Helfant, R. H., Scherlag, B. J., and Damato, A. N.,** Diphenylhydantoin prevention of arrhythmias in the digitalis-sensitized dog after direct-current cardioversion, *Circulation,* 37, 424, 1968.
139. **Eddy, J. D. and Singh, S. P.,** Treatment of cardiac arrhythmias with phenytoin, *Br. Med. J.,* 4, 270, 1969.

140. **Helfant, R. H., Seuffert, G. W., Patton, R. D., Stein, E., and Damato, A. N.,** The clinical use of diphenylhydantoin (Dilantin) in the treatment and prevention of cardiac arrhythmias, *Am. Heart J.,* 77, 315, 1969.
141. **Sirohiya, M. K., Bhatnagar, H. N. S., Shah, D. R., and Narang, N. K.,** Phenytoin sodium in cardiac arrhythmias, *J. Indian Med. Assoc.,* 64, 329, 1975.
142. **Stone, N., Klein, M. D., and Lown, B.,** Diphenylhydantoin in the prevention of recurring ventricular tachyarrhythmias, *Circulation,* 43, 420, 1971.
143. **Bigger, J. T., Jr., Schmidt, D. H., and Kutt, H.,** Relationships between the plasma level of diphenylhydantoin sodium and its cardiac antiarrhythmic effect, *Circulation,* 38, 363, 1968.
144. **Jalling, B., Barens, L. O., Rane, A., and Sjöquist, F.,** Plasma concentrations of diphenylhydantoin in young infants, *Pharmacol. Clin. (Berlin),* 2, 200, 1970.
145. **Dawson, K. P. and Jamieson, A.,** Value of blood diphenylhydantoin estimation in the management of childhood epilepsy, *Arch. Dis. Child.,* 46, 386, 1971.
146. **Svensmark, O. and Buchtal, F.,** Diphenylhydantoin and phenobarbital levels in children, *Am. J. Dis. Child.,* 108, 82, 1964.
147. **Lambie, D. C. and Caird, F. I.,** Phenytoin dosage, in the elderly, *Age Ageing,* 6, 133, 1977.
148. **Gibberd, F. B. and Webley, M.,** Studies in man of phenytoin absorption and its implications, *J. Neurol. Neurosurg. Psychiatry,* 38, 219, 1975.
149. **Dill, W. A., Kazenko, A., Wolf, L. M., and Glazko, A. J.,** Studies on 5,5'-diphenylhydantoin (Dilantin) in animals and man, *J. Pharmacol. Exp. Ther.,* 118, 270, 1956.
150. **Gugler, R., Manion, C. V., and Azarnoff, D. L.,** Phenytoin: pharmacokinetics and bioavailability, *Clin. Pharmacol. Ther.,* 19, 135, 1976.
151. **Arnold, K., Gerber, N., and Levy, G.,** Absorption and dissolution studies on sodium diphenylhydantoin capsules, *Can. J. Pharm. Sci.,* 5, 89, 1970.
152. **Furlanut, M., Benetello, P., Testa, G., and DaRonch, A.,** The effects of dose, age and sex on the serum levels of phenobarbital and diphenylhydantoin in epileptic patients, *Pharmacol. Res. Comm.,* 10, 85, 1978.
153. **Sherwin, A. L., Loynd, J. S., and Bock, G. W.,** Effects of age, sex, obesity and pregnancy on plasma diphenylhydantoin levels, *Epilepsia,* 15, 507, 1974.
154. **Kutt, H.,** Biochemical and genetic factor regulating dilantin metabolism in man, in *Drug Metabolism in Man,* Vessell, E. S., Ed., *Ann. N.Y. Acad. Sci.,* 179, 704, 1971.
155. **Hayes, M. J., Langman, H. J. S., and Short, A. H.,** Changes in drug metabolism with increasing age. II. Phenytoin clearance and protein binding, *Br. J. Clin. Pharmacol.,* 2, 73, 1975.
156. **Houghton, G. W., Richens, A., and Leighton, M.,** Effects of age, height, weight and sex on serum phenytoin concentrations in epileptic patients, *Br. J. Clin. Pharmacol.,* 2, 251, 1975.
157. **Porter, R. J. and Layzer, R. B.,** Plasma albumin concentration and diphenylhydantoin binding in man, *Arch. Neurol.,* 32, 298, 1975.
158. **Lightfoot, R. W., Jr. and Christina, C. L.,** Serum protein binding of thyroxine and diphenylhydantoin, *J. Clin. Endocrinol.,* 26, 305, 1966.
159. **Reidenberg, M. M., Odar-Cederlöf, I., von Bahr, C., Borgå, O., and Sjöquist, F.,** Protein binding of diphenylhydantoin and desmethylimipramine in plasma from patients with poor renal function, *N. Engl. J. Med.,* 285, 264, 1971.
160. **Ehrnebo, M. and Odar-Cederlöf, I.,** Binding of amobarbital, pentobarbital and diphenylhydantoin to red blood cells and plasma proteins in healthy volunteers and uraemic patients, *Eur. J. Clin. Pharmacol.,* 8, 445, 1975.
161. **Hooper, W. D., Bochner, F., Eadie, M. J., and Tyrer, J. H.,** Plasma protein binding of diphenylhydantoin, *Clin. Pharmacol. Ther.,* 19, 135, 1976.
162. **Odar-Cederlöf, I. and Borgå, O.,** Lack of relationship between serum free fatty acids and impaired plasma protein binding of diphenylhydantoin in chronic renal failure, *Eur. J. Clin. Pharmacol.,* 10, 403, 1976.
163. **Odar-Cederlöf, I. and Borgå, O.,** Impaired plasma protein binding of phenytoin in uremia and displacement effect of salicylic acid, *Clin. Pharmacol. Ther.,* 20, 36, 1976.
164. **Shoeman, D. W. and Azarnoff, D. L.,** The alternation of plasma proteins in uremia as reflected by their ability to bind digitoxin and diphenylhydantoin, *Pharmacology,* 7, 169, 1972.
165. **Glazko, A. J., Chang, T., Baukema, J., Dill, W. A., Goulet, J. R., and Buchanan, R. A.,** Metabolic disposition in normal human subjects following intravenous administration, *Clin. Pharmacol. Ther.,* 10, 498, 1960.
166. **Svensmark, O., Schiller, P. J., and Buchtal, F.,** 5,5'-diphenylhydantoin (Dilantin) blood levels after oral or intravenous dosage in man, *Acta Pharmacol. Toxicol.,* 16, 331, 1960.
167. **Maynert, E. W.,** The metabolic fate of diphenylhydantoin in the dog, rat and man, *J. Pharmacol. Exp. Ther.,* 130, 275, 1960.
168. **Svendsen, T. L., Kristensen, M. B., Mølholm Hansen, J., and Skovsted, L.,** The influence of disulfiram on the half-life and metabolic clearance of diphenylhydantoin and tolbutamide in man, *Eur. J. Clin. Pharmacol.,* 9, 439, 1976.

169. **Travers, R., Reynolds, E. H., and Gallagher, B.,** Variations in response to anticonvulsants in a group of epileptic patients, *Arch. Neurol.,* 27, 29, 1972.

170. **Eadie, M. J., Tyrer, J. H., and Hooper, W. D.,** Diphenylhydantoin dosage, *Proc. Aust. Assoc. Neurol.,* 10, 53, 1973.

171. **Bochner, F., Hooper, W. D., Tyrer, J. H., and Eadie, M. J.,** The renal handling of diphenylhydantoin and 5(p-hydroxyphenyl-5-phenylhydantoin), *Clin. Pharmacol. Ther.,* 14, 791, 1973.

172. **Blumsohn, D. and Seabrook, M.,** Oral diphenylhydantoin sodium and cardiovascular toxicity, *S. Afr. Med. J.,* 44, 11, 1970.

173. **Zoneraich, S., Zoneraich, O., and Siegel, J.,** Sudden death following intravenous sodium diphenylhydantoin, *Am. Heart J.,* 91, 375, 1976.

174. **Bivins, B. A., Rapp, R. P., Griffin, W. O., Jr., Blouin, R., and Bustrack, J.,** Dopamine-phenytoin interaction, a cause of hypotension in the critically ill, *Arch. Surg.,* 113, 245, 1978.

175. **Sullivan, J. M. and Solomon, H. S.,** Transient hypotensive effect of phenytoin in man, *J. Clin. Pharmacol.,* 17, 607, 1977.

176. **Rasmussen, S. and Kristensen, M.,** Choreoiathetosis during phenytoin treatment, *Acta Med. Scand.,* 201, 239, 1977.

177. **Palmer, K. T., Smith, A. E., and Taylor, B. B.,** Anticonvulsant osteomalacia, *Age Ageing,* 6, 228, 1977.

178. **Permin, H. and Sestoff, L.,** Deposits of plasma protein in the skin during treatment with carbamazepine and diphenylhydantoin, *Acta Med. Scand.,* 202, 113, 1977.

179. **Singh, B. N. and Jewitt, D. E.,** β-adrenoceptor blocking drugs in cardiac arrhythmias, in *Cardiovascular Drugs,* Vol. 2, β-adrenoceptor Blocking Drugs, Avery, G. S., Series Ed., University Park Press, Baltimore, 1977, 119.

180. **Gibson, D. and Sowton, E.,** The use of β-adrenergic receptor blocking drugs in dysrhythmias, *Progr. Cardiovas. Dis.,* 12, 16, 1969.

181. **Parmley, W. W. and Braunwald, E.,** Comparative myocardial depressant and antiarrhythmic properties of propranolol, d-propranolol and quinidine, *J. Pharmacol. Exp. Ther.,* 158, 11, 1967.

182. **Vaughn-Williams, E. M.,** Mode of action of beta receptor antagonists on cardiac muscle, *Am. J. Cardiol.,* 18, 399, 1966.

183. **Pitt, W. A. and Cox, A. R.,** The effect of the beta adrenergic antagonist propranolol in rabbit atrial cells with the use of the ultramicroscope technique, *Am. Heart J.,* 76, 242, 1968.

184. **Kleinfeld, M. and Stein, E.,** Propranolol on sinoatrial pacemaker cells, *Circulation,* 40, 123, 1969.

185. **Whitsett, L. S. and Lucchesi, B. R.,** Effects of beta receptor blockade and glucagon on the atrioventricular system in the dog, *Circ. Res.,* 13, 585, 1968.

186. **Berkowitz, W. D., Wit, A. L., Lau, S. H., Steiner, C., and Damato, A. N.,** The effects of propranolol on cardiac conduction, *Circulation,* 40, 855, 1969.

187. **Davis, L. D. and Temte, J. V.,** Effects of propranolol on the transmembrane potentials of ventricular muscle and Purkinje fibers of the dog, *Circ. Res.,* 12, 661, 1968.

188. **Rosati, R. A., Alexander, J. A., and Wallace, A. G.,** Failure of beta-adrenergic blockade to alter ventricular fibrillation threshold in the dog, *Circ. Res.,* 19, 721, 1966.

189. **Gettes, L. S. and Surawicz, B.,** Long term prevention of paroxysmal arrhythmias with propranolol therapy, *Am. J. Med. Sci.,* 254, 257, 1967.

190. **Stern, S. and Eisenberg, S.,** The effect of propranolol (Inderal) on the electrocardiogram of normal subjects, *Am. Heart J.,* 77, 192, 1969.

191. **Conway, J.,** The effect of age on the response to propranolol, *Int. J. Clin. Pharmacol.,* 4, 148, 1970.

192. **Castleden, C. M., Kaye, C. M., and Parson, R. I.,** The effect of age on plasma levels of propranolol and practolol in man, *Br. J. Clin. Pharmacol.,* 2, 303, 1975.

193. **Shand, D. G., Nuckolls, E. M., and Oates, J. A.,** Plasma propranolol levels in adults. With observations in four children, *Clin. Pharmacol. Ther.,* 11, 112, 1970.

194. **Paterson, J. W., Conolly, M. E., Dollery, C. T., Hayes, A., and Cooper, R. G.,** The pharmacodynamics and metabolism of propranolol in man, *Pharmacol. Clin.,* 2, 127, 1970.

195. **Evans, G. H. and Shand, D. G.,** Disposition of propranolol. V. Drug accumulation and steady state concentrations during oral administration in man, *Clin. Pharmacol. Ther.,* 14, 487, 1973.

196. **Evans, G. H. and Shand, D. G.,** Disposition of propranolol. VI. Independent variation in steady-state circulating drug concentrations and half-life as a result of plasma drug binding in man, *Clin. Pharmacol. Ther.,* 14, 494, 1973.

197. **Shand, D. G. and Rangno, R. E.,** The disposition of propranolol. I. Elimination during oral absorption in man, *Pharmacology,* 7, 1959, 1972.

198. **Kornhauser, D. M., Wood, A. J. J., Vestal, R. E., Wilkinson, G. R., Branch, R. A., and Shand, D. G.,** Biological determinants of propranolol disposition in man, *Clin. Pharmacol. Ther.,* 23, 165, 1978.

199. **Piafsky, K. M., Borgå, O., Odar-Cederlöf, O., Johansson, C., and Sjöquist, F.,** Increased plasma binding of propranolol and chlorpromazine mediated by disease-induced elevations of plasma α_1 acid glycoproteins, *N. Engl. J. Med.,* 299, 1435, 1978.

200. **Shand, D. G., Evans, G. H., and Nies, A. S.,** The almost complete hepatic extraction of propranolol during intravenous administration in the dog, *Life Sci.,* 10, 1417, 1971.

201. **Hayes, A. and Cooper, R. G.,** Studies on the absorption, distribution and excretion of propranolol in rat, dog and monkey, *J. Pharmacol. Exp. Ther.,* 176, 302, 1971.

202. **Walle, T. and Gaffney, T. E.,** Propranolol metabolism in man and dog: mass spectrometric identification of six new metabolites, *J. Pharmacol. Exp. Ther.,* 182, 83, 1972.

203. **Fitzgerald, J. D. and O'Donnell, S. R.,** Pharmacology of 4-hydroxypropranolol, a metabolite of propranolol, *Br. J. Pharmacol.,* 43, 222, 1971.

204. **Walle, T., Ishizaki, T., and Gaffney, T.,** Isopropylamine, a biologically active deamination product of propranolol in dogs: identification of deuterated and unlabeled isopropylamine by gas chromatography-mass spectrometry, *J. Pharmacol. Exp. Ther.,* 183, 508, 1972.

205. **Branch, R. A. and Shand, D. G.,** Propranolol disposition in liver disease: a physiological approach, *Clin. Pharmacokinet.,* 1, 264, 1976.

206. **Bianchetti, G., Graziani, G., Broncaccio, D., Morganti, A., Leonetti, G., Manfrin, M., Sega, R., Gomeni, R., Ponticelli, C., and Morselli, P. L.,** Pharmacokinetics and effects of propranolol in terminal uraemic patients and in patients undergoing regular dialysis treatment, *Clin. Pharmacokinet.,* 1, 373, 1976.

207. **Thompson, F. D., Joekes, A. M., and Foulkes, D. M.,** Pharmacodynamics of propranolol in renal failure, *Br. Med. J.,* 2, 434, 1972.

208. **Bauer, J. H., Pape, B., Zajicek, J., and Groshong, T.,** Propranolol in human plasma and breast milk, *Am. J. Cardiol.,* 43, 860, 1979.

209. **Gianelly, R. E. and Harrison, D. C.,** The antiarrhythmic properties of lidocaine and propranolol: a review, *Geriatrics,* 25, 120, 1970.

210. **Greenblatt, D. J. and Koch-Weser, J.,** Clinical toxicity of propranolol and practolol: a report from the Boston Collaborative Drug Surveillance Program, in *Cardiovascular Drugs,* Vol. 2, β-adrenoceptor Blocking Drugs, Avery, G. S., Series Ed., University Park Press, Baltimore, 1977, 179.

211. **Bauer, J. H. and Brooks, C. S.,** The long-term effect of propranolol on renal function, *Am. J. Med.,* 66, 405, 1979.

212. **Podolsky, S. and Pattavina, C. G.,** Hyperosmolar non-ketotic diabetic coma: a complication of propranolol therapy, *Metabolism,* 22, 685, 1973.

213. **Martin, C. M., Southwick, E. G., and Maibach, H. L.,** Propranolol-induced alopecia, *Am. Heart J.,* 86, 236, 1973.

214. **Voltolina, E. J., Thompson, S. I., and Tisue, J.,** Acute organic brain syndrome with propranolol, *Clin. Toxicol.,* 4, 357, 1971.

215. **Frohlich, E. D., Tarazi, R. C., and Dustan, H. P.,** Peripheral arterial insufficiency. A complication of beta-adrenergic blocking therapy, *J.A.M.A.,* 208, 2471, 1969.

216. **Robson, R. H.,** Recurrent migraine after propranolol, *Br. Heart J.,* 39, 1157, 1977.

217. **Tangsrud, S. E. and Golf, S.,** Cheilostomatitis associated with propranolol therapy, *Br. Med. J.,* 2, 1385, 1977.

218. **Alderman, E. L., Coltart, J., Wettach, G. E., and Harrison, D. C.,** Coronary artery syndromes after sudden propranolol withdrawal, *Ann. Intern. Med.,* 81, 625, 1974.

219. **Myers, M. G., Freeman, M. R., Juma, Z. A., and Wisenberg, G.,** Propranolol withdrawal in angina pectoris: a retrospective study, *Am. Heart J.,* 97, 298, 1979.

220. **Shiroff, R. A., Mathis, J., Zelis, R., Schneck, D. W., Babb, J. D., Leaman, D. M., and Hayes, A. D., Jr.,** Propranolol rebound — a retrospective study, *Am. J. Cardiol.,* 41, 778, 1978.

221. **Melville, I. I., Shister, H. E., and Huq, S.,** Iproveratril experimental data on coronary dilatation and antidysrhythmic action, *Can. Med. Assoc. J.,* 90, 761, 1964.

222. **Brichard, G. and Zimmerman, P. E.,** Verapamil in cardiac dysrhythmias during anaesthesia, *Br. J. Anaesth.,* 42, 1005, 1970.

223. **Schamroth, L.,** Immediate effects of intravenous verapamil on atrial fibrillation, *Cardiovasc. Res.,* 5, 419, 1971.

224. **Gotsman, M. S., Lewis, B. S., Bakst, A., and Mihta, A. S.,** Verapamil in life-threatening arrhythmias, *S. Afr. Med. J.,* 46, 2017, 1972.

225. **Schamroth, L., Krikler, D. M., and Garrett, C.,** Immediate effects of intravenous verapamil in cardiac arrhythmias, *Br. Med. J.,* 1, 660, 1972.

226. **Slome, R.,** The use of intravenous verapamil in cardiac arrhythmias, *S. Afr. Med. J.,* 47, 913, 1973.

227. **Storstein, O. and Landmark, K. H.,** Verapamil in the treatment of atrial tachycardia with block, *Acta Med. Scand.,* 198, 483, 1975.

228. **Heng, M. K., Singh, B. N., Roche, A. H. G., Norris, R. N., and Mercer, C. J.,** Effects of verapamil on cardiac arrhythmias and on the electrocardiogram, *Am. Heart J.,* 90, 487, 1975.

229. **Härtel, G. and Hartikainen, M.,** Comparison of verapamil and practolol in paroxysmal tachycardia, *Eur. J. Cardiol.,* 4, 87, 1976.
230. **Pattak, L., Iyengar, M., and Shah, S. J.,** Verapamil in supraventricular tachycardia, *Indian Heart J.,* 30, 163, 1978.
231. **Soler-Soler, J., Sagristá-Sauleda, J., Cabrera, A., Sauleda-Parés, J., Iglesias-Berengué, J., Permanyer-Miralda, G., and Roca-Llop, J.,** Effect of verapamil in infants with paroxysmal supraventricular tachycardia, *Circulation,* 59, 876, 1979.
232. **Breithardt, G., Seipel, L., Wiebringhaus, E., and Loogen, F.,** Effects of verapamil on sinus node function in man, *Eur. J. Cardiol.,* 8, 379, 1978.
233. **Carrasco, H. A., Fuenmayer, A., Barboza, J. S., and Gonzalez, G.,** Effects of verapamil on normal sinoatrial node function and on sick sinus syndrome, *Am. Heart J.,* 96, 760, 1978.
234. **Garvey, H. L.,** The mechanism of action of verapamil on the sinus and AV nodes, *Eur. J. Pharmacol.,* 8, 159, 1969.
235. **Singh, B. N. and Vaughn Williams, E. M.,** A fourth class of antidysrhythmia? Effects of verapamil on ouabain toxicity on atrial and ventricular intracellular potentials, and on other features of cardiac function, *Cardiovasc. Res.,* 6, 109, 1972.
236. **Cranefield, P. F., Aronson, R. S., and Wit, A. L.,** Effect of verapamil on the normal action potential and on a calcium-dependent slow response of canine cardiac Purkinje fibers, *Circ. Res.,* 34, 204, 1974.
237. **Husaini, M. H., Kvasnicka, J., Rydên, L., and Holmberg, S.,** Action of verapamil on sinus node, atrioventricular and intraventricular conduction, *Br. Heart J.,* 35, 734, 1973.
238. **Schomerus, M., Spiegelhalder, B., Steiren, B., and Eichelbaum, M.,** Physiological disposition of verapamil in man, *Cardiovasc. Res.,* 10, 605, 1976.
239. **Singh, B. N.,** Rational basis of antiarrhythmic therapy: clinical pharmacology of commonly used antiarrhythmic drugs, *Angiology,* 29, 206, 1978.

ANTIANGINAL AGENTS

Peter S. Chan and Peter Cervoni

INTRODUCTION

Angina pectoris is a frequent symptom in the aged. Its prevalence in the noninstitutionalized population of the U.S. reaches a peak of 106 episodes per 1000 in males at age 65, and then declines to 66 per 1000 between ages 75 and 79. In females, the prevalence is lower at earlier ages, but it reaches a peak of 120 per 1000 at 75 to 79 years.[1,2] Angina pectoris is a clinical syndrome and a manifestation of myocardial ischemia, in which the myocardial demand for oxygen exceeds the supply. The dominant underlying cause in the majority of cases is coronary atherosclerosis.[3,4] The occurrence of variant angina, induced by coronary artery spasm, is comparatively small. The cardinal feature of angina is recurrent substernal or precardial chest pain radiating down the left arm, brought on, particularly after meals, by effort or by emotional distress.

In patients with severe coronary atherosclerosis and obstruction, the typical electrocardiographic changes during the anginal attack brought on by effort is ST-segment depression. The severity of the coronary artery disease appears to be directly proportional to the degree of ST-segment depression. It is a common finding that ischemic symptoms occur when the coronary artery lumen is occluded more than 75%. The severity of ischemia in patients with equal degrees of occlusion depends on the extent of collateral circulation development and utilization of compensatory mechanisms, such as the opening of the venous-arterial bypass and capillaries to the ischemic area.[6,7] It appears that the longer it takes to form the atheromatous plaque, the better the development of the collateral vascular network distal to the plaque.[8] Occurrence of classical angina pectoris in the absence of any specific angiographic changes in coronary arteries has been reported in some patients.[9,10] It has been suggested that in these patients the major coronary disease may be in the smaller vessels, which are not clearly delineated by coronary angiography.[11] Another explanation is that angina may be caused by alteration of the neurohumoral regulation of the coronary circulation.[12]

In skeletal muscle, the extraction of oxygen from arterial blood is 25% of the amount available, 75% is not extracted and appears in the venous blood. Any increase in work is compensated by an increase in oxygen extraction, not by a rise in blood flow. Unlike skeletal muscle, cardiac muscle, at rest, extracts and utilizes 75% of the oxygen in arterial blood.[13] This is why the coronary oxygen reserve is very low. When myocardial work increases and demand for oxygen rises, the demand is met by increasing coronary flow, up to fivefold in a healthy heart. The ability to increase blood flow whenever demand increases is due to autoregulation. In a coronary artery with atherosclerotic plaques, arteriolar autoregulation is greatly impaired. After maximal coronary blood flow is reached, additional demand for oxygen has to be met by additional extraction of oxygen, up to 95%.[13] When coronary blood flow cannot be increased significantly due to atherosclerosis of the coronary artery, and maximal extraction of oxygen cannot meet the oxygen demand, myocardial ischemia occurs and leads to an anginal attack.

If anoxia occurs in the myocardium, blood vessels in the ischemic area are dilated maximally and extraction of oxygen is maximal. It is believed that no vasodilator can cause further dilation of these vessels.[23] This is one of the reasons why the so-called nonspecific classical coronary vasodilators that increase total coronary blood flow, and agents that increase oxygen dissociation from hemoglobin, are not efficacious in angina pectoris.

After failure of the classical coronary vasodilators such as dipyridamole in the treatment of angina pectoris, recent extensive hemodynamic studies on the heart have advanced the understanding of the myocardial nutritional circulation, and the concept of decreasing the workload of the heart (decrease of oxygen requirement) to alleviate angina.

Blood is supplied to the ventricular wall by extramural epicardial coronary arteries. These arteries branch off to the epicardium, and perpendicularly, to the endocardium. They finally connect to form the subendocardial plexus just below the endocardial surface. The branches ultimately divide into arterioles and then into capillaries.[4] The arterioles and precapillary sphincters provide a good regulatory mechanism for maintaining an adequate oxygen supply to the various layers of the myocardium. Precapillary sphincters are sensitive to intertitial oxygen tension and are continually opening and closing to regulate tissue oxygenation and nutrition.[4,14-16] This has been called the nutritional circulation, part of the autoregulation system. In the normal myocardium, the ratio of blood flow in the epicardium to blood flow in the endocardium usually approaches unity.[4]

The demand for oxygen in the myocardium depends on: (1) cardiac fiber length, (2) diastolic wall tension (end-diastolic ventricular volume and pressure-preload), (3) systolic pressure and wall tension (intraventricular pressure-afterload), (4) contractile force, and (5) heart rate.[4,17,18] During systole of the cardiac cycle, intramyocardial pressure in the endocardium is higher than the perfusion pressure of the coronary arteries; therefore, perfusion does not take place. Blood flow to the endocardium occurs only during diastole, at which time diastolic intramyocardial pressure (equals left ventricular end-diastolic pressure) is only about 5 mmHg.[19-22] The effective perfusion period depends on: (1) the subendocardial blood flow and (2) the duration of diastole. Due to the greater intramyocardial pressure and tension, the subendocardium is more prone to ischemia and is more vulnerable to reduction of coronary perfusion, compared to the epicardium.[22]

During a myocardial ischemic attack, end-diastolic ventricular pressure and volume increase, cardiac size increases, and diastolic perfusion pressure distal to the atherosclerotic obstruction is reduced.[24-36,45] It has been estimated that during an anginal attack, the end-diastolic ventricular pressure increases from 5 to 30 mmHg and the systemic diastolic blood pressure decreases from 80 to 40 mmHg. Therefore, the pressure gradient does not favor adequate perfusion of the endocardium, thus resulting in ischemia.[22]

The failure of dipyridamole in the treatment of angina pectoris may be attributed to any of the following:

1. Even though dipyridamole can increase total coronary blood flow up to sixfold, it mainly dilates healthy arteries in normal regions because vessels in the ischemic regions have already been maximally dilated by anoxia. The excessive dilation in the non-diseased regions will divert blood flow from the ischemic regions and produce "coronary steal".[37-39] This is detrimental to the ischemic tissues.
2. Dipyridamole abolishes autoregulation.
3. Dipyridamole dilates small resistance vessels instead of large conducting vessels.[40]

Before antianginal therapy is instituted, it is important to exclude the following causes that can induce transient myocardial ischemia. They are hypertension, thyrotoxicosis, anemia, paroxysmal tachyarrhythmias, left ventricle failure, methemoglobinemia, carboxyhemoglobin, aortic stenosis and insufficiency, and pulmonary hypertension.[41] Antianginal agents should act by decreasing the work of the heart, or by increasing the blood supply specifically to the ischemic zone rather than to the entire myocardium nondiscriminately.

The main categories of antianginal drugs available are (1) nitroglycerin and other nitrates and (2) β-adrenergic blocking agents (β-blockers). The concomitant use of nitrates and β-adrenoceptor blocking agents is significantly more effective than either class of agent alone.

It is a common finding that a placebo may relieve the anginal pain in 35 to 60% of the patients.[11,42] In addition, the anginal attack is of short duration, usually less than 2 min after cessation of effort, and is relieved promptly by rest. This makes the study of any agent for its ability to abolish the acute anginal attack difficult.

NITROGLYCERIN AND OTHER NITRATES

It is generally agreed that nitroglycerin, given sublingually, is more effective than a placebo in abolishing the anginal symptoms.[43-45] However, nitroglycerin given orally is generally not efficacious. Nitroglycerin delays significantly the onset of cardiac pain and ECG signs of ischemia during exercise tests; it increases the time required for pain appearance in the anoxemia test by 50%.[46]

According to current concepts, the antianginal effects of nitroglycerin are mainly due to its effects on the peripheral systemic circulation. Effects here result in decreasing the workload of the heart by venous pooling, with a subsequent reduction in venous return, thus decreasing left ventricular end-diastolic pressure (preload). This is followed by reduction of left ventricular end-diastolic volume, cardiac size, and ventricular wall tension, all of which are important determinants of myocardial oxygen consumption. Reducing cardiac work decreases oxygen requirement, and eventually abolishes ischemia. Moreover, when left ventricular end-diastolic pressure decreases, intramyocardial pressure around the endocardial vessels drops; this facilitates blood flow through the endocardial region.[47-66] The traditional view of the direct effects of nitroglycerin on the coronary circulation appears to be of secondary importance. This has been demonstrated by many investigators, particularly by Ganz and Marcus,[67] who studied the effects of nitroglycerin in pacing-induced angina by monitoring coronary blood flow, circulatory hemodynamic changes, and pain in patients with coronary heart disease. They found that nitroglycerin, administered directly through a catheter into the left coronary artery in a dose capable of increasing coronary blood flow in normal individuals, did not relieve pacing-induced anginal pain in spite of an increase in coronary blood flow. In contrast, nitroglycerin given intravenously relieved anginal pain in spite of a decrease of coronary blood flow. The relief of pain was preceded by a decrease of left ventricular end-diastolic pressure. It has also been found that mild phlebotomy (about 276 mℓ of blood), which effectively relieved anginal attack, produced the same preload reduction as produced by nitroglycerin.[68] Nevertheless, there are voluminous data on the direct effects of nitroglycerin on the coronary circulation. Even though nitroglycerin does not increase total coronary blood flow significantly, blood flow through the nutritional circulation is increased.[69] This will increase blood supply to the endocardium which is the area most vulnerable to ischemia in patients with coronary heart disease. Nitroglycerin causes dilation of the large conducting blood vessels[37] and does not abolish coronary arteriolar autoregulation.[40] Through the dilation of the intramural arterial network, nitroglycerin causes favorable redistribution of blood flow to the endocardium and subendocardium,[37] and indications are that nitroglycerin improves blood perfusion in regions of ischemic myocardium.[46] Nitroglycerin also reduces systemic arterial blood pressure (afterload).[28,66] These direct effects of nitroglycerin on heart and systemic blood pressure probably contribute to its antianginal efficacy.

Nitroglycerin ointment,[70] for percutaneous administration, has been found to be efficacious in angina pectoris and has a prolonged duration of action useful in prophylaxis.

The side effects of nitroglycerin are: headache, dizziness, weakness, and postural hypotension.

Long-acting nitrates, such as pentaerythritol tetranitrate, isosorbide dinitrate, and erythrityl tetranitrate, have been on the market for a long time, but their oral (excluding sublingual) use for angina pectoris remains controversial. Well-designed, double-blind studies have found these oral nitrates disappointing, on the whole, and no more effective than a placebo in the prevention of angina.[71,72] This may be due partly to rapid inactivation of the nitrates in the gastrointestinal tract and liver.

β-ADRENOCEPTOR BLOCKING AGENTS

β-Adrenoceptor blocking agents (β-blockers) have become an important and efficacious class of drugs in the management of angina pectoris.[73-78] After an adequate β-adrenoceptor blockade, patients can increase their workload 30 to 40% before anginal pain occurs. They also experience less frequent and less severe anginal attacks in their daily life. The major therapeutic effects of β-blockers derive from their ability to decrease the physiological responses to exercise, viz., cardioacceleration, increased contractility and blood pressure. Antagonism of these responses by β-blockers diminishes the increased work of the heart and its hemodynamic changes. β-Blockers lengthen the period of diastole of the cardiac cycle as a result of reduction in heart rate, so that better perfusion of the endocardium and subendocardium is achieved. Heart rate is decreased in normal individuals and in patients with angina pectoris, both at rest and during exercise. A heart rate of 55 to 60 beats per minute (bpm) in the standing position at rest or 70 bpm during mild exercise should be attained. The cardiac output at rest and during exercise is decreased by β-blockers. The greater the reduction in heart rate, the greater the reduction in cardiac output. Stroke volume is unchanged. However, the reduction in cardiac output is not entirely due to the decrease in heart rate. β-Blockers reduce the peak rate of rise of left ventricular pressure (peak dP/dt) at rest and during exercise. β-Blockade may alter the contractility of the myocardium independently of end-diastolic fiber length by antagonizing the positive inotropic effects of sympathetic activity and circulating catecholamines. The mean systolic ejection rate (i.e., stroke volume divided by ejection time) during exercise is reduced by β-blockade. There is a small reduction of arterial blood pressure and plasma volume. All these actions on preload and afterload of the heart tend to decrease cardiac work and therefore decrease myocardial oxygen consumption. However, β-blockade increases ventricular end-diastolic pressure and volume as well as ventricular wall tension. Coronary blood flow is decreased and the coronary vascular resistance is increased by β-blockade. Undoubtedly, these effects counteract part of the overall antianginal action of the β-blockers.

Cardioselective β-blockers such as atenolol[79] and metoprolol[80] have been shown to be equally effective as cardio-nonselective β-blockers in the treatment of stable angina pectoris and cause less bronchoconstriction and airway obstruction.

β-Blockers may precipitate heart failure in patients with poor cardiac reserve; their cardiac output depends largely on the elevated sympathetic activity. Only cardioselective β-blockers should be used in patients with asthma.

Withdrawal of β-blockers should be gradual over a period of many days to avoid the precipitation of severe anginal attacks and possible myocardial infarction. There is suggestive evidence to show that β-blockers may significantly lower the incidence of transmural infarction of severe arrhythmias and of delayed heart failure in patients who had previously experienced an infarct.

Concomitant use of β-blockers and sublingual nitrates produces additive beneficial effects on subendocardial perfusion, and has been shown to be more effective than either class of agent alone.

REFERENCES

1. **Rodstein, M.,** Coronary artery disease in the aged, *Bull. N.Y. Acad. Med.,* 49, 1124, 1973.
2. Mortality from angina pectoris, *Stat. Bull. Metrop. Life Insur. Co.,* 53, 2, 1972.
3. **Charlier, R.,** Antianginal drugs, in *Handbook of Experimental Pharmacology,* Vol. 31, Eichler, O., Farah, A., Herken, H., and Welch, A. D., Eds., Springer-Verlag, Berlin, 1971, 7.

4. **Winbury, M. M.,** Experimental coronary disease — models and methods of drug evaluation, in *Handbook of Experimental Pharmacology,* Vol. 16 (Part 3), Schmier, J. and Eichler, O., Eds., Springer-Verlag, New York, 1975, 1.

5. **Roberts, W. C.,** Coronary heart disease: a review of abnormalities observed in the coronary arteries, *Cardiovasc. Med.,* 2, 29, 1977.

6. **McGregor, M. and Fam, W.,** Regulation of coronary blood flow, *Bull. N.Y. Acad. Med.,* 42, 940, 1966.

7. **Coffman, F. D. and Gregg, D. E.,** Reactive hyperemia characteristics of the myocardium, *Am. J. Physiol.,* 199, 1143, 1960.

8. **Schaper, W.,** *The Collateral Circulation of the Heart,* Elsevier, Amsterdam, 1971.

9. **Hellstrom, H. R.,** Vasopressor in ischemic heart disease — a hypothesis, *Perspect. Biol. Med.,* 16, 427, 1973.

10. **Kemp, H. G., Elliott, W. C., and Gorlin, R.,** The anginal syndrome with normal coronary arteriography, *Trans. Assoc. Am. Physicians,* 80, 59, 1967.

11. **DeGraff, A. C.,** Drugs for diseases of the heart, in *Drugs of Choice, 1978-1979,* Modell, W., Ed., C.V. Mosby, St. Louis, 1978, chap. 24.

12. **Kaverina, N. V. and Chumburidze, V. B.,** Antianginal drugs, *Pharmacol. Ther.,* 4, 109, 1979.

13. **Charlier, R.,** Antianginal drugs, in *Handbook of Experimental Pharmacology,* Vol. 31, Eichler, O., Farah, A., Herken, H., and Welch, A. D., Eds., Springer-Verlag, Berlin, 1971, chap. 2.

14. **Winbury, M. M., Howe, B. B., and Weiss, H. R.,** Effect of nitroglycerin and dipyridamole on epicardial and endocardial oxygen tension. Further evidence for redistribution of myocardial blood flow, *J. Pharmacol. Exp. Ther.,* 176, 184, 1971.

15. **Howe, B. B. and Winbury, M. M.,** Effect of pentrinitrol, nitroglycerin and propranolol on small vessel blood content of the canine myocardium, *J. Pharmacol. Exp. Ther.,* 187, 465, 1973.

16. **Weiss, H. R. and Winbury, M. M.,** Nitroglycerin and chromonar on small-vessel blood content of the ventricular walls, *Am. J. Physiol.,* 226, 838, 1974.

17. **Hood, W. B., Jr.,** Pathophysiology of ischemic heart disease, *Progr. Cardiovasc. Dis.,* 14, 297, 1971.

18. **Ross, R. S.,** Pathophysiology of coronary circulation, *Br. Heart J.,* 33, 173, 1971.

19. **Becker, L. and Pitt, B.,** Regional myocardial blood flow, ischemia and antianginal drugs, *Ann. Clin. Res.,* 3, 353, 1971.

20. **Buckberg, G. D., Fixler, D. E., Archie, J. P., and Hoffman, J. I. E.,** Experimental subendocardial ischemia in dogs with normal coronary arteries, *Circ. Res.,* 30, 67, 1972.

21. **Parratt, J. R.,** Pharmacological approaches to the therapy of angina, in *Advances in Drug Research,* Vol. 9, Simmonds, A. B., Ed., Academic Press, London, 1974, 103.

22. **Parratt, J. R.,** Recent advances in the pathophysiology and pharmacology of angina, *Gen. Pharmacol.,* 6, 247, 1975.

23. **Weisse, A. B. and Regan, T. J.,** The current status of nitrites in the treatment of coronary artery disease, *Progr. Cardiovasc. Dis.,* 12, 72, 1969.

24. **Weiner, L., Dwyer, E. M., and Cox, J. W.,** Left ventricular hemodynamics in exercise-induced angina pectoris, *Circulation,* 38, 240, 1968.

25. **Linhard, J. W., Hildner, F. J., Barold, S. S., Lister, J. W., and Samet, P.,** Left heart hemodynamics during angina pectoris induced by arterial pacing, *Circulation,* 40, 483, 1969.

26. **Levine, J. H. and Wagman, R. J.,** Energetics of the human heart, *Am. J. Cardiol.,* 9, 372, 1962.

27. **Kirk, E. S. and Honig, C. R.,** Nonuniform distribution of blood flow and gradients of oxygen tension within the heart, *Am. J. Physiol.,* 207, 661, 1964.

28. **Hoeschen, R. J., Bousvaros, G. A., Klassen, G. A., Fam, W. M., and McGregor, M.,** Haemodynamic effects of angina pectoris, and of nitroglycerin in normal and anginal subjects, *Br. Heart J.,* 28, 221, 1966.

29. **Dwyer, E. M.,** Left ventricular pressure-volume alteration and regional disorders of contraction during myocardial ischemia induced by atrial pacing, *Circulation,* 42, 1111, 1970.

30. **Braunwald, E.,** Control of myocardial oxygen consumption: physiologic and clinical considerations, *Am. J. Cardiol.,* 27, 416, 1971.

31. **Braunwald, E.,** The determinants of myocardial oxygen consumption, *Physiologist,* 12, 65, 1969.

32. **Parker, J. O., DiGiorgi, S., and West, R. O.,** A hemodynamic study of acute coronary insufficiency precipitated by exercise, *Am. J. Cardiol.,* 17, 479, 1966.

33. **Parker, J. O., West, R. O., and DiGiorgi, S.,** The hemodynamic response to exercise in patients with healed myocardial infarction without angina, *Circulation,* 36, 734, 1967.

34. **Parker, J. O.,** The effect of ischemia on myocardial function, in *Effect of Acute Ischaemia on Myocardial Function,* Oliver, M. F., Julian, D. G., and Donald, K. W., Eds., Churchill Livingstone, Edinburgh, 1972, 288.

35. **Marshall, R. H. and Parratt, J. R.,** Drug-induced changes in blood flow in the acutely ischemic canine myocardium; relationship to subendocardial driving pressure, *Clin. Exp. Pharmacol. Physiol.,* 1, 99, 1974.

36. **Moss, A. J.,** Intramyocardial oxygen tension, *Cardiovasc. Res.,* 3, 314, 1968.

37. **Winbury, M. M., Howe, B. B., and Hefner, M. A.,** Effects of nitrates and other coronary dilators on large and small coronary vessels. An hypothesis for the mechanism of action of nitrates, *J. Pharmacol. Exp. Ther.,* 168, 70, 1969.
38. **Rowe, G. G.,** Inequalities of myocardial perfusion in coronary artery disease ("coronary steal"), *Circulation,* 42, 193, 1970.
39. **Wilcken, D. E. L., Pavloni, H. J., and Eikens, E.,** Evidence for i.v. dipyridamole (Persantin) producing a "coronary steal" effect in the ischemic myocardium, *Austr. N.Z. J. Med.,* 1, 8, 1971.
40. **Nickerson, M.,** Vasodilator drugs, in *The Pharmacological Basis of Therapeutics,* 5th ed., Goodman, L. S. and Gilman, A., Eds., Macmillan, New York, 1975, chap. 34.
41. **Mudge, G. H.,** Angina pectoris, in *Current Therapy,* Conn, H. F., Ed., W. B. Saunders, Philadelphia, 1979, 168.
42. **Folli, G., Radice, M., Beltrami, A., Potenza, S., and Mariotti, G.,** Placebo effect in the treatment of angina pectoris, *Acta Cardiol. (Brux),* 33, 231, 1978.
43. **Kay, H. B.,** Angina pectoris: getting the most from drug therapy, *Drugs,* 13, 276, 1977.
44. **Aronow, W. S.,** Medical treatment of angina pectoris. III. Pharmacology of sublingual nitrates as antianginal drugs, *Am. Heart J.,* 84, 273, 1972.
45. **Warren, S. E. and Francis, G. S.,** Nitroglycerin and nitrate esters, *Am. J. Med.,* 65, 53, 1978.
46. **Charlier, R.,** Antianginal drugs, in *Handbook of Experimental Pharmacology,* Vol. 31, Eichler, O., Farah, A., Herken, H., and Welch, A. D., Eds., Springer-Verlag, Berlin, 1971, chap. 5.
47. **Sonnenblick, E. H. and Skelton, C. L.,** Myocardial energetics: basic principles and clinical implications, *N. Engl. J. Med.,* 285, 668, 1971.
48. **Robin, E., Cowan, C., Puri, P., Ganguly, S., DeBoyrie, E., Martinez, M., Stock, T., and Bing, R. J.,** A comparative study of nitroglycerin and propranolol, *Circulation,* 36, 175, 1967.
49. **Najmi, M., Griggs, D. M., Kasparian, H., and Novack, P.,** Effects of nitroglycerin on hemodynamics during rest and exercise in patients with coronary insufficiency, *Circulation,* 35, 46, 1967.
50. **Greenberg, H., Gwyer, E. M., Jr., Jameson, A. G., and Pinkernell, B. H.,** Effects of nitroglycerin on the major determinants of myocardial oxygen consumption. An angiographic and hemodynamic assessment, *Am. J. Cardiol.,* 36, 426, 1975.
51. **Parker, J. O., West, R. O., and DiGeorgi, S.,** The effect of nitroglycerin on coronary flow and the hemodynamic response to exercise in coronary artery disease, *Am. J. Cardiol.,* 27, 59, 1971.
52. **Frick, M. H., Balcon, R., Cross, D., and Sowton, E.,** Hemodynamic effect of nitroglycerin in patients with angina pectoris studied by an arterial pacing method, *Circulation,* 37, 160, 1968.
53. **Fam, W. M. and McGregor, M.,** Effects of nitroglycerin and dipyridamole on regional coronary resistance, *Circ. Res.,* 22, 649, 1968.
54. **Dumesnil, J. G., Ritman, E. L., Davis, G. D., Grau, G. T., Rutherford, B. D., and Frye, R. L.,** Regional left ventricular wall dynamics before and after sublingual administration of nitroglycerin, *Am. J. Cardiol.,* 36, 419, 1975.
55. **DeMaria, A. N., Vismara, L. A., Auditore, K., Amsterdam, E. A., Zelis, R., and Mason, D. T.,** Effects of nitroglycerin on left ventricular cavity size and cardiac performance determined by ultrasound in man, *Am. J. Med.,* 57, 754, 1974.
56. **Campion, B., Frye, R., and Zitnick, R.,** Peripheral venous pooling: a major hemodynamic effect of nitroglycerin, *Clin. Res.,* 17, 233, 1969.
57. **Burggraf, G. W. and Parker, J. O.,** Left ventricular volume changes after amyl nitrate and nitroglycerin in man as measured by ultrasound, *Circulation,* 49, 136, 1974.
58. **Brandt, J. L., Caccese, A., and Dock, W.,** Slit-Kymographic evidence that nitroglycerine decreases heart volume and stroke volume while increasing the amplitude of ballistocardiographic waves, *Am. J. Med.,* 12, 650, 1952.
59. **Bernstein, L., Friesinger, G. C., Lichtlen, P. R., and Ross, R. S.,** The effect of nitroglycerin on the systemic and coronary circulation in man and dogs. Myocardial blood flow measurement with xenon[133], *Circulation,* 33, 107, 1966.
60. **Arborelius, M., Lecerof, H., Malm, A., and Malmborg, R. O.,** Acute effect of nitroglycerin on haemodynamics of angina pectoris, *Br. Heart J.,* 30, 407, 1968.
61. **Aronow, W. S.,** Medical treatment of angina, *Am. Heart J.,* 85, 132, 1973.
62. **Reddy, S. P., Curtiss, E. I., O'Toole, J. D., Matthews, R. G., Salerni, R., Leon, D. F., and Shaver, J. A.,** Reversibility of left ventricular asynergy by nitroglycerin in coronary artery disease, *Am. Heart J.,* 90, 479, 1975.
63. **McAnulty, J. H., Hattenhauer, M. T., Rosch, J., Kloster, F. E., and Rahimtoola, S. H.,** Improvement in left ventricular wall motion following nitroglycerin, *Circulation,* 51, 140, 1975.
64. **Mason, D. T., Zelis, R., and Amsterdam, E. A.,** Actions of nitrites on the peripheral circulation and myocardial oxygen consumption; significance in the relief of angina pectoris, *Chest,* 59, 296, 1971.

65. **Zelis, R., Mason, D. T., Spann, J. F., and Amsterdam, E. A.,** The mechanism of action in the relief of angina pectoris. Reduction of myocardial oxygen requirements by extracoronary vasodilation and its attenuation by the chronic administration of isosorbide dinitrate, *Ann. Intern. Med.,* 72, 779, 1970.

66. **Williams, J. K., Glick, G., and Braunwald, E.,** Studies on cardiac dimensions in intact unanesthetized man. Effects of nitroglycerin, *Circulation,* 32, 767, 1965.

67. **Ganz, W. and Marcus, H. S.,** Failure of intracoronary nitroglycerin to alleviate pacing-induced angina, *Circulation,* 46, 880, 1972.

68. **Parker, J. O., Case, R. B., Khaja, F., Ledwich, J. R., and Armstrong, P. W.,** The influence of changes in blood volume in angina pectoris. A study of the effect of phlebotomy, *Circulation,* 41, 593, 1970.

69. **Winbury, M. M.,** Redistribution of left ventricular blood flow produced by nitroglycerin, *Circ. Res.,* 28(Suppl. 1), 140, 1971.

70. **Francis, G. S. and Hagan, A. D.,** Nitroglycerin ointment: a review, *Angiology,* 28, 873, 1977.

71. **Aronow, W. S.,** Medical treatment of angina pectoris. III. Long-acting nitrites as antianginal drugs, *Am. Heart J.,* 84, 706, 1972.

72. **Goldstein, R. E. and Epstein, S. E.,** Nitrates in the prophylactic treatment of angina pectoris, *Circulation,* 58, 917, 1973.

73. **Prichard, B. N. C.,** β-Adrenoceptor blocking drugs in angina pectoris, in *Cardiovascular Drugs,* Vol. 2, β-Adrenoceptor Blocking Drugs, Avery, G. S., Ed., University Park Press, Baltimore, 1978, chap. 4.

74. **Sostman, H. D. and Langou, R. A.,** Contempory medical management of stable angina pectoris, *Am. Heart J.,* 95, 775, 1978.

75. **Gibson, D. G.,** Pharmacodynamic properties of β-adrenergic receptor blocking drugs in man, *Drugs,* 7, 8, 1974.

76. **Frishman, W. and Silverman, R.,** Clinical pharmacology of the new beta-adrenergic blocking drugs. 3. Comparative clinical experience and new therapeutic applications, *Am. Heart J.,* 98, 119, 1979.

77. **McDevitt, D. G.,** Adrenoceptor blocking drugs, clinical pharmacology and therapeutic use, *Drugs,* 17, 267, 1979.

78. **Short, D.,** The management of the patient with angina, *Am. Heart J.,* 94, 135, 1977.

79. **Heel, R. C., Brogden, R. N., Speight, T. M., and Avery, G. S.,** Atenolol: a review of its pharmacological properties and therapeutic efficacy in angina pectoris and hypertension, *Drugs,* 17, 425, 1979.

80. **Brogden, R. N., Heel, R. C., Speight, T. M., and Avery, G. S.,** Metoprolol: a review of its pharmacological properties and therapeutic efficacy in hypertension and angina pectoris, *Drugs,* 14, 321, 1977.

ANTIHYPERTENSIVE AGENTS

Peter S. Chan and Peter Cervoni

INTRODUCTION

Hypertension is a serious mass public health problem affecting the elderly. Based on World Health Organization criteria, anyone whose systolic blood pressure is 160 mmHg or greater and/or whose diastolic blood pressure is 95 mmHg or greater is considered hypertensive. In the U.S. and most western countries, about 11 to 13% of the population is over 65 years of age.[1,2] In the National Health Examination Survey carried out by the U.S. Public Health Service between 1960 and 1962, 27% of white men and 66% of black men, and 49% of white women and 71% of black women, in the age range of 65 to 74 years, had systolic blood pressures of at least 160 mmHg or diastolic blood pressures of 95 mmHg. Between the ages of 75 and 79 years, 40% of the white men, 60% of the black men, 45% of the white women, and 69% of the black women had hypertension.[3,4] Arterial blood pressure in industrialized countries increases with age.[4,5] Of deaths due to cardiovascular diseases in the U.S., 3/4 are in the age group of 65 and over.[6]

Hypertension is the single most important identifiable factor that affects other cardiovascular diseases such as congestive heart failure, stroke, myocardial infarction, kidney failure, and the acceleration of atherosclerosis.[4,7,8]

In the elderly, systolic hypertension is very prevalent.[4,5,9,10] While the incidence of diastolic hypertension tends to remain stable from late middle-age on, systolic hypertension continues to mount even in the 7th decade of life and beyond.[4,7,11] The probable cause of systolic hypertension in the elderly is the increasing rigidity of the large arterial blood vessels.[12] Systolic hypertension has serious prognostic implications. Chronic systolic hypertension causes loss of aortic distensibility and aortic volume, increases the incidence of atheroma and thrombi formation, and increases arterial deterioration and degeneration.[13] The Framingham studies indicate that cardiac enlargement, heart failure, coronary arterial disease, and strokes were all more closely related to systolic than to diastolic blood pressure levels.[14,15,16] Life insurance data clearly demonstrate a linear relationship between the level of systolic blood pressure and increased cardiovascular mortality and morbidity.[8,17] Other studies indicate that the incidence of cerebral hemorrhage and aneurysms also appear to be directly proportional to systolic pressure.[18-20]

Diastolic hypertension in the elderly arises from the same pathologic conditions as in younger people, but it compromises circulation to the brain, heart, and kidneys more severely in the elderly than in the young. Diastolic hypertension in the aged is characterized by normal cardiac output and increased total peripheral resistance. Effective reduction of blood pressure retards the progression of vascular deterioration and renal insufficiency.[9]

Regardless of the patient's age, systolic blood pressure above 160 mmHg and diastolic blood pressure above 95 mmHg should be treated.[4,5,7,9] Antihypertensive treatment benefits the elderly as much as the younger population.[21-25] Antihypertensive therapy is not contraindicated in patients with a history of cerebrovascular accidents.[22,26,27] Available evidence indicates that antihypertensive treatment prevents hemorrhagic and thrombotic strokes.[9,10,13] Control of high systolic blood pressure is particularly important when evidence of target organ damage is present.[10]

The prime goal of therapy is conservation of heart, brain, and kidney functions, which are most often damaged by prolonged hypertension.[9] Antihypertensive treatment should effect the least possible impairment of organ function.[5,9,13,21] In the elderly, the arteries supplying the brain undergo atherosclerotic changes.[9,13] Impaired cerebral blood flow due to atherosclerosis alters brain functions and autonomic reflexes.[9] In the aged, the cerebral blood flow may decrease 20 to 30% due to the combined factors of advancing age and atherosclerosis.[28]

Orthostatic hypotension is more frequent and severe in the elderly following the use of agents that will normally aggravate orthostatic hypotension. This is primarily due to decreased baroreceptor sensitivity and a reduction in peripheral venous tone.[29-33] Agents that inhibit autonomic activity must be used with great care.[34]

Renal functions, such as renal blood flow and the glomerular filtration rate, decrease 50% in the elderly.[35] The ability of the renal tubules to concentrate or dilute the urine in the elderly is diminished.[36-39] As renal function progressively diminishes with increasing age, rapid and excessive reduction of blood pressure may severely compromise glomerular filtration rate. The propensity of antihypertensives to cause retention of electrolytes and water in the elderly, therefore, is great.

Incidence of coronary artery disease is higher in hypertensive patients over age 60 than in younger patients. Therefore, the need for therapeutic caution must be emphasized to avoid anginal attacks.

High blood pressure in the elderly should be reduced to the desired level slowly, over many weeks and cautiously, so that blood flow to vital organs such as brain, heart, and kidneys is not impaired. Gradual reduction of arterial pressure allows time for adaptive processes, particularly with regard to readjustment of autoregulatory mechanisms controlling blood flow. Cerebral blood flow is usually kept constant within a certain range of arterial blood pressure. Abrupt reduction of pressure in hypertension may strain the limits of autoregulation. Below a certain level of arterial pressure, cerebral blood flow will vary directly with blood pressure. Slow and cautious lowering of arterial pressure allows time for resetting of autoregulatory levels, and allows pressure control without interference with the stability of cerebral flow. It is best to start therapy with low doses, to avoid abrupt or rapid lowering of arterial pressure.

APPROACHES TO THE TREATMENT OF HYPERTENSION

Most physicians follow the stepped care approach as recommended by the Joint National Committee on Detection, Evaluation, and Treatment of High Blood Pressure,[40] and endorsed by the American Heart Association and many medical societies:

Step 1. The patient is started on a thiazide or a thiazide-like diuretic.
Step 2. If a sufficient hypotensive response is not achieved, either propranolol, reserpine, methyldopa, clonidine, or prazosin is added.
Step 3. If the response to two drugs is insufficient, a vasodilator like hydralazine is added.
Step 4. If the desired blood pressure level is not achieved with three drugs, then guanethidine is added.

Laragh et al. advocate that before treatment starts, a renin profile should be obtained on each patient.[41-44] According to this approach, if the plasma renin activity (PRA) is high or normal, a β-adrenoceptor blocker or an angiotensin I converting enzyme inhibitor, captopril, should be tried first. If the PRA is low, a diuretic should be used first. Laragh claims that a β-adrenoceptor blocker or a converting enzyme inhibitor combined with a diuretic should normalize 70% of all hypertensive patients. If blood pressure lowering is not achieved by using a β-adrenoceptor blocker or a converting enzyme inhibitor plus a diuretic, then either a vasodilator, clonidine, or methyldopa is added.

Antihypertensive drugs can be grouped broadly into the following categories:

1. Diuretics
   A. General diuretics: hydrochlorothiazide and other thiazides, quinethazone, chlorthalidone, metolazone and ticrynafen (discussed below as thiazide-like group of diuretics)
   B. High-ceiling loop diuretics: furosemide and ethacrynic acid
   C. Aldosterone antagonists: spironolactone
   D. Potassium-sparing diuretics: triamterene and amiloride
2. Drugs affecting the autonomic nervous system (see Dr. Roberts' chapter in this handbook)
   A. α-Adrenoceptor blockers: phentolamine, prazosin
   B. β-Adrenoceptor blockers: propranolol, metoprolol
   C. Adrenergic neuronal blocking agents: guanethidine, bethanidine, debrisoquine
   D. Catecholamine depleting agents: reserpine
   E. Ganglionic blocking agents: trimethaphan
   F. Monoamine oxidase inhibitor: pargyline
3. Centrally acting drugs: α-methyldopa, clonidine, reserpine
4. Vasodilators: hydralazine, prazosin, diazoxide, minoxidil, nitroprusside
5. Renin-angiotensin system antagonists: captopril

DIURETICS

General Diuretics

Except in high-renin patients, a thiazide-like diuretic should be the first drug to be used for treatment of mild to moderate hypertension in ambulatory patients. Diuretics are the cornerstone of all antihypertensive regimens and they alone can normalize over 50% of all essential hypertensive cases, including most of the low-renin hypertensive elderly. This is because the diuretics not only exert blood pressure lowering effects through extracellular fluid volume contraction, but also prevent or counteract the side effects of sodium and fluid retention produced by almost all other marketed antihypertensives except the β-blockers. The prevention of sodium and fluid retention will enhance the blood pressure lowering effect of other antihypertensive agents in most patients.

Diuretics cause about a 10% decrease in plasma volume in the acute phase.[45,46] Cardiac output is reduced and the calculated total peripheral resistance is increased. After several months of continuous diuretic treatment, most clinical studies show that a persistent reduction of plasma volume of about 5% is maintained.[47-49] Diuretics generally do not reduce the blood pressure of normotensive subjects.

The usual decrease of blood pressure treated with thiazide-like diuretics for over 3 weeks is about 21 mmHg in systolic pressure and 10 mmHg in diastolic pressure.[50] A persistent reduction of peripheral resistance on long-term treatment was observed despite the fact that cardiac output was restored.[49] In response to sodium loss, PRA and angiotensin II levels increased. The blood pressure in the recumbent and standing positions was reduced equally by diuretics, so orthostatic or postural hypotension seldom occurred. This is particularly important to the elderly. The hypotensive effect was maintained during exercise. The antihypertensive effect of the diuretics was maintained in long-term therapy without development of tolerance.

Thiazide-like diuretics cause a maximal excretion of 10 to 15% of the filtered sodium load. A longer-acting diuretic, such as chlorthalidone, metolazone, or polythiazide is a better choice for the elderly since better compliance can be achieved for a once-daily dosing regimen. The prolonged action of chlorthalidone is due to its greater lipid solubility and its preferential and prolonged binding to renal tissues. The hypotensive effect is mainly due to the reduction in extracellular fluid volume secondary to blood volume reduction and sodium loss.[51-53]

The following effects caused by diuretics are considered less important as a mechanism of their antihypertensive action: (1) direct vasodilatory action on blood vessels, (2) decrease of the vasoconstricting effects of circulating norepinephrine and angiotension II, and (3) increased sodium efflux from blood vessels. The thiazide or thiazide-like diuretics produce relatively mild side effects. The major ones are hypokalemia, hyperuricemia, and hyperglycemia. Hypokalemia occurs because potassium excretion increases as increased amounts of sodium (due to inhibition of reabsorption) are presented to the more distal Na^+-K^+ ion exchange site in the tubule. The degree of potassium excretion caused by a diuretic varies directly with the circulating aldosterone level. At adequate doses, the thiazides, chlorthalidone, quinethazone, metolazone, and the new diuretic, ticrynafen, exert approximately the same degree of blood pressure lowering despite the diversified chemical structures. Ticrynafen produces uricosuria and hypouricemia[54,55] and is considered an advantage in patients predisposed to gout, but the long-term benefit of plasma uric acid reduction remain to be seen.

High-Ceiling Loop Diuretics

High-ceiling loop diuretics, such as furosemide and ethacrynic acid, are generally not considered as the first diuretic to be used for the treatment of hypertension in the elderly because of their tendency to produce rapid electrolyte imbalance and dehydration. High-ceiling loop diuretics are used: (1) when renal function is impaired, (2) as an adjunct in hypertensive crisis or emergency, and (3) in resistant hypertension where thiazides cannot effectively eliminate the sodium and water retention problem. Furosemide is more widely used than ethacrynic acid. Excessive loss of water and sodium may result in dehydration and reduction in blood volume, with possible circulatory collapse in the elderly. In mild hypertension, most clinical studies indicate that thiazides produce a greater decrease in blood pressure than furosemide in hypertensive patients with normal renal function.[50] In addition to hypokalemia, hyperglycemia, and hyperuricemia, high doses of furosemide or ethacrynic acid may cause ototoxicity.[56-58]

Aldosterone Antagonists

Spironolactone is a competitive antagonist of aldosterone. By counteracting the sodium-retaining and potassium-losing effects of aldosterone at the Na^+-K^+ exchange sites of the renal distal tubules, spironolactone increases sodium and water excretion and normalizes plasma potassium level. Spironolactone is efficacious in lowering the elevated blood pressure in patients with primary hyperaldosteronism and in many patients with essential hypertension, even if the aldosterone level is not elevated.[59] The exact mechanism whereby spironolactone works in essential hypertension with normal aldosterone is not clear. However, spironolactone is more efficacious in patients with low PRA.[60,61] Spironolactone enhances blood pressure lowering effects of other antihypertensives, including the thiazide-like diuretics. Spironolactone prevents hypokalemia in patients on thiazide, furosemide, or ethacrynic acid. However, potassium supplementation should not be concomitantly given with spironolactone. Hyperkalemia and elevated blood urea nitrogen may occur in the elderly patients with impaired renal function. Gynecomastia may be associated with the use of spironolactone and is usually reversible upon withdrawal of the drug.

Potassium-Sparing Diuretics

Triamterene and amiloride are either potassium-sparing or potassium-retaining diuretics, acting at the Na^+-K^+ exchange sites in the renal distal tubules, independent of aldosterone. Their action is not through competitive antagonism of aldosterone. Triamterene and amiloride by themselves produce only slight blood pressure reductions, but are useful as an adjunct to the thiazide-like diuretics and furosemide to prevent and to treat hypokalemia. Potassium supplementation should not be used concomitantly with triamterene or amiloride. Hyperkalemia may occur in elderly patients, particularly those with renal impairment. Amiloride has been marketed in the U.S.

DRUGS AFFECTING THE AUTONOMIC NERVOUS SYSTEM

See Dr. Roberts' chapter in this handbook.

CENTRALLY ACTING DRUGS

Methyldopa

Methyldopa (α-methyldopa) is one of the most widely prescribed drugs for treatment of hypertension. Methyldopa is converted to α-methyl-norepinephrine in central and peripheral neurons. The antihypertensive effect of methyldopa is abolished by centrally acting dopa decarboxylase inhibitors,[62,63] but not by inhibitors acting only peripherally.[64] Therefore, it is concluded that methyldopa must be decarboxylated centrally for its antihypertensive activity and that the peripheral action is a minor mechanism.[65] The central hypotensive effects require the activation of the α-adrenoceptors,[65-67] probably located in the lower brainstem at the level of the nucleus tractus solitarii.

Methyldopa used alone reduces blood pressure by about 20/13 and 38/22 mmHg in mild, and moderate, or severe hypertension, respectively.[50] Sodium and water retention, weight gain, and edema usually occur in patients receiving methyldopa alone for several months. A thiazide-like diuretic is usually needed to overcome such side effects. Combinations of methyldopa and a thiazide-like diuretic lower blood pressure better than either one used alone. Methyldopa does not decrease renal blood flow or glomerular filtration rates, so it can be used in patients with renal impairment without further deterioration of renal function. However, in long-term therapy, a thiazide-like diuretic or furosemide may be required to augment the antihypertensive effects of methyldopa.

The blood pressure reduction induced by methyldopa is as effective in the recumbent as in the standing position. Therefore, risk or aggravation of orthostatic hypotension is less of a problem in the elderly than in younger groups.

Methyldopa inhibits the renin release from the kidney and may contribute partly to the antihypertensive effect in some high-renin patients. Methyldopa can be used in moderate, severe, and complicated hypertension; its antihypertensive effect is maintained as long as the therapy continues, provided that the salt and water retention problem is prevented by the use of a diuretic. Methyldopa decreases total peripheral resistance by 30%. Renal vascular resistance is also decreased by methyldopa.[68] Animal studies show that methyldopa prevents cardiac hypertrophy associated with hypertension.

The major adverse effects of methyldopa are drowsiness, sedation (particularly in the elderly), nasal congestion, dry mouth, and salt and fluid retention. More serious side effects, such as hemolytic anemia, positive direct antiglobulin (Coomb's) test, drug-induced fever, and hepatitis have been reported.

Clonidine

Clonidine is a centrally acting, potent hypotensive. Its principal action is the activation of the central α-adrenoceptors in the brainstem vasomotor center.[67,69,70] α-Adrenoceptor blocking agents abolish its hypotensive action and its peripheral α-adrenoceptor agonist effect. Intravenous clonidine produces an initial transient hypertensive response by activation of the peripheral α-adrenoceptors, and is followed by a prolonged hypotensive response as a result of the excitation of the central α-adrenoceptors.

Although clonidine alone has been used successfully for the treatment of hypertension, clonidine is more commonly added to a diuretic to enhance its control of blood pressure. Clonidine is in the same efficacy range as methyldopa. Clonidine decreases renin and aldosterone secretion. Orthostatic hypotension is not common, since clonidine lowers blood pressure equally in the standing and supine positions. Patients undergoing clonidine therapy have normal hemodynamic responses to exercise. Clonidine decreases heart rate and total peripheral resistance, but exerts no significant effect on renal blood flow or glomerular filtration rate. When clonidine is withdrawn abruptly, some patients may experience a rebound phenomenon, whereby blood pressure rises rapidly to a level higher than the predrug level, and the patient experiences symptoms of tachycardia, agitation, headache and nervousness. Therefore, if withdrawal of clonidine is desired, the dose should be reduced gradually over 2 weeks. If rebound phenomena occur, resumption of clonidine therapy or administration of phentolamine intravenously will reduce the blood pressure.

The common adverse effect of clonidine are drowsiness, sedation, dry mouth, fatigue, and dizziness.

Reserpine

Reserpine is the most active purified alkaloid derived from *Rauwolfia serpentina*. Reserpine is efficacious in mild, moderate, and severe hypertension. When used in combination with hydrochlorothiazide, reserpine was found to be more efficacious than hydrochlorothiazide plus propranolol or hydralazine plus propranolol in mild hypertension. The major antihypertensive effect of reserpine is primarily due to depletion of catecholamines from the peripheral adrenergic nerves. However, depletion of norepinephrine from the vasomotor centers also plays a role in its action. Both norepinephrine and serotonin are depleted in the brain, myocardium, blood vessels, and adrenergic nerve endings. The most serious adverse effect is mental depression, which sometimes may be severe enough to cause suicide. Reserpine should never be administered to patients with a history of depression.

The frequent adverse effects of reserpine are: depression (particularly at high dose), nasal congestion, drowsiness, sedation, lethargy, sodium and fluid retention, decreased libido, impotence, nightmares, excessive gastric secretion, and activation of peptic ulcer.

VASODILATORS

Vasodilators referred to here are those agents that act directly on the vasculature without interfering with the autonomic nervous system, with the exception of prazosin. It is desirable to reduce the total peripheral resistance by relaxing the arteriolar smooth muscle. The advantages of most vasodilators in the treatment of hypertension are: (1) they are generally free from central effects and (2) they do not induce fatigue or diminished vigilance.

Hydralazine

Hydralazine lowers arterial blood pressures by vasodilation in all species studied, including man. The vasodilation is due to direct action on the vascular smooth muscle.[71] Vasodilation occurs in major vascular beds, such as the renal, carotid, coronary, mesenteric, and femoral. Hydralazine has more pronounced effects on the capacitance blood vessels than the resistance vessels.[71] In the face of hypotension, hydralazine has the ability to increase renal blood flow. Cardiac output is usually increased. Due to reflex sympathetic activation, tachycardia accompanies hypotension.[72] Hydralazine increases PRA and causes sodium and water retention.

Due to tachycardia and increased cardiac output, as well as sodium and water retention, hydralazine is usually added to a regimen of a diuretic and methyldopa, clonidine, β-adrenoceptor blocker, or reserpine. In such a triple combination, a 30/20 mmHg lowering of blood pressure can be achieved. Myocardial stimulation can cause myocardial ischemia and should be used cautiously in patients with coronary insufficiency.

The common adverse effects are headache, tachycardia, flushing, salt and water retention, dizziness; also anginal attacks in patients with ischemic heart disease. At doses higher than 200 mg/day, a lupus erythematosus-like syndrome may occur in some patients.

Prazosin

Prazosin appears to produce its major antihypertensive effect by post synaptic α-adrenoceptor blockade.[73,74] The peripheral arterioles are selectively relaxed. Prazosin causes minor direct relaxation of the arteriolar vascular smooth muscle. Unlike the conventional α-adrenoceptor blockers, prazosin rarely produces tachycardia. Postural dizziness and lightheadedness are very common after the first dose of prazosin. For this reason, the first dose of prazosin is recommended to be given at bedtime. Prazosin, when used with a diuretic, has approximately the same efficacy range as methyldopa plus a diuretic. Prazosin lowers arterial blood pressure at rest and during exercise. Heart rate, cardiac index, and stroke volume are not significantly altered and PRA is reduced in hypertensive patients. The most important hemodynamic effect of prazosin in humans is an impressive reduction in total peripheral resistance. Its antihypertensive effect is greatly enhanced by the concomitant administration of either a diuretic or a β-adrenoceptor blocker.

The common adverse effects are headache, drowsiness, postural hypotension, weakness, palpitation, nausea, and vomiting. Syncope with sudden loss of consciousness occurs in less than 0.2% of the patients.

Diazoxide

Diazoxide is a potent vasodilator, closely related chemically to the thiazide diuretics, but devoid of diuretic activity. As a matter of fact, diazoxide produces severe electrolyte and water retention and subsequent edema formation. Diazoxide in its intravenous form is approved only for use in hypertensive emergencies and refractory hypertension.[75,76] Due to rapid protein binding, diazoxide has to be administered at a dose of 5 mg/kg by rapid (less than 20 sec) intravenous bolus injection, in order to deliver adequate drug concentrations to the arterial smooth muscles. The duration of action is usually between 6 to 8 hr. If the initial dose is not effective, another dose can be given 30 min later. The disadvantage of intravenous rapid bolus injection of this long acting and potent vasodilator is that a sudden drastic reduction of arterial blood pressure may precipitate cerebral ischemia in patients with impaired cerebral circulation, and myocardial ischemia in patients with limited coronary reserve. Diazoxide causes severe tachycardia, it increases cardiac output and PRA. A high-ceiling loop diuretic, such as furosemide should be concomitantly used to counteract salt and water retention. Due to the release of catecholamines and the suppression of insulin release from the pancreas, diazoxide produces hyperglycemia.

Sodium Nitroprusside

Sodium nitroprusside is a potent vasodilator, used only in hypertensive crisis.[50,75,76] It dilates the arterial and venous vascular beds. It has to be given by a constant intravenous infusion; the onset of action is within seconds, and it can bring the blood pressure to any desired level. Nitroprusside is indicated and is effective in virtually all hypertensive crises. It is also effective in acute pulmonary edema and refractory congestive heart failure because it reduces preload and afterload. Unlike other vasodilators, the increase in heart rate in hypertensive patients is slight to moderate. As with other vasodilators, PRA activity is increased and total peripheral resistance is greatly reduced. Blood pressure begins to rise immediately after the intravenous infusion is stopped. The frequent adverse effects are headache, anorexia, nausea, abdominal cramps, dizziness, weakness, and restlessness. Cyanide poisoning can occur.

Minoxidil

Minoxidil is a potent, orally active vasodilator; the vasodilation obtainable is much greater than with hydralazine.[50,75] Minoxidil selectively concentrates in the arterial vasculature and as a result it has a long duration of action. Minoxidil provokes a marked reduction of vascular resistance and severe tachycardia. It also causes severe sodium and water retention, as well as a pronounced increase in cardiac output and PRA. Most clinical trials of minoxidil have been carried out in severe, malignant, and refractory hypertension patients. Remarkable results have been obtained when it is used concomitantly with a β-adrenoceptor blocker, propranolol, and a diuretic, either hydrochlorothiazide or furosemide. It is effective where other antihypertensives have failed. Many nephrectomies have been avoided due to the good antihypertensive efficacy of minoxidil. The frequent adverse effects are tachycardia, sodium and water retention, and hirsutism.

RENIN-ANGIOTENSIN SYSTEM ANTAGONISTS

Captopril

Captopril (SQ 14,225) is a potent, orally active inhibitor of the angiotensin I converting enzyme system which catalyzes the formation of angiotensin II from its inactive precursor, angiotensin I. This enzyme is believed to be identical with kininase II, which catalyzes the degradation of bradykinin. Angiotensin II is known to be an extremely potent vasoconstrictor and stimulator of the release of aldosterone. Bradykinin is a very potent vasodilator. By inhibiting the converting enzyme, the angiotensin II level should decrease in the circulation, and the tissue bradykinin level should increase.

Laragh et al.[77] found that among all patients with essential hypertension about 16% are in the high, 57% in the normal, and 27% in the low renin subgroups. Laragh et al.[41-43,78,79] found that in patients with renal hypertension and in patients with high and normal renin, essential hypertension responded well to (1) the β-adrenoceptor blocker, propranolol; (2) saralasin and angiotensin II antagonists; (3) teprotide (SQ 20,881), a nonapeptide; and (4) the new, orally active angiotensin converting enzyme inhibitor, captopril (an amino acid derivative). The degree of blood pressure reduction was correlated with: (1) the level of pretreatment PRA, (2) the induced suppression of urinary aldosterone excretion, and (3) the subsequent changes in potassium balance and serum potassium.

Gavras et al.,[80] Larochelle et al.,[81] and Brunner et al.[82,83] also found captopril efficacious in patients with renal hypertension and in patients with essential hypertension. The finding that captopril is efficacious in patients with essential hypertension certainly widens the spectrum of its utility. Whether the bradykinin buildup after captopril contributes to its antihypertensive activity is unclear. It has been suggested that part of the antihypertensive activity of captopril may be due to mechanisms other than inhibition of synthesis of angiotensin II.

Adverse effects reported for captopril are skin rash (particularly at high doses) and modification of the sense of taste.

REFERENCES

1. Population Estimates and Projections, 1977, Series P-25, No. 734, Bureau of the Census, U.S. Department of Commerce, Washington, D.C., 1978.
2. Population Estimates, 1975, Population Division of the United Nations, Library, United Nations, New York, 1975.
3. Heart Disease in Adults, United States, 1960—1962, National Center for Health Statistics, Series 11, No. 6, Public Health Service, U.S. Department of Health, Education and Welfare, Washington, D.C., 1964.
4. **Stamler, J.,** High Blood Pressure in the United States, An Overview of the Problem and the Challenge, Publ. No. (NIH) 73-486, U.S. Department of Health, Education and Welfare, Washington, D.C., 1973.

5. **Dyer, A. R., Stamler, J., Shekelle, R. B., Schoenberger, J. A., and Farinaro, E.,** Hypertension in the elderly, *Med. Clin. North Am.,* 61, 513, 1977.
6. **Marx, J. L. and Kolata, G. B.,** Combating the #1 killer, *The Science Report on Heart Research,* American Association for the Advancement of Science, Washington, D.C., 1978, 4.
7. **Stamler, J.,** *Lectures on Preventive Cardiology,* Grune & Stratton, New York, 1967.
8. *Build and Blood Pressure Study, 1959,* Vol. 1, Society of Actuaries, Chicago, 1959.
9. **Chrysant, S. G., Frohlich, E., and Papper, S.,** Why hypertension is so prevalent in the elderly and how to treat it, *Geriatrics,* 31, 101, 1976.
10. **Adanopoulos, P. N., Chrysanthakopoulis, S. G., and Frolich, E. D.,** Systolic hypertension: nonhomogeneous disease, *Am. J. Cardiol.,* 36, 697, 1975.
11. **Stamler, J., Stamler, R., Riedlinger, W. F., Algera, G., and Roberts, R. H.,** Hypertension screening of 1 million Americans: Community Hypertension Evaluation Clinic (CHEC) Program, 1973 through 1975, *J. Am. Med. Assoc.,* 235, 2299, 1976.
12. **Onesti, G. and Moyer, J. H.,** Hypertension past 60, *Geriatrics,* 22, 192, 1967.
13. **Harris, R.,** Treatment of hypertension in geriatric patients, *Clin. Med.,* 83, 9, 1976.
14. **Kannel, W. B., Gordon, T., and Schwartz, M. J.,** Systolic versus diastolic blood pressure and risk of coronary heart disease, the Framingham study, *Am. J. Cardiol.,* 27, 335, 1971.
15. **Kannel, W. B. and Sorlie, P.,** Hypertension in Framingham, in *Epidemiology and Control of Hypertension,* Paul, O., Ed., Symposia Specialists, Miami, Fla., 1975, 553.
16. **Koch-Weser, J.,** Correlation of pathophysiology and pharmacology in primary hypertension, *Am. J. Cardiol.,* 32, 499, 1973.
17. Actuarial Society of America, *Supplement of Blood Pressure Study,* Actuarial Society of America, Chicago, 1941, 6.
18. **Kannel, W. B., Wolf, D., and Dawber, T. R.,** Hypertension and cardiac impairments increase stroke risk, *Geriatrics,* 33, 71, 1978.
19. **Colandrea, M. A., Friedman, G. D., Nichaman, M. Z., and Lynd, C. N.,** Systolic hypertension in the elderly. An epidemiologic assessment, *Circulation,* 41, 239, 1970.
20. **Shekelle, R., Ostfeld, A., and Klawans, H.,** Hypertension and risk of stroke in the elderly population, *Stroke,* 5, 71, 1974.
21. **Finnerty, F. A.,** Hypertension in the elderly, special considerations in treatment, *Postgrad. Med.,* 65, 119, 1979.
22. **Tarazi, R. C.,** Should you treat systolic hypertension in elderly patients?, *Geriatrics,* 33, 25, 1978.
23. **Freis, E. D.,** The value of treatment of hypertension, *Univ. Mich. Med. Cent J.,* 44, 120, 1978.
24. Veterans Administration Cooperative Study Group on Antihypertensive Agents, Effects of treatment on morbidity in hypertension. Results in patients with diastolic blood pressures averaging 115 through 129 mmHg, *J. Am. Med. Assoc.,* 202, 116, 1967.
25. Veterans Administration Cooperative Study Group on Antihypertensive Agents, Effects of treatment on morbidity in hypertension. III. Influence of age, diastolic pressure, and prior cardiovascular disease; further analysis of side effects, *Circulation,* 45, 991, 1972.
26. **Carter, A. B.,** Hypotensive therapy in stroke survivors, *Lancet,* 1, 485, 1970.
27. **Marshall, J.,** A trial of long term hypotensive therapy in cerebrovascular disease, *Lancet,* 1, 10, 1974.
28. **Bender, A. D.,** The effect of increasing age on the distribution of peripheral blood flow in man, *J. Am. Geriatr. Soc.,* 13, 192, 1965.
29. **Bristow, J. D., Honour, A. J., Pickering, G. W., Sleight, P., and Smyth, H. S.,** Diminished baroreflex sensitivity in high blood pressure, *Circulation,* 39, 48, 1969.
30. **Appenzeller, O. and Descaries, L.,** Circulating reflexes in patients with cerebrovascular disease, *N. Engl. J. Med.,* 271, 820, 1964.
31. **Gribbin, B., Pickering, T. G., Sleight, P., and Peto, R.,** Effect of age and high blood pressure on baroreflex sensitivity in man, *Circ. Res.,* 29, 424, 1971.
32. **Caird, F. I., Andrews, G. R., and Kennedy, R. D.,** Effect of posture on blood pressure in the elderly, *Br. Heart J.,* 35, 527, 1973.
33. Drugs causing postural hypotension, *Med. Lett.,* 20, 15, 1978.
34. Drugs in the elderly, *Med. Lett.,* 21, 43, 1979.
35. **Rowe, J. W., Andres, R., Tobin, J. D., Norris, A. H., and Shock, N. W.,** The effect of age on creatinine clearance in men, a cross-sectional and longitudinal study, *J. Gerontol.,* 31, 155, 1976.
36. **Papper, S.,** The effects of age in reducing renal function, *Geriatrics,* 28, 83, 1973.
37. **Pelz, K. S., Gottfried, S. P., and Paz, E.,** Kidney function studies in old men and women, *Geriatrics,* 20, 145, 1965.
38. **Wollam, G. L. and Gifford, R. W., Jr.,** The kidney as a target organ in hypertension, *Geriatrics,* 31, 71, 1976.
39. **Vestal, R. E.,** Drug use in the elderly, a review of problems and special considerations, *Drugs,* 16, 358, 1978.

40. Report of the Joint National Committee on Detection, evaluation and treatment of high blood pressure, Publ. No. (NIH) 77-1088, U.S. Department of Health, Education and Welfare, Washington, D.C., 1977.
41. **Laragh, J. H.,** Modern system for treating high blood pressure based on renin profiling and vasoconstriction — volume analysis. A primary role for beta blocking drugs such as propranolol, *Am. J. Med.,* 61, 797, 1976.
42. **Case, D. B., Atlas, S. A., Laragh, J. H., Sealey, J. E., Sullivan, P. A., and McKinstry, D. N.,** Clinical experience with blockade of renin-angiotensin-aldosterone system by an oral converting-enzyme inhibitor (SQ 14,225), captopril in hypertensive patients, *Progr. Cardiovasc. Dis.,* 21, 159, 1978.
43. **Laragh, J. H.,** The renin system in high blood pressure, from disbelief to reality. Converting-enzyme blockade for analysis and treatment, *Progr. Cardiovasc. Dis.,* 21, 159, 1978.
44. **Laragh, J. H., Letcher, R. L., and Pickering, T. G.,** Renin profiling for diagnosis and treatment of hypertension, *J. Am. Med. Assoc.,* 241, 151, 1979.
45. **Wilson, I. M. and Freis, E. D.,** Relationship between plasma and extracellular fluid volume depletion and the antihypertensive effect of chlorothiazide, *Circulation,* 20, 1028, 1959.
46. **Hansen, J.,** Hydrochlorothiazide in the treatment of hypertension, *Acta Med. Scand.,* 183, 317, 1968.
47. **Tarazi, R. C., Dustan, H. P., and Frohlich, E. D.,** Long-term thiazide therapy in essential hypertension. Evidence for persistent alteration in plasma volume and renin activity, *Circulation,* 41, 709, 1970.
48. **Leth, A.,** Changes in plasma and extracellular fluid volumes in patients with essential hypertension during long-term treatment with hydrochlorothiazide, *Circulation,* 42, 479, 1970.
49. **Lund-Johansen, P.,** Hemodynamic changes in long term diuretic therapy of essential hypertension, *Acta Med. Scand.,* 187, 509, 1970.
50. **McMahon, F. G.,** *Management of Essential Hypertension,* Futura, Mount Kisco, New York, 1978.
51. **Tarazi, R. C.,** Diuretic drugs, mechanism of antihypertensive action, in *Hypertension: Mechanism and Management,* Onesti, G., Kim, K. E., and Moyer, J. H., Eds., Grune & Stratton, New York, 1973, 251.
52. **Shah, S., Khatri, I., and Freis, E. D.,** Mechanism of antihypertensive effect of thiazide diuretics, *Am. Heart J.,* 95, 611, 1978.
53. **Dirks, J. H.,** Mechanisms of action and clinical uses of diuretics, *Hosp. Pract.,* 99, 99, 1979.
54. **Nemati, M., Kyle, M. C., and Freis, E. D.,** Clinical study of ticrynafen. A new diuretic, antihypertensive, and uricosuric agent, *J. Am. Med. Assoc.,* 237, 652, 1977.
55. **de Carvalho, J. H., Dunn, F. G., Chrysant, S. G., and Frohlich, E. D.,** Tricrynafen, a novel uricosuric antihypertensive natriuretic agent, *Arch. Intern. Med.,* 138, 53, 1978.
56. **Cooperman, I. B. and Rubin, I. L.,** Toxicity of ethracrynic acid and furosemide, *Am. Heart J.,* 85, 831, 1973.
57. **Quick, C. A. and Hoppe, W.,** Permanent deafness associated with furosemide administration, *Ann. Otol. Rhinol. Laryngol.,* 84, 94, 1975.
58. **Bourke, E.,** Furosemide, bumetamide, and ototoxicity, *Lancet,* 1, 917, 1976.
59. **Crane, M. G. and Harris, J. J.,** Effects of spironolactone in hypertensive patients, *Am. J. Med. Sci.,* 260, 311, 1970.
60. **Spark, R. F. and Melby, J. C.,** Hypertension and low plasma renin activity, presumptive evidence for mineralocorticoid excess, *Ann. Intern. Med.,* 75, 831, 1971.
61. **Ferguson, R. K., Turek, D. M., and Ronner, D. R.,** Spironolactone and hydrochlorothiazide in normal-renin and low-renin essential hypertension, *Clin. Pharm. Ther.,* 21, 62, 1977.
62. **Day, M. D., Roach, A. G., and Whiting, R. L.,** The mechanism of the antihypertensive action of α-methyldopa in hypertensive rats, *Eur. J. Pharmacol.,* 21, 271, 1973.
63. **Henning, M.,** Interaction of dopa decarboxylase inhibitors with the effect of alpha-methyldopa on blood pressure and tissue monoamines in rats, *Acta Pharmacol. Toxicol.,* 27, 137, 1969.
64. **Henning, M.,** Studies on the mode of action of α-methyldopa, *Acta Physiol. Scand.,* Suppl. 322, 1, 1969.
65. **Henning, M. and Rubenson, A.,** Evidence that the hypotensive action of methyldopa is mediated by central actions of methylnoradrenaline, *J. Pharm. Pharmacol.,* 23, 407, 1971.
66. **Heise, A. and Kroneberg, G.,** Central nervous α-adrenergic receptors and the mode of action of α-methyldopa, *Naunyn-Schmeidebergs Arch. Pharmacol.,* 279, 285, 1973.
67. **Haeusler, G. and Finch, L.,** On the nature of the central hypotensive effect of clonidine and α-methyldopa, *J. Pharmacol. (Paris),* 3, 544, 1972.
68. **Gifford, R. E., Jr., Ed.,** *Methyldopa in the Management of Hypertension,* Merck, Sharp & Dohme, West Point, Pa., 1972.
69. **Kobinger, W.,** Pharmacologic basis of the cardiovascular actions of clonidine, in *Hypertension: Mechanisms and Management,* Onesti, G., Kim, K. E., and Moyer, J. H., Eds., Grune & Stratton, New York, 1973, 369.
70. **Schmitt, H., Schmitt, H., and Fenard, S.,** Evidence for an alpha-sympathomimetic component in the effects of Catapresan on vasomotor centres: antagonism by piperoxan, *Eur. J. Pharmacol.,* 14, 98, 1971.

71. **Ablad, B. and Mellander, J.,** Comparative effects of hydralazine, sodium nitrite and acetylcholine on resistance and capacitance blood vessels and capillary filtration in skeletal muscle in the cat, *Acta Physiol. Scand.,* 58, 319, 1963.

72. **Gross, F.,** Drugs acting on arteriolar smooth muscle (vasodilator drugs), in *Antihypertensive Agents: Handbook of Experimental Pharmacology,* Vol. 39, Gross, F., Ed., Springer-Verlag, Berlin, 1977, chap. 8.

73. **Commarato, M. A., Langley, A. E., Dugan, D. H., Lattime, E. C., Smith, R. D., Tessman, D. K., and Kaplan, H. R.,** Prazosin and phentolamine: comparative cardiovascular and autonomic profiles, *Clin. Exp. Hyperten.,* 1, 191, 1978.

74. **Brogden, R. N., Heel, R. C., Speight, T. M., and Avery, G. S.,** Prazosin: a review of its pharmacological properties and therapeutic efficacy in hypertension, *Drugs,* 14, 163, 1977.

75. **Oates, J. A., Conolly, M. E., Prichard, B. N. C., Shand, D. G., and Schapel, G.,** The clinical pharmacology of antihypertensive drugs, in *Antihypertensive Agents; Handbook of Experimental Pharmacology,* Vol. 39, Springer-Verlag, Berlin, 1977, chap. 13.

76. **Gifford, R. W., Jr.,** Management and treatment of malignant hypertension and hypertensive emergencies, in *Hypertension: Physiopathology and Treatment,* Genest, J., Koiw, E., and Kuchel, O., Eds., McGraw-Hill, New York, 1977, chap. 31.2.

77. **Laragh, J. H.,** An approach to the classification of hypertensive states, in *Hypertension-Mechanisms, Diagnosis and Management,* Davis, J. O., Laragh, J. R., and Selwyn, A., Eds., H. P. Publishing Co., New York, 1977.

78. **Atlas, S. A., Case, D. B., Sealey, J. E., Sullivan, P. M., and Laragh, J. H.,** Involvement of renin-angiotensin-aldosterone axis in antihypertensive action of captopril (SQ 14,225), *Circulation,* 58(2), 143, 1978.

79. **Case, D. B., Atlas, S. A., Sullivan, P., and Laragh, J. H.,** Successful acute and chronic treatment of severe and malignant hypertension with oral converting enzyme inhibitor, captopril, *Circulation,* 60(2), 130, 1979.

80. **Gavras, H., Brunner, H. R., Turini, G. A., Kershaw, G. R., Tifft, C. R., Cuttelod, S., Gavras, I., Vukovich, R. A., and McKinstry, D. N.,** Antihypertensive effect of the oral angiotensin converting enzyme inhibitor, SQ 14,225 in man, *N. Engl. J. Med.,* 298, 991, 1978.

81. **Larochelle, P., Genest, J., Kuchel, O., Boucher, R., Gufkowska, Y., and McKinstry, D.,** Effect of captopril (SQ 14,225) on blood pressure, plasma renin activity and angiotensin I converting enzyme activity, *Can. Med. Assoc. J.,* 121, 309, 1979.

82. **Brunner, H. R., Wauters, J. P., McKinstry, D., Waeber, B., Turini, G., and Gavras, H.,** Inappropriate renin secretion unmasked by captopril (SQ 14,225) in hypertension of chronic renal failure, *Lancet,* 2, 704, 1978.

83. **Brunner, H. R., Gavras, H., Turini, G. A., Waeber, B., and Wauters, J. P.,** Long-term angiotensin blockade in hypertensive patients with chronic renal failure, *Clin. Res.,* 26, 459A, 1978.

ANTIATHEROSCLEROTIC AGENTS

Peter S. Chan and Peter Cervoni

INTRODUCTION

Atherosclerosis is a complex disease of the arteries in which deposits of plaques (atheromas) containing cholesterol, other lipoid material, connective tissue, smooth muscle cells, and calcified tissues are formed within the intima and inner media of the artery, causing the lumen to narrow. Among the many hypotheses that have been put forth for the cause and pathogenesis of atherosclerosis, the response-to-injury hypothesis draws the most attention.[1] According to this hypothesis, when the arterial endothelial lining is injured either mechanically, chemically, by immunologic reactions, or by other causes, while such injuries are in the process of repair, the following events occur: (1) platelets aggregate and release platelet factors, (2) smooth-muscle cells proliferate, (3) lipids infiltrate and accumulate, particularly cholesterol;[2] (4) connective tissue accumulates, and (5) calcium is deposited. Through many years of growth of a plaque or atheroma, the lumen of the artery narrows continuously. If the narrowing is more than 75%, the tissues or organs supplied by such a partially occluded artery will suffer from ischemia whenever demand for oxygen increases.[3] If the narrowing occurs in the coronary arteries, angina pectoris will be manifested. Myocardial infarction and stroke will result if ulceration occurs in the atheroma, causing an arterial thrombus to form, which occludes the rest of the lumen of the arteries supplying the heart and brain, respectively.

Atherosclerosis is the most ubiquitous, disabling, and devastating disease of older people in American society. The disease is very prevalent.[4] For years it has been assumed to be an unavoidable concomitant of the aging process. A growing body of evidence is now available to show that it is neither a natural nor a necessary component of aging.[5-10]

CHARACTERISTICS AND RISK FACTORS

Atherosclerosis is the most important underlying factor that provokes myocardial and cerebral ischemia, arrhythmias, and sudden coronary death. Hence, it is one of the most important factors contributing to death from cardiovascular diseases, and accounts for more deaths than cancer, diabetes, all infections, and accidents combined.[11,12] In the U.S. alone, the economic loss from cardiovascular diseases is more than $28 billion each year.[11]

Studies in the U.S. on men who died from accidental causes or in the Korean and Vietnam wars[13-14] have shown that atherosclerosis starts shortly after the childhood years and that clinically significant lesions begin to appear in the 3rd decade of life. In the elderly years, atherosclerosis in most patients has progressed to the complicated, organized, atheromatous plaque stage and elderly patients suffer various forms of ischemia. There is a 5-fold increase in the incidence of atherosclerosis from age 30 to age 65 in white males. Over 80% of persons age 65 and older have atherosclerotic cardiovascular diseases.[6] It is too late to prevent the initiation of atherosclerosis in the elderly, but current concepts indicate that the progression of atherosclerosis can be significantly slowed and that even substantial regression is possible.[15-20]

The following risk factors have been recognized as important for the pathogenesis of atherosclerosis and coronary heart diseases:[21-23]

1. Increased total serum cholesterol
2. Elevated low-density lipoprotein (LDL)

3. Decreased high-density lipoprotein (HDL)
4. Hypertension
5. Smoking
6. Obesity
7. Diabetes
8. Lack of physical exercise
9. Familial lipid metabolism disorders
10. Elevated very-low-density lipoprotein (VLDL)
11. Elevated triglycerides

Population comparisons suggest that mass hyperlipidemia is a prime requisite for mass atherosclerosis. Habitually incorrect diet is the chief factor leading to mass hyperlipidemia.[5]

The plasma lipids, such as cholesterol and triglycerides, are transported and circulated in a water-soluble form as lipoprotein complexes.[24-36] Lipoproteins can be separated either by ultracentrifugation or electrophoresis. By the ultracentrifugation technique, lipoproteins can be divided into four main classes:

1. Chylomicrons
2. VLDL
3. LDL
4. HDL

The major apoprotein components of lipoproteins are usually called ApoA I and II, ApoB, and ApoC I, II, and III. By the electrophoresis technique, the lipoproteins can be classified into prebeta, beta, and alpha types, corresponding to VLDL, LDL, and HDL, respectively. The characteristics of human plasma lipoproteins are shown in Table 1.

Werner et al.,[28] Keys et al.,[29] and others[30-32] have shown increasing plasma cholesterol levels with increasing age in both men and women. Plasma triglyceride and LDL levels also increase with age.[33,34] The plasma HDL cholesterol usually falls with increasing age.[31]

In North America, HDL cholesterol levels drop sharply and substantially in men after age 14, from 53 to 44 to 46 mg/100 mℓ. Women have 30% higher HDL cholesterol than men in middle age.[35] However, Glueck et al.[36] studying the octogenarian kindreds, found a preponderance of elevated HDL. Therefore, elevated HDL levels may be correlated with longevity. Crouse et al.[37] found that in humans, tissue cholesterol and cholesterol ester increased with age; in particular, human aortic cholesterol and cholesterol esters increased with age.[38] Higher cholesterol esters were found in the atherosclerotic portions of the aorta than in the healthy segments.[39]

Many studies have shown that aging affects lipid metabolism in animals.[40] Blood and tissue lipid levels rose in aging Sprague-Dawley rats,[41] but not in Fischer 344 rats.[40,42] Cholesterol synthesis, turnover, and excretion decreased in aging rats.[43-45] Accumulation of lipids in most tissues was found to be increased in aged rabbits.[46] The effects of age on lipid metabolism and body lipid constituents in humans and laboratory animals are summarized in Table 2.

During the past 2 decades, plasma total cholesterol and triglyceride were considered important risk factors for coronary heart disease (CHD).[23] Hypolipidemic agents were developed in the hope of reducing the morbidity and mortality of CHD. Using the lipoprotein fractionation techniques, it was found that patients who had CHD commonly had elevated VLDL and LDL, but low HDL. Elevated LDL and total cholesterol were drawing the most attention. The significance of the finding of low HDL was largely ignored until 1975, when Miller and Miller proposed that HDL is involved in normal tissue cholesterol synthesis and that low HDL cholesterol was associated with increased risk of CHD.[47] Many recent studies

Table 1
CHARACTERISTICS OF HUMAN PLASMA LIPOPROTEINS

		Classification		
	Chylomicrons	VLDL[a]	LDL[a]	HDL[a]
Chemical composition (%)				
Protein	0.5—1.0	5—15	25	45—55
Major apoproteins	Apo A-I	Apo B	Apo B	Apo A-I
	Apo B (Apo LDL)	Apo C-I		Apo A-II
	Apo C	Apo C-II		
		Apo C-III		
		Apo E		
Lipids				
Free cholesterol	3	6	8	2
Esterfied cholesterol	6	16	39	17
Triglyceride	>85	50—70	5—10	2—4
Phospholipids	3—6	10—20	20—25	30
Physical properties				
Density (g/mℓ)	<0.95	0.95—1.006	1.006—1.063	1.063—1.125 (HDL$_2$)
				1.125—1.210 (HDL$_3$)
S$_f$ (ultracentrifuge)[b]	>400	20—400	0—20	—
Mobility (paper electrophoresis)	Origin	prebeta (pre β)	beta (β)	alpha (α)
Molecular weight	10^3—$10^4 \times 10^6$	5—10×10^6	2—3×10^6	0.2—0.4×10^6
Size (Å)	750—10,000	300—800	215—220	75—100

[a] VLDL = very low density lipoprotein; LDL = low density lipoprotein; HDL = high density lipoprotein.

[b] S$_f$ = lipoprotein flotation rate in Svedburg units (10^{-13} cm/sec/dyne/g) in a sodium chloride solution of density 1.063 g/mℓ (26°C).

Table 2
CHANGES IN LIPID CONSTITUENTS AND METABOLISM IN THE AGED

Species	Lipid constituents and metabolism	Changes in the aged	Ref.
Humans	Plasma cholesterol	Increased	28—32
	Plasma triglyceride	Increased	33, 34
	Plasma LDL	Increased	33, 34
	Tissue cholesterol	Increased	37, 38
	Tissue cholesterol esters	Increased	37, 38
	Plasma HDL	Decreased	31
Rats (Sprague-Dawley)	Tissue lipids	Increased	41
Rats (Sprague-Dawley, Wistar)	Cholesterol synthesis, turnover, excretion	Decreased	43—45
Rats (Fischer 344)	Tissue lipids	No change	40, 42

present convincing evidence that HDL cholesterol had a high predictive power for future CHD. Gordon et al.[48] reported on data from 1025 men and 1445 women, aged 49 to 82 years, in Framingham, Mass. They found that the incidence of CHD per 1000 subjects increased from 25 to 100 in men, and from 14 to 164 in women, as plasma HDL cholesterol decreased from the range of 64 to 74 to the range of 24 to 34 mg/100 mℓ. The association was independent of plasma LDL cholesterol, plasma triglyceride, blood pressure, cigarette consumption, and relative body weight. The predictive power of plasma HDL cholesterol for future CHD was estimated to be approximately fourfold greater than that of LDL cholesterol, and eightfold greater than that of plasma total cholesterol.

In the Tromso (Norway) Heart Study of 6595 men aged 20 to 49 years, the CHD risk was found to be inversely related to the HDL cholesterol level and directly related to the LDL and VLDL cholesterol levels.[49] Castelli et al.[50] reported that in a study of 6859 men and women, ages 40 years or older, in 5 locations in the U.S., persons with low plasma HDL cholesterol had a higher incidence of CHD than persons with higher HDL concentrations. Other studies reported similar findings.[51-53] Walker and Walker found, in a village of South African blacks, that the elderly who had high HDL cholesterol levels were free of CHD.[54] A 10 mg/mℓ decrease in HDL cholesterol increased the CHD risk 2-fold. Jenkins et al.[55] found that people with low plasma HDL levels had more severe coronary atherosclerosis than those with higher levels. Patients with familial Tangier disease,[56] in which HDL is nearly absent, had large cholesterol deposits in their tissues, including their arterial tissues.

Factors known to increase plasma HDL are[57,58] (1) female sex, (2) high physical activity, (3) estrogenic hormones, (4) alcohol, (5) chlorinated hydrocarbons, (6) heparin, (7) weight loss, (8) phenytoin, and (9) familial hyper-HDL-emia. Factors known to decrease plasma HDL are[57,58] (1) male sex, (2) short-term high carbohydrate diet, (3) insulin deficiency and resistance, (4) uremia, (5) liver disease, (6) biliary obstruction, (7) hyperlipoproteinemia type I or IV, (8) Tangier disease, (9) familial hypo-HDL-emia, (10) obesity, and (11) hypertriglyceridemia.

It has been postulated that HDL may be an important factor in preventing cholesterol influx and in facilitating cholesterol efflux from tissues, thereby reducing tissue cholesterol levels, hence decreasing deposition therein.[59] Miller and Miller suggested that plasma HDL is a transport mechanism for carrying cholesterol from peripheral tissues,[47,60] including arterial walls, to the plasma and then to the liver for catabolism and excretion. Another mode of action of HDL is believed to be through its ability to inhibit uptake and degradation of LDL, thereby depressing net increase in the arterial wall.[61,62] It has been suggested that HDL may play a role in triglyceride metabolism. HDL levels are markedly decreased in subjects with exogenous hypertriglyceride. HDL apoprotein catabolism is enhanced by the increased triglyceride flux in patients with nephrotic syndrome and in normal individuals on short-term carbohydrate diets.[58] HDL levels are lower in humans than in some animal species, such as dog, sheep, and rat, which are resistant to atherosclerosis. Therefore, HDL may act as an antiatherogenic agent.[63] High plasma HDL cholesterol is protective against CHD.[55,63,64] It is known that the ratio of the subfractions HDL_2 to HDL_3 is higher in females than in males, that it is increased by estrogen, and is decreased in patients who have survived a myocardial infarction. Feeding of high cholesterol diets to men decreased the HDL_2 to HDL_3 ratio and induced the appearance of an abnormal HDL called HDL_c. HDL_c is known to cause cellular accumulation of cholesterol.[65]

It has been suggested that HDL retards atherosclerosis by inhibiting tissue cholesterol and LDL uptake into extrahepatic cells, owing to the binding of HDL to the cell membrane. Therefore, HDL prevents the accumulation of cholesterol in the arterial wall.[62]

In the elderly, plasma total cholesterol per se is not a good risk predictor for CHD.[48] Current concepts indicate that patients with elevated LDL cholesterol and low HDL cholesterol are prone to CHD; therefore, LDL cholesterol and HDL cholesterol are better predictors of future CHD.

There is substantial convincing evidence that a low level of HDL cholesterol is associated with a high risk of CHD. However, whether raising the HDL cholesterol levels can decrease the risk of CHD remains to be seen. Therefore, the data most urgently needed are those which would demonstrate that raising HDL protects against atherosclerosis and CHD in animals and humans. Since the HDL concept has been advanced only in the last few years, no new program has been initiated at this time to search specifically for drugs that will elevate plasma HDL protein concentration or HDL cholesterol levels. Most of the existing hypolipidemic agents have been, or are being, tested for their ability to influence the HDL cholesterol. Except for estrogen and nicotinic acid[65] and possibly gemfibrozil,[66] most of the current hypolipidemic agents do not raise HDL levels above normal.[67]

Despite the fact that plasma total cholesterol and triglyceride levels are comparatively inferior predictors of future CHD, and despite the rather disappointing results of current hypolipidemic agents on secondary prevention of recurrent CHD,[68] hypolipidemic drugs still have their place in lowering the elevated plasma lipids, particularly in the atherogenic LDL fraction,[69] in hyperlipoproteinemia. Hyperlipoproteinemia may cause disturbing xanthomas, recurring pancreatitis, and CHD. Until the results of well-designed studies on the primary prevention of CHD by hypolipidemic drugs are known, it is probably beneficial to continue to lower the plasma VLDL and LDL fractions of patients at high risk. According to the current hypothesis, hypolipidemic agents which will lower the HDL protein or HDL cholesterol should be avoided.

Hyperlipoproteinemia (HLP) has been classified into five major types:[70,71]

Type I	Chylomicrons present in fasting plasma (hyperchylomicronemia)
Type IIa	Increased LDL concentration with normal VLDL
Type IIb	Increased LDL concentration with increased VLDL
Type III	Increased lipoprotein intermediate forms
Type IV	Increased VLDL
Type V	Increased chylomicrons and VLDL

Type I is rare. Types IIb and Type IV are common. Type III and Type V are common. Type I HLP is characterized by an increase in chylomicra. There is a marked increase in triglycerides; however, cholesterol levels are normal. Increased triglycerides are due to a deficiency in extrahepatic lipoprotein lipase. Type IIa HLP is usually seen with familial combined hyperlipidemia. Type III may be associated with a familial disorder, or may be secondary to myxedema or to dysproteinemia. A decreased ability to transform the intermediate lipoprotein into LDL appears to be the underlying factor. Type IV is usually seen with familial hypertriglyceridemias and familial combined hyperlipidemias, also associated with hypothyroidism, renal failure and diabetes mellitus. Type V is quite frequently seen secondary to insulin-dependent diabetes mellitus, alcoholism, and nephrosis. Types IIa, IIb, and IV abnormalities involve VLDL and LDL for which there is a positive correlation between plasma concentration and the incidence of atherosclerosis.

TREATMENT

Most experts agree that an appropriate diet is the treatment of choice for HLP. Drugs should be used only as an adjunct when the patient cannot adhere to a prescribed diet or when insufficient correction of HLP occurs.

Nicotinic Acid (Niacin)

Nicotinic acid is a potent lipid-lowering drug, but troublesome side effects limit its use. In the Coronary Drug Project,[72,73] nicotinic acid, 3 g/day, was administered to men on a chronic basis. It reduced the plasma cholesterol and triglyceride concentrations by 10 and 25%, respectively. Nicotinic acid, when used above 3 g/day, is effective in Types IIa, IIb, III, IV, and V HPL. Nicotinic acid is used in Type II HPL only when an appropriate diet plus cholestyramine or colestipol (the drugs of choice for Type II HPL) cannot reduce the lipids to the desired levels, as is the case in extremely elevated LDL cholesterol concentration in familial Type IIa HPL. With use of nicotinic acid, an additional fall of 30% in plasma cholesterol has been reported.[71,74] Although nicotinic acid is effective in Type III HPL, clofibrate is the drug of choice and should be used first.

The data from the Coronary Drug Project yielded no evidence that nicotinic acid influenced the mortality of survivors of myocardial infarction, although there was evidence of a slight beneficial effect in protecting patients from recurrent myocardial infarction. The study disclosed a high incidence of cardiac arrhythmias and gastrointestinal problems among the men who were studied.

Plasma free fatty acids (FFA) are a major source of plasma VLDL synthesis in man. Nicotinic acid is a potent inhibitor of the release of FFA from adipose tissues.[75-78] As a result, plasma FFA and the elevated VLDL triglyceride concentrations decrease. Due to the limiting FFA supply, VLDL synthesis decreases. Since VLDL is the major precursor of LDL, LDL also decreases due to reduction in synthesis.[74,79] Nicotinic acid has been reported to increase the catabolism of VLDL.[80] If the pretreatment HDL cholesterol level is low, a small increase in HDL cholesterol can be achieved by nicotinic acid therapy.[65,81]

The side effects noted with nicotinic acid are intense cutaneous flushing, pruritus, nausea, vomiting, diarrhea, peptic ulceration, abnormal liver function, hyperglycemia, hyperuricemia, and cardiac arrhythmias.[71,72] Flushing and pruritus occur in most patients during the first few weeks of therapy, but the intensity decreases in the majority of patients within a few weeks.

Clofibrate

Clofibrate is very effective in lowering plasma triglyceride-rich VLDL, but has less effect in lowering cholesterol.[71,82-88] The lowering is typified by the findings of the Coronary Drug Project trial, in which clofibrate, 1.8 g/day, lowered plasma cholesterol by 6.5% and triglyceride by 22%.[72] In one study, clofibrate was found to be without effect in lowering triglycerides in an older group of senile and brain-damaged women.[89]

Clofibrate is always effective in Type III HLP and less effective in Types II and IV HLP.[71] Co-administration of clofibrate and a bile acid sequestering resin to patients with Types II and IV HLP produces additional lowering in VLDL and LDL cholesterol. It has been reported that clofibrate increased the LDL cholesterol instead of decreasing it, in some of the Type IV and Type V HLP.[90] In these patients, clofibrate may increase rather than decrease atherogenic risk.

Clofibrate inhibits cholesterol synthesis and increases fecal excretion of neutral sterols.[91] Its triglyceride-lowering effect results from a decrease in hepatic synthesis and in release of triglycerides.[92] Clofibrate may reduce VLDL by increasing the activity of lipoprotein lipase in adipose tissue, thereby increasing the clearance of VLDL.

The Coronary Drug Project provides no evidence to indicate that the total mortality or cause-specific mortality was reduced by clofibrate.[72,93] In the recent primary prevention trial carried out in Edinburgh, Budapest, and Prague by Oliver et al.,[94] in over 10,000 individuals over a period of 4 to 8 years, clofibrate lowered plasma cholesterol by 8.8% and triglyceride by 20%. Clofibrate did not influence the incidence of CHD deaths, but the incidence of major nonfatal CHD was reduced by 20%. Mortality due to all causes, including mortality due to cancer, increased 37% in the group using clofibrate.

Clofibrate has been shown to reduce the rate of nonfatal CHD, independent of serum lipid lowering.[95-97] Clofibrate did not influence the rate of progress of CHD in patients with coronary bypass, after 1 year of therapy. Although it is generally well accepted by patients, clofibrate use in the Coronary Drug Project resulted in statistically significant increased incidence of gallstones, thromboembolism, intermittent claudication, angina pectoris, and cardiac arrhythmia.

Cholestyramine

Cholestyramine resin, which is a bile acid sequestering agent, is not digested in nor absorbed from the gastrointestinal tract. Its mechanism of action is believed to be the exchange of its chloride ions for bile acids in the intestine. The bound bile acids are thus excreted in the feces. The removal of bile acids (up to three to eight times normal) increases the conversion of cholesterol to bile acids in the liver. Over 90% of cholesterol leaves the body daily in the feces, in the form of bile acids. Bile acids are required for the intestinal absorption and enterohepatic reabsorption of cholesterol. The removal of bile acids will decrease the absorption of cholesterol and other sterols; thus it will increase cholesterol excretion.[98,99]

Cholestyramine is the most efficacious LDL-cholesterol-lowering drug; the decrease can be 25 to 30% at a dose of 16 to 32 g/day.[100-103] Cholestyramine is the drug of choice for Type IIa HLP, where it is highly efficacious.[71,104] Only LDL cholesterol concentrations are reduced in Type IIb HLP by cholestyramine. It is not recommended to be used in Types III, IV, or V HLP because it may increase plasma triglyceride concentrations. Cholestyramine increases the catabolism of LDL.[105] HDL may be decreased by cholestyramine.[81]

Cholestyramine has been shown to cause regression of advanced atherosclerosis in non-human primates.[16,20] A 7-year multicenter, primary prevention trial of cholestyramine in atherosclerosis and CHD involving 4000 hypercholesterolemic males is in progress.[100]

Side effects of cholestyramine are nausea and vomiting, abdominal cramps and distension, and constipation. Constipation is very common in the elderly, so a stool softener should be used concomitantly. Cholestyramine may interfere with absorption of fat-soluble vitamins, chlorothiazide, digitalis, and warfarin anticoagulants.

Colestipol

Colestipol resin, like cholestyramine, is also a bile acid sequestering agent. Its mode of action in lowering plasma cholesterol is identical to that of cholestyramine. In a study involving 2278 hypercholesterolemic patients, colestipol, 15 g/day lowered plasma cholesterol about 20%.[106] Other studies also showed good efficacy.[107-109] Side effects of colestipol are similar to those of cholestyramine.

d-Thyroxine

d-Thyroxine has one tenth the metabolic effect of l-thyroxine. d-Thyroxine increases conversion of cholesterol to bile acids and increases excretion of sterol in the feces.[110-113] It was reported that d-thyroxine increases cholesterol synthesis in the liver, but the increased synthesis was usually less than the increased excretion. In the Coronary Drug Project trial, d-thyroxine, 6 mg/day, decreased serum cholesterol by 12% and serum triglyceride by 20%. The primary decrease was in the LDL fraction; VLDL is relatively unchanged. d-Thyroxine was discontinued in the middle of the Coronary Drug Project trial due to increased cardiovascular mortality and a high rate of nonfatal myocardial infarction.[114]

Estrogen

Large doses of ethinyl estradiol (1 mg/day), given to male patients with elevated LDL, lowered plasma cholesterol by 50% and LDL concentration by 30% while HDL concentration almost doubled.[115]

In the Coronary Drug Project trial, conjugated estrogen was used in a dose of 2.5 and 5 mg/day in 2 groups of patients. At the higher dose, the cholesterol-lowering effect was modest but serum triglyceride was elevated significantly.[114] Nonfatal myocardial infarctions, thrombophlebitis, and pulmonary embolism were significantly more frequent than in the placebo group. Patient compliance was poor because of feminizing side effects. Administration of the higher dose of conjugated estrogens was discontinued after about 18 months. At the low dose, the cholesterol-lowering effect was slight and serum triglyceride tended to increase. Excessive incidence of venous thromboembolism and mortality from all causes was observed. This study was also discontinued after 56 months.[116]

Various estrogen-progestogen oral contraceptive preparations have been studied for their effects on lipid metabolism. It was generally found that the estrogen component caused elevation of serum triglyceride concentrations;[117,118] oral contraceptives may accelerate atherogenesis in women prone to CHD.

The effects of estrogen on the HDL_2 to HDL_3 ratio have not been studied in recent years. In view of its inevitable feminizing side effects and the triglyceride elevating effects, the prospects of estrogen treatment of patients with atherosclerosis appears to be poor.[119]

Probucol

Probucol has been approved recently for marketing in the U.S. as a cholesterol-lowering agent. Probucol is primarily indicated for treatment of Type IIa and Type IIb HLP. Its main effect is lowering serum cholesterol by about 21%; it has no significant effect on serum triglyceride concentrations.[120-124] Probucol does not seem to inhibit cholesterol synthesis in the later stages, because no desmosterol or 7-dehydrocholesterol accumulation was found.[100,125,126] Probucol increases excretion of bile acids in the feces. Its side effects are nausea and vomiting, diarrhea, and abdominal pain.

REFERENCES

1. **Ross, R. and Glomset, J. A.,** The pathogenesis of atherosclerosis, *N. Engl. J. Med.,* 295, 420, 1976.
2. **Small, D. M.,** Cellular mechanisms for lipid deposition in atherosclerosis, *N. Engl. J. Med.,* 297, 893 and 924, 1977.

3. **Roberts, W. C.,** Coronary heart disease: a review of abnormalities observed in the coronary arteries, *Cardiovasc. Med.,* 2, 29, 1977.

4. **Kagan, A. R.,** Focus on atherosclerosis, *WHO (W.H.O.) Chron.,* 31, 167, 1977.

5. **Blackburn, H.,** How nutrition influences mass hyperlipidemia and atherosclerosis, *Geriatrics,* 33, 42, 1978.

6. **Bierman, E. L.,** Atherosclerosis and aging, *Fed. Proc., Fed. Am. Soc. Exp. Biol.,* 37, 2832, 1978.

7. **Bierman, E. L. and Ross, R.,** Aging and atherosclerosis, in *Atheroscleros's Reviews,* Paoletti, R. and Grotto, A. M., Jr., Eds., Raven Press, New York, 1977, 79.

8. **Roberts, J. C., Jr. and Strauss, L., Eds.,** *Comparative Atherosclerosis,* Harper & Row, New York, 1965.

9. **Eggen, D. A. and Solberg, L. A.,** Variation of atherosclerosis with age, *Lab. Invest.,* 18, 571, 1968.

10. **Goldrick, R. B., Sinnett, P. F., and Whyte, H. M.,** An assessment of coronary heart disease and coronary risk factors in a New Guinea Highland population, in *Atherosclerosis II,* Jones, R. J., Ed., Springer-Verlag, New York, 1970, 366.

11. Heart Facts, American Heart Association, New York, 1977.

12. Arteriosclerosis: A report by the National Heart and Lung Institute Task Force on arteriosclerosis, Vol. 2, Publ. No. (NIH) 72-219, U.S. Department of Health, Education, and Welfare, Washington, D.C., 1971.

13. **Enos, W. F., Holmes, R. H., and Beyer, J.,** Coronary disease among United States soldiers killed in action in Korea, *J. Am. Med. Assoc.,* 152, 1090, 1953.

14. **McNamara, J. J., Malot, M. A., Stremple, J. F., and Cutting, R. T.,** Coronary artery disease in combat casualties in Vietnam, *J. Am. Med. Assoc.,* 216, 1185, 1971.

15. **Schettler, G., Stange, E., and Wissler, R. W., Eds.,** Atherosclerosis — Is It Reversible? *Springer-Verlag,* Berlin, 1977.

16. **Wissler, R. W. and Vesselinovitch, D.,** Studies of regression in advanced atherosclerosis in experimental animals and man, *Ann. N.Y. Acad. Sci.,* 275, 363, 1976.

17. **Wissler, R. W. and Vesselinovitch, D.,** Regression of atherosclerosis in experimental animals and man, *Modern Concepts Cardiovasc. Dis.,* XLVI (6), 27, 1977.

18. **Blankenhorn, D. H.,** Reversibility of latent atherosclerosis, *Modern Concepts Cardiovasc. Dis.,* XLVII (5), 79, 1978.

19. **Blankenhorn, D. H., Brooks, S. H., Selzer, R. H., and Barndt, R., Jr.,** The rate of atherosclerosis change during treatment of hyperlipoproteinemia, *Circulation,* 57, 355, 1978.

20. **Wissler, R. W.,** Evidence for regression of advanced atherosclerotic plaques, *Artery,* 5, 398, 1979.

21. **Connor, W. E.,** The relationship of hyperlipoproteinemia to atherosclerosis: the decisive role of dietary cholesterol and fat, in *The Biochemistry of Atherosclerosis,* Scanu, A. M., Ed., Marcel Dekker, New York, 1979, chap. 16.

22. **Farcot, J-C., Hashimoto, K., Meerbaum, S., and Corday, E.,** Do risk factor interventions prevent or reverse arteriosclerosis?, *Cardiovasc. Clin.,* 8, 1, 1977.

23. **Kannel, W. B., Castelli, W. P., Gordon, T., and McNamara, P. M.,** Serum cholesterol, lipoproteins, and the risk of coronary heart disease: the Framingham study, *Ann. Intern. Med.,* 74, 1, 1971.

24. **Smellie, R. M. S., Ed.,** *Plasma Lipoproteins,* Academic Press, London, 1971.

25. **Kent, S.,** Lipoprotein metabolism and atherosclerosis, *Geriatrics,* 33, 93, 1978.

26. **Morrisett, J. D., Jackson, R. L., and Gotto, A. M., Jr.,** Lipidprotein interactions in the plasma lipoproteins, *Biochem. Biophys. Acta,* 472, 93, 1977.

27. **Smith, L. C., Pownall, H. J., and Gotto, A. M., Jr.,** The plasma lipoproteins: structure and metabolism, *Ann. Rev. Biochem.,* 47, 751, 1978.

28. **Werner, M., Tolls, R. E., Hultin, J. V., and Mellecker, J.,** Influence of sex and age on the normal range of eleven serum constituents, *Z. Klin. Chem. Klin. Biochem.,* 8, 105, 1970.

29. **Keys, A., Mickelsen, O., Miller, E. V. O., Hayes, E. R., and Todd, R. L.,** The concentration of cholesterol in the blood serum of normal men and its relation to age, *J. Clin. Invest.,* 29, 1347, 1950.

30. **Pincherle, G.,** Factors affecting the mean serum cholesterol, *J. Chronic Dis.,* 24, 289, 1971.

31. **Slack, J., Noble, N., Meade, T. W., and North, W. R. S.,** Lipid and lipoprotein concentrations in 1604 men and women in working populations in North West London, *Br. Med. J.,* 2, 353, 1977.

32. **Kornerup, V.,** Concentrations of cholesterol, total fat and phospholipid in serum of normal men, *Arch. Intern. Med.,* 85, 398, 1950.

33. **Bloch, K., Borek, E., and Rittenberg, D.,** Synthesis of cholesterol in surviving liver, *J. Biol. Chem.,* 162, 441, 1946.

34. **Benjamin, W., Gellhorn, A., Wagner, M., and Kundel, H.,** Effects of aging in lipid composition and metabolism in the adipose tissues of the rat, *Am. J. Physiol.,* 201, 540, 1961.

35. **Rifkind, B. M., Tamir, I., and Heiss, G.,** Preliminary high density lipoprotein findings. The lipid research clinic, in *High Density Lipoproteins and Atherosclerosis,* Gotto, A. M., Jr., Miller, E. R., and Oliver, M. F., Eds., Elsevier/North-Holland, Amsterdam, 1978, 109.

36. **Glueck, C. J., Gartside, P. S., Steiner, P. M.,** Hyperalpha- and hypobetalipoproteinemia in octogenarian kindreds, *Atherosclerosis,* 27, 387, 1977.

37. **Crouse, J. R., Grundy, S. M., and Ahrens, E. J., Jr.,** Cholesterol distribution in the bulk tissues of man: variation with age, *J. Clin. Invest.,* 51, 1292, 1972.

38. **Bottcher, C. J. F.,** Lipids of the lumen arterial wall, in *Drugs Affecting Lipid Metabolism,* Garattini, S. and Paoletti, R., Eds., Elsevier, Amsterdam, 1961, 54.

39. **Smith, E. B.,** The influence of age and atherosclerosis on the chemistry of aortic intima. I. The lipids, *J. Atheroscler. Res.,* 5, 224, 1965.

40. **Kritchevsky, D.,** Diet, lipid metabolism, and aging, *Fed. Proc., Fed. Am. Soc. Exp. Biol.,* 38, 2001, 1979.

41. **Carlson, L. A., Froberg, S. O., and Nye, E. R.,** Effect of age on blood and tissue lipid levels in the male rat, *Gerontologia,* 14, 65, 1968.

42. **Story, J. A., Tepper, S. A., and Kritchevsky, D.,** Age-related changes in the lipid metabolism of Fischer 344 rats, *Lipids,* 11, 623, 1976.

43. **Hruza, Z.,** Effect of endocrine factors on cholesterol turnover in young and old rats, *Exp. Gerontol.,* 6, 199, 1971.

44. **Hruza, Z. and Zbuzkova, V.,** Decrease of excretion of cholesterol during aging, *Exp. Gerontol.,* 8, 29, 1973.

45. **Yamamoto, M. and Yamamura, Y.,** Changes of cholesterol metabolism in the aging rat, *Atherosclerosis,* 13, 365, 1971.

46. **Hrachovec, J. P. and Rockstein, M.,** Age changes in lipid metabolism and their medical implications, *Gerontologia,* 3, 305, 1959.

47. **Miller, G. J. and Miller, N. E.,** Plasma-high-density-lipoprotein concentration and development of ischemic heart disease, *Lancet,* 1, 16, 1975.

48. **Gordon, T., Castelli, W. P., Hjortland, M. C., Kannel, W. B., and Dawber, T. R.,** High density lipoprotein as a protective factor against coronary heart disease, the Framingham study, *Am. J. Med.,* 62, 707, 1977.

49. **Miller, N. E., Forde, O. H., Thelle, D. S., and Mjos, O. D.,** The Tromso heart study. High-density lipoprotein and coronary heart disease: a prospective case-control study, *Lancet,* 1, 965, 1977.

50. **Castelli, W. P., Cooper, G. R., Doyle, J. T., Garcia-Palmieri, M., Gordon, T., Hames, C., Hulley, S. B., Kagan, A., Kuchmak, M., McGee, D., and Vicic, W.,** Distribution of triglyceride and total LDL and HDL cholesterol in several populations: a cooperative lipoprotein phenotyping study, *J. Chron. Dis.,* 30, 147, 1977.

51. **Castelli, W. P., Doyle, J. T., Gordon, T., Hames, C. G., Hjortland, M. C., Hulley, S. B., Kagan, A., and Zukel, W. J.,** HDL cholesterol and other lipids in coronary heart disease. The cooperative lipoprotein phenotyping study, *Circulation,* 55, 767, 1977.

52. **Kannel, W. B., Castelli, W. P., and Gordon, T.,** Cholesterol in the prediction of atherosclerosis disease, new perspectives based on the Framingham study, *Ann. Intern. Med.,* 90, 85, 1979.

53. **Castelli, W. P., Doyle, J. T., Gordon, T., Hames, C., Hulley, S. B., Kagan, A., McGee, D., Vicic, W. J., and Zukel, W. J.,** HDL cholesterol levels (HDLC) in coronary heart disease. A cooperative lipoprotein phenotyping study, *Circulation,* 52, II-97, 1975.

54. **Walker, A. R. P. and Walker, B. F.,** High high-density lipoprotein cholesterol in African children and adults in a population free of coronary heart disease, *Br. Med. J.,* 2, 1336, 1978.

55. **Jenkins, P. J., Harper, R. W., and Nestel, P. J.,** Severity of coronary atherosclerosis related to lipoprotein concentration, *Br. Med. J.,* 2, 388, 1978.

56. **Fredrickson, D. S., Gotto, A. M., Jr., and Levy, R. I.,** Familial lipoprotein deficiency (Tangier disease), in *The Metabolic Basis of Inherited Disease,* 3rd ed., Stanbury, J. S., Wyngaarten, J. B., and Fredrickson, D. S., Eds., McGraw-Hill, New York, 1972, 513.

57. **Nikkila, E. A.,** Metabolic and endocrine control of plasma high density lipoprotein, in *High Density Lipoprotein and Atherosclerosis,* Gotto, A. M., Jr., Miller, N. E., and Oliver, M. E., Eds., Elsevier/North-Holland, Amsterdam, 1978, 177.

58. High density lipoproteins, *Med. Lett.,* 21, 2, 1979.

59. **Glomset, J. A.,** Physiological role of lecithin-cholesterol acetyltransferase, *Am. J. Clin. Nutr.,* 23, 1129, 1970.

60. **Miller, G. J. and Miller, N. E.,** Do high density lipoproteins protect against coronary atherosclerosis?, in *High Density Lipoprotein and Atherosclerosis,* Gotta, A. M., Jr., Miller, N. E., and Oliver, M. F., Eds., Elsevier/North Holland, Amsterdam, 1978, 95.

61. **Carew, T. E., Hayes, S. B., Kochinsky, T., and Steinberg, D.,** A mechanism by which high density lipoproteins may slow the atherogenic process, *Lancet,* 1, 1315, 1976.

62. **Bondjers, G., and Bjorkerud, S.,** HDL dependent elimination of cholesterol from human arterial tissue, *Proc. Eur. Soc. Clin. Invest.,* 9, 51, 1975.

63. **Miller, N. E.,** The evidence for the antiatherogenicity of high density lipoprotein in man, *Lipids,* 13, 914, 1978.

64. **Miller, G. J.,** Editorial: high-density lipoprotein, low-density lipoprotein and coronary heart disease, *Thorax,* 33, 137, 1978.

65. **Gotto, A. M., Jr., Miller, N. E., and Oliver, M. F., Eds.,** *High Density Lipoprotein and Atherosclerosis,* Elsevier/North Holland, Amsterdam, 1978.

66. **Manninen, V. and Tuomilehto, J.,** Treating lipid disorders, *Am. Heart J.,* 97, 674, 1979.

67. **Levy, R. I.,** High density lipoproteins, 1978 — an overview, *Lipids,* 13, 911, 1978.

68. **Ahrens, E. H.,** The management of hyperlipidemia: whether rather than how, *Ann. Intern. Med.,* 85, 87, 1976.

69. **Steinberg, D.,** Editorial: the rediscovery of high density lipoprotein: a negative risk factor in atherosclerosis, *Eur. J. Clin. Invest.,* 8, 107, 1978.

70. **Fredrickson, D. S. and Lees, R. S.,** A system for phenotyping hyperlipoproteinemia, *Circulation,* 31, 321, 1965.

71. **Levy, R. I. and Rifkind, B. M.,** Lipid lowering drugs and hyperlipidaemia, in *Cardiovascular Drugs,* Vol. 1, Antiarrhythmic, Antihypertensive and Lipid Lowering Drugs, Avery, G. S., Ed., University Park Press, Baltimore, 1978, chap. 1.

72. Coronary Drug Project Research Group: clofibrate and niacin in coronary heart disease, *J. Am. Med. Assoc.,* 231, 360, 1975.

73. Coronary Drug Project Report on clofibrate and niacin, *Atherosclerosis,* 30, 241, 1978.

74. **Levy, R. I. and Langer, T.,** Hypolipidemic drugs and lipoprotein metabolism, *Adv. Exp. Med. Biol.,* 26, 155, 1972.

75. **Vik-Mo, H. and Mjos, O. D.,** Mechanisms for inhibition of free fatty acid mobilization by nicotinic acid and sodium salicylate in canine subcutaneous adipose tissue *in situ, Scand. J. Clin. Lab. Invest.,* 38, 209, 1978.

76. **Peterson, M. J., Hillman, C. C., and Ashmore, J.,** Nicotinic acid: studies on the mechanism of its antilipolytic activity, *Mol. Pharmacol.,* 4, 1, 1968.

77. **Carlson, L. A.,** Studies on the effect of nicotinic acid on catecholamine stimulated lipolysis in adipose tissue *in vitro, Acta Med. Scand.,* 173, 719, 1963.

78. **Kudchodkar, B. J., Sodhi, H. S., Horlick, L., and Mason, D. T.,** Mechanisms of hypolipidemic action of nicotinic acid, *Clin. Pharmacol. Ther.,* 24, 354, 1978.

79. **Fleischmajer, R.,** Pathophysiology and treatment of hyperlipidemias, in *Clinical Therapeutics,* Lowenthal, D. T. and Major, D. A., Eds., Grune & Stratton, New York, 1978, chap. 1.

80. **Carlson, L. A., Olsson, A. G., Oro, L., Rossner, S., and Walldius, G.,** Effects of hypolipodemic regimens on serum lipoprotein, in *Atherosclerosis III,* Springer-Verlag, Berlin, 1974, 768.

81. **Carlson, L. A. and Olsson, A. G.,** Effect of hypolipodemic drugs on serum lipoproteins, *Progr. Biochem. Pharmacol.,* 15, 238, 1979.

82. **Witiak, D. T., Newman, H. A. I., and Feller, D. R.,** *Clofibrate and Related Analogs — A Comprehensive Review,* Marcel Dekker, New York, 1977, 3.

83. **Hunninghake, D. B., Tucker, D. R., and Azarnoff, D. L.,** Long-term effect of clofibrate (Atromid-S) on serum lipid in man, *Circulation,* 39, 675, 1969.

84. **Best, M. M. and Duncan, C. H.,** Reduction of serum triglycerides and cholesterol by ethyl-*p*-chlorphenoxyisobutyrate (CPIB), *Am. J. Cardiol.,* 15, 230, 1965.

85. **Harrison, M. T. and Goldberg, D. M.,** The effect of Atromid in essential hyperlipemia, *J. Atheroscler. Res.,* 3, 561, 1963.

86. **Hellman, L., Zumoff, B., Kessler, G., Kara, E., Rubin, I. L., and Rosenfeld, R. S.,** Reduction of cholesterol and lipids in man by ethyl-*p*-chlorphenoxyisobutyrate, *Ann. Intern. Med.,* 59, 477, 1963.

87. **Azarnoff, D. L.,** Individualization of treatment of hyperlipoproteinemic disorders, *Med. Clin. North Am.,* 58, 1129, 1974.

88. **Brown, H. B., Lewis, L. A., and Page, I. H.,** Effects of clofibrate and a fat-modified diet on serum lipids, *Clin. Pharmacol. Ther.,* 17, 171, 1975.

89. **Kallio, V. and Sourander, L. B.,** Effect of ethyl chlorophenoxyisobutyrate on serum lipid in aged women, *Gerontol. Clin.,* 8, 349, 1966.

90. **Lees, R. S. and Wilson, D. E.,** Reciprocity of plasma low and very low density lipoprotein concentrations in lipemia, *J. Clin. Invest.,* 49, 56A, 1970.

91. **Grundy, S. M., Ahrens, E. H., Jr., Salen, G., and Quintao, E.,** Mode of action of Atromid-S® on cholesterol metabolism in man, *J. Clin. Invest.,* 48, 33a, 1969.

92. **Yeshurun, D. and Gotto, M. J., Jr.,** Drug treatment of hyperlipidemia, *Am. J. Med.,* 60, 379, 1976.

93. Editorial: clofibrate: a final verdict?, *Lancet,* 2, 1131, 1978.

94. **Oliver, M. F., Heady, J. A., Morris, J. N., and Cooper, G. R.,** A co-operative trial in the primary prevention of ischemic heart disease using clofibrate, report from the Committee of Principal Investigators, *Br. Heart J.,* 40, 1069, 1978.

95. **Krasno, L. R. and Kidera, G. J.,** Clofibrate in coronary heart disease. Effect on morbidity and mortality, *J. Am. Med. Assoc.,* 219, 845, 1972.

96. Physicians of Newcastle upon Tyne Region, Trial of clofibrate in the treatment of ischemia heart disease, *Br. Med. J.*, 4, 767, 1971.

97. Research Committee of the Scottish Society of Physicians, Ischaemic heart disease: a secondary prevention trial using clofibrate, *Br. Med. J.*, 4, 775, 1971.

98. **Tennent, D. M., Siegel, H., Zaretti, M. E., Kuron, G. W., Ott, W. H., and Wolf, F. J.,** Plasma cholesterol lowering action of bile acid binding polymers in experimental animals, *J. Lipid Res.*, 1, 467, 1960.

99. **Garbutt, J. T. and Kenney, T. S.,** Effect of cholestyramine on bile acid metabolism in normal man, *J. Clin. Invest.*, 51, 2781, 1972.

100. **Martz, B. L.,** Drug management of hypercholesterolemia, *Am. Heart J.*, 97, 389, 1979.

101. **Howard, R. P., Brusco, O. J., and Furman, R. H.,** Effect of cholestyramine administration on serum lipids and on nitrogen balance in familial hypercholesterolemia, *J. Lab. Clin. Med.*, 68, 12, 1966.

102. **Hashim, S. A. and Van Itallie, T. B.,** Cholestyramine resin therapy for hypercholesterolemia, *J. Am. Med. Assoc.*, 192, 289, 1965.

103. **Glueck, C. J., Ford, S., Jr., and Scheel, D.,** Colestipol and cholestyramine resin comparative effects in familial Type II hyperlipoproteinemia, *J. Am. Med. Assoc.*, 222, 676, 1972.

104. **Levy, R. I., Fredrickson, D. S., Schulman, R., and Bilheimer, D. W.,** Dietary and drug treatment of primary hypolipoproteinemia, *Ann. Intern. Med.*, 77, 267, 1972.

105. **Lewis, B.,***The Hyperlipidemias — Clinical and Laboratory Practice*, J. B. Lippincott, Philadelphia, 1976, 353.

106. **Dorr, A. E., Gundersen, K., Schneider, J. C., Jr., Spencer, T. W., and Martin, W. B.,** Colestipol hydrochloride in hypercholesterolemic patients — effect on serum cholesterol and mortality, *J. Chronic Dis.*, 31, 5, 1978.

107. **Cooper, E. E. and Michel, A. M.,** Colestipol hydrochloride, a new hypolipidemic drug. A two-year study, *South. Med. J.*, 68, 303, 1975.

108. **Harvengt, C. and Desager, J. P.,** Colestipol in familial Type II hyperlipoproteinemia: a three-year trial, *Clin. Pharmacol. Ther.*, 20, 310, 1976.

109. **Fellin, R., Briani, G., Balestrieri, P., Baggio, G., Baiocchi, M. R., and Crepaldi, G.,** Long-term effects of colestipol (U-26,597A) on plasma lipids in familial Type II hyperbeta-lipoproteinemia, *Atherosclerosis*, 22, 431, 1975.

110. **Owen, W. R.,** Dextrothyroxine, in *Treatment of the Hyperlipidemic State*, Casdorph, H. R., Ed., Charles C Thomas, Springfield, Ill., 1971, 297.

111. **Kritchevsky, D.,** Influence of thyroid hormone and related compounds on cholesterol biosynthesis and degradation. A review, *Metabolism*, 9, 984, 1962.

112. **Boyd, G. S. and Oliver, M. F.,** The effect of certain thyroxin analogs on the serum lipids in human subjects, *J. Endocrinol.*, 21, 33, 1960.

113. **Engelberg, H.,** Effect of sodium D-thyroxine on serum cholesterol and low-density lipoproteins in man, *Geriatrics*, 17, 711, 1962.

114. **Stamler, J.,** The Coronary Drug Project — findings with regard to estrogen, dextrothyroxine, clofibrate and niacin, in *Atherosclerosis — Metabolic, Morphologic and Clinical Aspects (Adv. Exp. Med. Biol.,)* Vol. 82, Manning, G. W. and Haust, M. D., Eds., Plenum Press, New York, 1977, 52.

115. **Russ, E. M., Eder, H. A., and Barr, D. P.,** Influence of gonadal hormone on protein-lipid relationships in human plasma, *Am. J. Med.*, 19, 4, 1955.

116. Coronary Drug Project Research Group: The Coronary Drug Project. Findings leading to discontinuation of the 2.5 mg/day estrogen group, *J. Am. Med. Assoc.*, 226, 652, 1973.

117. **Roessner, S., Larsson-Cohn, U., Carlson, L. A., and Boberg, J.,** Effect of oral contraceptive agent on plasma lipids, plasma lipoproteins, the intravenous fat tolerance and the postheparin lipoprotein lipase activity, *Acta Med. Scand.*, 190, 301, 1971.

118. **Kekki, M. and Nikkilae, E. A.,** Plasma triglyceride turnover during use of oral contraceptives, *Metab. Clin. Exp.*, 20, 878, 1971.

119. **Oliver, M. F.,** Hormones, in *Atherosclerosis*, Schettler, F. G. and Boyd, G. S., Eds., Elsevier, Amsterdam, 1969, 865.

120. **Polachek, A. A., Katz, H. M., Sack, J., Selig, J., and Littman, M. L.,** Probucol in the long-term treatment of hypercholesterolemia, *Curr. Med. Res. Opin.*, 1, 323, 1973.

121. **Barnhart, J. W., Rytter, D. J., and Molello, J. A.,** An overview of the biochemical pharmacology of probucol, *Lipids*, 12, 29, 1977.

122. **Murphy, B. F.,** Probucol (Lorelco) in treatment of hyperlipemia, *J. Am. Med. Assoc.*, 238, 2537, 1977.

123. **Heel, R. C., Brogden, R. N., Speight, T. M., and Avery, G. S.,** Probucol: a review of its pharmacological properties and therapeutic use in patients with hypercholesterolaemia, *Drugs*, 15, 409, 1978.

124. **Parsons, W. B., Jr.,** Effect of probucol in hyperlipidemic patients during two years of administration, *Am. Heart J.*, 96, 213, 1978.

125. **Barnhart, J. W., Sefranka, J. A., and McIntosh, D. D.,** Hypercholesterolemic effect of 4,4-(isopropylidenedithio)bis(2,6-di-t-butylphenol-(probucol), *Am. J. Clin. Nutr.,* 23, 1229, 1970.
126. **Davignon, J.,** Clofibrate and DH-581 in the long term treatment of primary hyperlipoproteinemia, in *Proc. 3rd Int. Symp. Atherosclerosis,* Springer-Verlag, Berlin, 1974, 794.

Drugs Acting on Different Components of the Nervous System

DRUGS FOR PSYCHIATRIC DISORDERS

Akira Horita and Richard C. Veith

INTRODUCTION

Our current understanding of the mechanism of action of psychotropic drugs is based largely on their effects on brain transmitter and modulator systems. Recent studies suggest that many of the neurochemical systems are altered in aging humans and animals. These findings, together with the known changes that take place in drug disposition in the elderly, are predictive of altered responsiveness of the aged to psychotropic drugs.

In order to fully appreciate how neurochemical changes might affect the pharmacology of psychotropic drug action we shall first briefly discuss the current status of several of the biogenic amine transmitters and how drugs act upon them. For this purpose the term "biogenic amines" will be limited to the catecholamines, norepinephrine (NE) and dopamine (DA), and the indoleamine 5-hydroxytryptamine (5HT, serotonin). However, we remind the reader that many other biogenic amines exist in the brain to function as possible neuroregulators.[1]

Norepinephrine is well known as the transmitter of the peripheral sympathetic nervous system. The biochemical pathways for its synthesis, degradation, and mechanisms of storage and release have been well defined. Much of the research on these peripheral neurons has been extended to central noradrenergic neurons, and, as expected, many common properties between the two systems have been found. Until about the mid-1950s, DA was considered mainly as a precursor of NE, but with its discovery in specific brain areas, DA has rapidly attained independent status as a neurotransmitter. The DA system appears to be crucial in the striatum and limbic systems in regulating motor function and certain behavioral activities. The psychopharmacology of the neuroleptic drugs is also based on their activity on these DA systems. Serotonin has been investigated extensively and is currently thought to play a role in the functions of sleep and sexual behavior, among others.

The drugs to be discussed in this chapter act at the level of the synapse of these monoaminergic neurons. Fluorescent histochemical methods have revealed the presence of nodules or "varicosities" arranged in chainlike fashion along the fine terminal branches of monoamine containing neurons. The varicosity, together with the postsynaptic cell, form the synaptic unit where transmission occurs and where drug action mechanisms can modify transmission.

Figure 1 illustrates diagrammatically a simplified model of a noradrenergic synapse. The varicosity is shown to contain those processes necessary for the biosynthesis, degradation, and release of the transmitter. It also depicts the regulation of NE synthesis by the end products, DA and NE, acting as inhibitors of tyrosine hydroxylase, the rate-limiting enzyme in the biosynthesis pathway. DA, synthesized from L-dopa, enters the granules to become hydroxylated to NE. Release of this newly synthesized NE occurs when nerve stimulation leads to the fusion of the granules with the cell membrane, resulting in the opening and extrusion of the transmitter into the synaptic cleft. Upon its release, NE may be involved in at least three different processes, including (1) interaction with postsynaptic receptors to initiate the postsynaptic response, (2) uptake back into the varicosity and into the granules, presumably to be reused in the transmission process, and (3) stimulation of presynaptic receptors which modulate the release of further NE into the synaptic cleft.

Upon interacting with postsynaptic receptors, NE may initiate a hyperpolarizing or de-

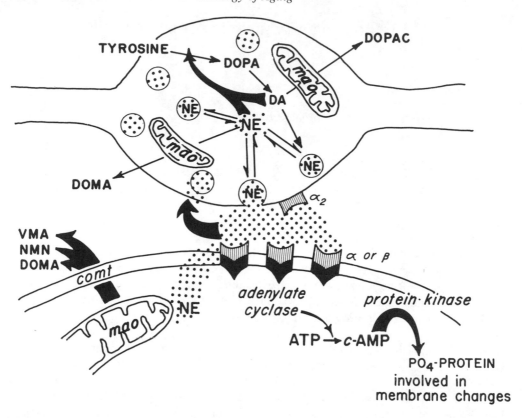

FIGURE 1.   Diagram representing the noradrenergic varicosity and its postsynaptic receptor site. Abbreviations used: ATP — aminotriphosphatase; COMT — catechol-*o*-methyltransferase; DA — dopamine; DOMA — dehydroxymandelic acid; DOPAC — dehydroxyphenylacetic acid; MAO — monoamine oxidase; NE — norepinephrine; NMN — normetanephrine; and VMA — vanillylmandelic acid.

polarizing influence on the postsynaptic cell. This event presumably involves alterations in membrane permeability to various ions, although the steps involved in the process are not entirely understood. In some instances the postsynpatic receptor is coupled to the adenylate cyclase system (as shown in Figure 1). Activation of postsynaptic receptors results in increased levels of adenosine 3',5'-cyclic monophosphate (cyclic AMP) which acts as a second messenger to activate protein kinase and protein phosphorylation. These latter events are thought to lead ultimately to the postsynaptic response. Catecholamines that enter the post-synaptic cell may also undergo degradation via deamination and/or *O*-methylation.

The reuptake of NE into the varicosity represents an active and specific process, the primary means by which the synaptic cleft is rapidly cleared of NE. The importance of the reuptake pump in terminating NE activity is illustrated by the potentiated response of tissues to neurally released or injected NE in the presence of reuptake blockers, such as cocaine or the tricyclic antidepressants.

The presynaptic receptor of the noradrenergic varicosity may be considered as a modified α-type receptor (sometimes referred to as the α_2 receptor).[2,3] Upon its stimulation by NE or certain other α-agonists, the varicosity responds with a decrease in NE release. In contrast, antagonism of the presynaptic receptors by α-antagonists, such as phentolamine or phenoxybenzamine, results in an increase in NE release. Thus, the presence of NE in the synaptic cleft can activate the presynaptic α-receptors, thereby modulating its own release. This represents another of the regulatory mechanisms for release of a transmitter from its stores. The concept of presynaptic receptors has become important in our current understanding of the mechanisms of antidepressant drug action, as we shall discuss in a later section.

The DA varicosity exhibits similar but not identical properties as the noradrenergic neurons. Upon entering the granules, DA is not converted to NE because the enzyme, dopamine β-hydroxylase, is absent. The reuptake mechanism is also different in that many of the NE uptake inhibitors are ineffective in blocking the DA pump. In brain, the major DA neurons are represented by the nigrostriatal, mesolimbic, and tuberoinfundibular pathways, although more recent studies suggest the presence of several other DA pathways.[4, 5] The neostriatum contains by far the greatest proportion of total brain DA.

Serotonin also shares many similarities with the NE system. The biosynthetic pathway, however, consists of an initial hydroxylation via tryptophan hydroxylase, followed by a decarboxylation to form the amine. As with the other monoamines, serotonin release and reuptake are specific processes. Deamination via monoamine oxidase, with the formation of 5-hydroxyindole acetic acid (5HIAA), represents its major degradation pathway.

ROLE OF BIOGENIC AMINES IN PSYCHOTROPIC DRUG ACTION

It is now clear that the mechanisms of action of neuroleptics, antidepressants, and psychomotor stimulants are associated with their influences on the monoaminergic synapse. The following descriptions, which are based partly on speculation and are intentionally oversimplified, will attempt to present the current views on the mechanism of action of the psychotropic drugs.

Antidepressant Drugs — Monoamine Oxidase Inhibitors (MAOI)

The discovery that the antidepressant property of iproniazid was related to its ability to inhibit brain MAO initiated the search for newer and more specific agents. Although many active MAOI were developed as antidepressants, they have lost their appeal because of undesirable side effects and the introduction of the tricyclic antidepressants. The mechanism by which MAOI exert their antidepressant effect is believed to be an increase of biogenic amines concentration in the synaptic cleft. By inhibiting intraneuronal MAO, these agents protect biogenic amines from being inactivated by deamination. The postsynaptic mechanisms by which antidepressant activity is initiated by MAOI are unknown, although recent evidence suggests that they may be similar to those whereby the tricyclic antidepressants produce their effects (see below). The inhibition of MAO protects not only NE, but also DA and serotonin from deamination, thus making it difficult to establish which of these amines is responsible for the clinical response.

Antidepressant Drugs — Tricyclic Antidepressants (TCA)

All of the clinically used TCA share the common property of inhibiting reuptake of NE by noradrenergic neurons. Some of them are also active as reuptake blockers of 5HT in serotonergic neurons. By blocking this mechanism, the normal removal of NE from the synaptic cleft is hindered, and the transmitter persists in the cleft to exert a more pronounced and prolonged effect on the postsynaptic receptors. Potentiated responses to NE have been demonstrated in peripheral organs in vitro and in vivo, and it is on the basis of such observation that the mechanism of antidepressant action of TCA was proposed. Later clinical investigations indicated that certain of these agents, such as desipramine, are more effective in patients with low urinary output of 3-methoxy-4-hydroxyphenylglycol (MHPG), a NE metabolite largely of CNS origin, whereas other agents, such as amitriptyline, are more effective in depressed patients excreting normal or high MHPG levels.[6-10] A reassessment of the TCA led to the discovery that amitriptyline possessed greater serotonin than NE reuptake blocking activity. These findings have led some investigators to postulate the existence of at least two subtypes of depressions, one associated with low MHPG output and responsive to TCA predominantly blocking NE reuptake, and the other associated with normal MHPG output but with low cerebrospinal fluid 5HIAA and responsive to agents that inhibit serotonin reuptake. This also implied that abnormalities in both the NE and serotonin systems might be factors in depression.

Regardless of the transmitter(s) involved in depression, there exists a serious inconsistency between the onset of blockade of amine reuptake and the onset of clinical efficacy of TCA in depressed patients. The former effect is demonstrable within minutes to hours after drug administration (depending upon the nature of the experiment), whereas the clinical response generally appears only after several days or weeks of treatment. This delay may be attributed partially to the time required to achieve optimal steady-state plasma levels of these drugs. However, this and other discrepancies as well as results from studies based on animals chronically treated with these drugs have forced investigators to seek other explanations of mechanisms of antidepression. Such studies are only recently beginning to provide newer answers as to possible mechanisms of action for TCA agents.

One school of thought[11-14] postulates that the TCA and MAOI produce an increase in synaptic NE, and the prolonged presence of higher concentrations of NE after chronic drug administration results in a desensitization (or down regulation) of noradrenergic postsynaptic receptors. This desensitization apparently results from a decreased number of receptors (as demonstrated by a decreased B_{max} in receptor binding assays) and/or from diminished NE-sensitive adenylate cyclase in brain tissue. These changes occurred only after chronic treatment of animals with the antidepressants and thus correlate better with the onset of the clinical effects of antidepressant drugs. If these data are to have meaning, the total concept of depression and its treatment by enhancing monoamine transmission processes requires reappraisal. These studies imply that the antidepressants are effective because they reduce the density of postsynaptic noradrenergic receptors and thereby inhibit noradrenergic transmission. It then follows that depression must be the result of a hypersensitivity or hyperactivity of central noradrenergic systems. The clinical findings that both mania and depression are characterized by a chronic state of hyperarousal lends support to such an hypothesis.[15,16] Thus, although the presynaptic reuptake blockade of NE still serves as the initial event associated with the antidepressant drugs, the eventual clinical response is now linked with changes that take place at the post-synaptic receptors.

A second view of the mechanisms of antidepressant action of TCA is based on the concept of altered presynaptic α-receptors which occurs with chronic, but not acute, drug treatment. As described above, the terminals of NE neurons possess presynaptic α-receptors which, when stimulated, reduce NE release from its varicosity. Crews and Smith demonstrated that electrically stimulated atrial strips taken from rats pretreated with desipramine for 3 weeks exhibited much greater release of ^{3}H-NE than preparations receiving the drug for only 1 day.[17] Blockade of presynaptic α-receptors with low concentrations of phenoxybenzamine produced further increases in ^{3}H-NE release in strips taken from animals receiving desipramine for 1 day, but not from animals pretreated for 3 weeks. These and other results led the authors to speculate that chronic desipramine treatment results in a gradual desensitization of the presynaptic α-receptors which leads to an enhanced release of NE into the synaptic cleft. They also postulated that a similar mechanism might mediate the antidepressant action of TCA in man where only after chronic administration are the drugs effective. Their hypothesis is supported in part by the work of Svensson and Usdin,[18] who reported that chronic treatment with TCA resulted in a reduced responsiveness of the presynaptic α-receptors in the locus coeruleus of rat brain.

Neuroleptic Drugs — Reserpine

This alkaloid of the Rauwolfia plant was one of the first active neuroleptics known. It is no longer employed as such, but an understanding of its mechanism of action has contributed much toward the amine hypothesis of mental disorders. Reserpine was found to deplete both the peripheral and central NE stores and the central stores of DA and 5HT. This depleting action occurs at the level of the granules of the monoaminergic neuron varicosity. By some as yet unknown mechanisms, reserpine irreversibly inhibits the granular uptake and storage system, thus preventing the maintenance of a normal level of amine for release. When sufficient doses of reserpine are administered, intraneuronal monoamine levels are reduced or depleted. The intensity of its pharmacological effect is related to the reduced functioning of these monoaminergic neurons. Since reserpine affects both catecholamines and serotonin, it was not clear at first which of these putative transmitters was involved in the antipsychotic activity. Now it appears that the decrease in catecholamines, in particular DA, is responsible for the neuroleptic property of reserpine.

Neuroleptic Drugs — Phenothiazines and Butyrophenones

Chlorpromazine was the first of the phenothiazines to be recognized as a truly neuroleptic agent. Since its discovery, a great many related compounds have been synthesized and about a dozen of these are available as useful phenothiazine neuroleptics. The butyrophenones, of which haloperidol is currently the only commercially available compound in the U.S., represent a departure from the phenothiazine molecule. However, both the phenothiazines and butyrophenones have in common the property of blocking DA receptors in the central nervous system. It is this property that appears to be responsible for the antipsychotic effect;[19-21] in fact, the newly developed receptor binding assays indicate a direct correlation between DA receptor binding affinities and the dosages of neuroleptics necessary to exert antipsychotic activity.[22-24]

Although some half-dozen DA neuronal systems have been described,[4-5] the two major pathways relevant to neuroleptic drugs are the nigrostriatal and mesolimbic pathways. The former is important in the normal control of motor systems; disorders therein result in disturbed motor functions such as are found in Parkinson's and Huntington's diseases. The extrapyramidal symptoms (EPS) frequently produced by the neuroleptic drugs are associated with the ability of these drugs to block DA receptors in the neostriatum. The mesolimbic system is normally associated with the regulation of emotional and behavioral functions. The neuroleptic-induced blockade of DA receptors in the limbic system is thought to be responsible for the antipsychotic activity of these agents. This implies then, that schizophrenia is characterized by excessive DA activity in the limbic system. The evidence to date suggests no increase in DA turnover in schizophrenia. However, some recent evidence that brains of schizophrenic patients may possess greater numbers of DA receptors supports the hypothesis of DA involvement in this disease. These are no doubt overly simplistic views on the genesis of schizophrenia, but they are of heuristic value toward our understanding of the disease and its pharmacotherapy.

If DA receptor blockade is the mechanism of the neuroleptic and EPS, one would expect a greater frequency of EPS with the more potent agents. This assumption has been confirmed; potent drugs, such as fluphenazine and haloperidol tend to produce greater frequencies of EPS than do the less active compounds. In addition, the incidence of EPS associated with the use of these agents seems to be inversely related to their potency in competing against potent muscarinic antagonists for muscarinic cholinergic receptors.[74]

There is currently a growing concern over another series of side effects associated with prolonged neuroleptic therapy. These effects, called "tardive dyskinesias", appear mainly during or after withdrawal from prolonged therapy. In contrast to the EPS which are related to blockade of neostriatal DA receptors, tardive dyskinesias are associated with a supersensitivity of DA receptors resulting from their prolonged blockade. Animal investigations have revealed that the number, but not binding affinities, of receptors in the striatum increases after chronic neuroleptic treatment, and that this appears to mediate an exaggerated response to a standard dose of DA agonist. Also, in contrast to EPS, anticholinergic drugs are ineffective in alleviating the symptoms of tardive dyskinesia. In fact, they may worsen the condition. Instead, drugs that increase cholinergic function, such as physostigmine or choline, are said to be helpful in reducing dyskinetic responses. Other agents, such as reserpine or tetrabenzine, which reduce DA function, are also employed to reduce this drug-induced disorder.

NEUROTRANSMITTERS AND DRUG EFFECTS IN THE AGING BRAIN

The preceding review of the monoaminergic systems and the effects of psychotropic drugs thereon was based on the mature nervous system. One may expect quantitative or qualitative differences in drug efficacy depending upon the nature and severity of neurochemical changes that occur during the aging process. In the following section we shall discuss some of the age-related neurochemical changes that might influence the activity of those drugs covered in this chapter. More inclusive reviews of other transmitter changes with aging may be found in other references.[25-27]

One of the most striking neurochemical changes that occurs in the aging brain is the progressive decrease in the enzymes, tyrosine hydroxylase,[28] and aromatic amino acid decarboxylase (DOPA decarboxylase),[26] which are essential in the biosynthesis of DA and NE. The rate of decline of these enzymes is much steeper than the fall in gamma-aminobutyric acid and acetylcholine biosynthesizing enzymes. As a result, the enzyme profiles of the elderly may progressively resemble those of the Parkinsonian patient. Interestingly, the aged in many instances do exhibit some of the signs and symptoms of Parkinsonism, and reference has been made to the possibility that similar mechanisms may play a role in the induction of Parkinsonism and in the process of aging.[29] Indeed, Barbeau has postulated that Parkinson's disease may represent "an accelerated aging phenomenon resulting from the selected atrophy of the heavily pigmented cells in the brainstem, from whence originate dopaminergic and noradrenergic pathways."[30]

Other investigators have also noted changes in brain levels of catecholamines or their associated enzymes in the elderly. Robinson and co-workers reported on the progressive increase in monoamine oxidase (MAO) activity in human hindbrain, platelets, and plasma.[31-33] Associated with this enzyme change in the elderly was a corresponding decrease in NE and increased 5HIAA levels. From these data the authors suggested that the age-related increase in brain MAO could represent a compensatory mechanism to increase amine turnover in order to make available newly synthesized monoamine for synaptic transmission. The possibility that such changes in enzyme activity might be predisposing factors to the development of depression in the aged was also considered. Gottfries et al.[34] and Adolfsson[35] confirmed the increased MAO activity and decreased DA and NE levels in brains of the elderly, but they also noted that the amine levels were even lower in several brain regions of Alzheimer's patients.

Considerable evidence from animal experiments indicates that biogenic amine systems and the effect of drugs acting on them are altered during aging. Prior to their findings in man, McGeer et al.[36] reported on the decrease of tyrosine hydroxylase activity in the striatum of aged rats. A decrease in activity of this enzyme may be the basis for the decreased DA levels and turnover reported by Finch.[37] Changes in brain NE levels, however, appear to exhibit a species dependency although in most animals a fall in hypothalamic NE was observed.[38-41] Joseph et al.[42] demonstrated that aging rats responded poorly to amphetamine on a motor test. Upon analyzing striatal DA levels, they found a significant decrease of this amine in the older animals. They also found that the number of DA receptors, as measured by the receptor binding assay, was decreased in older animals, whereas the binding affinities, represented by the K_d, were unchanged. Interestingly, although receptor concentrations were changed, the animal's response to a direct acting agonist, apomorphine, was unchanged. In contrast, Govoni et al.[43] also observed a 40% reduction of ^{3}H-haloperidol binding to striatal membranes from brains of older rats, but their Scatchard plots indicated that this reduction was the consequence of a decreased affinity rather than a decrease in the number of receptors. In addition, Saunders et al.[44] found that amphetamine exerted greater locomotor activity in older (9 month) than in younger (2.5 month) rats. They also found that the intensity of chlorpromazine-induced hypothermia and morphine-induced vocalization were both greater in the older group of rats. The brain levels of chlorpromazine at 2.5 hr in both groups of animals were not significantly different, indicating that older animals were more sensitive to the drug effects. However, it must be noted that these authors employed 9-month-old rats as their ''old'' rats, whereas most other aging studies employ 24 to 29-month-old animals as the senescent model.

It is apparent that some inconsistencies exist between changes in receptors and drug-induced responses in the aging animal. However, the recent neurochemical studies of Weiss et al.[45] clearly demonstrated the loss of receptor regulating capacity in the aging brain. Aged animals exhibited a reduced density of β-receptors but no change in binding affinity for ^{3}H-dihydroalprenolol. Moreover, in older animals, the ability to develop β-receptor subsensitivity with chronic desipramine administration was still present but their ability to increase receptor density after chronic reserpine treatment was severely diminished in several brain regions. The authors suggested that this decline in adaptive capacity, that is, the inability to increase receptor density in the face of reduced adrenergic input, may explain the reduced physiological responsiveness of aged tissue to adrenergic stimuli. Makman et al.[46] also observed decreased monoamine receptor densities in selected areas of aging rabbit brain. Furthermore, in the striatum they found that the decreased numbers of receptors corresponded to a decline in activation of DA-sensitive adenylate cyclase. This is consistent with the data of Puri and Volicer.[47] In contrast to earlier findings in mice and rats by other workers,[37,42] it is reported by Makman et al.[46] that rabbit striata did not exhibit an age-related decrease in DA levels, indicating that no loss of the presynaptic component of the DA system occurred in this species. Although the mechanisms of the selective decline of striatal DA receptors is unknown, the authors suggested that such losses with aging might contribute to the functional deterioration in Parkinson's disease and to the increased incidence of extrapyramidal effects of the neuroleptics in the elderly.

The selective loss of DA neuron function in aging was also evident from the data of Jonec and Finch,[48] who found that DA, but not NE, uptake was reduced in synaptosomes from aged mouse brain. The decreased DA uptake was characterized by an increase in K_m with no change in V_{max}. From these and other observations, Finch suggested that the catecholamine neurons which regulate hormone secretions might act as pacemakers of aging for cells elsewhere in the body.[49]

Of the biogenic amines discussed in this chapter, serotonin has been least studied in aged animals or man. Meek et al.[50] compared the age-related changes in acetylcholine and serotonin content and synthesis in different brain nuclei. They observed that while serotonin levels and tryptophan hydroxylase activities were reduced in all brain areas investigated, acetylcholine contents were unchanged, and choline acetyltransferase (CAT) activity decreased only in the caudate nucleus. These results suggest a general degeneration of serotonergic neurons in aging, with much less degeneration in the cholinergic system. In human brains, Shih and Young found changes in both affinity and density of serotonin receptors.[51] Membranes from cerebral cortex of aged humans displayed an increased number of binding sites but a markedly lowered affinity.

CLINICAL USE OF PSYCHOTROPIC DRUGS IN THE AGED

It is now recognized that psychoactive agents are among the most commonly prescribed drugs for the elderly.[52,53] Both the use of psychoactive drugs[52,53,55,57,58] and the incidence of adverse effects[59-64] appear to increase with age. Although reviews of psychoactive drug use in the elderly have appeared recently,[65-70] our knowledge of the pharmacokinetics related to these drugs in the aged is limited. Systematic investigation of pharmacokinetic changes in the elderly, utilizing recent technological advances that permit measurement of plasma levels of many psychoactive agents, has proceeded only to a limited extent. Moreover, existing reports of clinical trials of the psychoactive medications are complicated by inadequacies of experimental design, confusion in the psychiatric diagnostic nomenclature, and heterogeneity of research populations. With these limitations in mind, we will attempt to provide some guidelines for the clinical use of three classes of CNS drugs in the elderly: antipsychotic drugs, antidepressant drugs, and the psychostimulants.

Antipsychotic Drugs — Clinical Use

The antipsychotic drugs are used to treat a multiplicity of conditions in the aged. Unfortunately, this situation, reflected in diagnostically heterogeneous patient populations, complicates the interpretation of the clinical studies of these drugs. A majority of the studies on the use of these agents have been uncontrolled and represent variably designed trials of drugs for the treatment of the whole spectrum of geriatric psychopathology. Chronic elderly schizophrenics, agitated, depressed patients, and patients with behavioral disturbances stemming from acute or chronic organic brain syndromes all receive these drugs and mixed populations have been included in even some of the otherwise well-controlled double-blind studies. It is not surprising that these studies have yielded conflicting results from which it is difficult to draw definitive conclusions.

Clinical investigations of the antipsychotic agents have primarily focused on treatment of elderly chronic schizophrenics and management of the behavioral problems associated with cognitively impaired elderly. Thioridazine[122-146] has been the most popular antipsychotic in clinical use, due to its sedative properties and reduced incidence of extrapyramidal adverse effects. Other antipsychotics studied have been chlorpromazine,[141,146-153,157,285] mesordazine,[154,155] acetophenazine,[156-159] fluphenazine,[73] trifluoperazine,[160-163] triflupromazine,[164] haloperidol,[142,143,146,165-169] thiothixene,[172-174] chlorprothixene,[229] perphenazine,[170,171] piperacetazine,[144] and loxapine.[175] There is no convincing evidence that the antipsychotics differ in terms of efficacy when used in comparable doses. These agents are clearly effective in the treatment of decompensated elderly chronic schizophrenics, and they provide symptomatic relief for some elderly patients who exhibit agitated and confused behavior associated with the organic brain syndromes. The late onset schizophreniform paranoid illness in the elderly, paraphrenia,[71] has been effectively treated with the antipsychotics.[72,73] It is also clear that the antipsychotic drugs do not exert any specific therapeutic effect on memory impairment or intellectual deterioration in patients with Alzheimer's disease, multi-infarct dementia, or other irreversible organic brain syndromes. The results of the double-blind, placebo-controlled or comparative studies of the antipsychotics in the elderly are summarized in Table 1.

Antipsychotic Drugs — Adverse Effects

Although there appears to be no difference in the efficacy of these drugs, there are clinically relevant differences in adverse effects in relation to patient age. The most significant adverse effects that would be more serious for the elderly include sedative, anticholinergic, extrapyramidal, and cardiovascular effects. Oral administration of the aliphatic and piperidine phenothiazines, particularly chlorpromazine and thioridazine, are more sedating than the other antipsychotics. However, even small doses by the parenteral route the more potent piperazine phenothiazines, thioxanthenes, and butyrophenones can produce marked sedative effects in the geriatric population. The sedative effect can be an asset when treating sleep disturbances in agitated patients, but it can also promote increasing confusion, disorientation, and agitation in the cognitively impaired elderly by further clouding consciousness. The propensity of these agents to reduce sedation is related to differences in their potency for blocking α-noradrenergic receptors.[120,121]

The peripheral and central anticholinergic properties of the antipsychotics create multiple problems in the aged. The less potent aliphatic and piperidine phenothiazines possess rel-

Table 1
DOUBLE-BLIND TRIALS OF ANTIPSYCHOTIC AGENTS IN THE ELDERLY

Drugs	Daily dose (mg)	Duration	N	Diagnoses	Results	Ref.
Thioridazine Haloperidol	50—500 1—4	12 weeks	50	Mixed[a]	Equally effective	143
Thioridazine Chlorpromazine	30—120 30—120	12 weeks	132	Schizophrenia OBS	Equally effective	141
Thioridazine Haloperidol	50—107.7 1—2.17	6 weeks	46	OBS, senile psychosis	Equally improved behavior Haloperidol superior in improving social interactions	142
Thioridazine Piperacetazine	30—45 15—90	30 days	50	OBS[b]	Equally effective Fewer adverse effects with piperacetazine	144
Chlorpromazine Placebo	70—225	8 weeks	48	Mixed	Chlorpromazine superior	150
Chlorpromazine Placebo	50—300	3 weeks	50	Mixed	Slight deterioration when placebo substituted	149
Acetophenazine Placebo	20—60	3—8 weeks	27	Mixed	Acetophenazine superior	156
Acetophenazine Chlorpromazine Placebo	20—120 25—150	8 weeks	45	Schizophrenia	Acetophenazine superior Chlorpromazine = placebo	157
Acetophenazine Trifluoperazine Imipramine Placebo	20—126 2—12 25—150	27 weeks	308	Schizophrenia	Acetophenazine and trifluoperaine equally effective and superior to imipramine and placebo	158
Trifluoperazine Placebo	4—8	8 weeks	27	OBS with psychosis	No significant difference	161
Thiothixene Placebo	6—15	4 weeks	42	OBS	No significant difference	173
Haloperidol Placebo	0.5—3	6 weeks	18	OBS	Haloperidol superior	165
Perphenazine Placebo	≤30	6 weeks	25	Paranoid delusions	Perphenazine superior	170

[a]   May include organic brain syndrome, schizophrenia, affective disease, alcoholism, medical illness.
[b]   OBS = organic brain syndrome.

atively greater anticholinergic properties than do the other antipsychotics.[74,75] Dry mouth, constipation, visual disturbances, urinary retention, and the possibility of precipitating glaucoma in susceptible individuals markedly reduce drug compliance. This complicates the clinician's attempt to achieve therapeutic doses of drugs in the patient. Not infrequently an agitated elderly patient receiving antipsychotic medication will become progressively more agitated, prompting the clinician to increase the dose of the antipsychotic only to find that the patient's condition becomes aggravated as the "atropine-psychosis" of central anticholinergic toxic delirium develops. Elderly patients appear to be particularly sensitive to the central anticholinergic effects of these drugs.[4,76-79]

The tendency for the antipsychotics to produce EPS has been largely responsible for the popularity of thioridazine use in geriatric patients. The propensity of various agents to produce EPS has been attributed to the degree of their inherent anticholinergic activity which offsets the imbalance imposed upon the extrapyramidal centers by the dopamine blocking action of these agents.[74,75] As an antipsychotic with great anticholinergic activity,[74,75] thioridazine rarely produces EPS. The piperazine phenothiazines and butyrophenones, which are relatively weak anticholinergic drugs but potent DA blockers, frequently produce Parkinsonism, akathisia, rigidity, tremor, and occasionally acute dystonias.[63,80,81] The common practice of using an anticholinergic medication in combination with these drugs to prevent or to treat EPS puts the elderly patient at risk of the anticholinergic toxicities noted above. The development of tardive dyskinesias is of particular concern for the elderly. Numerous reports suggest that age, age at onset of antipsychotic treatment, or age and the use of high doses of antipsychotic drugs are contributing etiological factors.[82-86] Surveys report a prevalence of tardive dyskinesia in 40 to 50% of patients under 70 years of age receiving these drugs, and as high as 75% in patients older than 70 years.[83]

The adverse cardiovascular effects of the antipsychotic drugs of particular concern in the elderly are postural hypotension, electrocardiographic changes, and arrhythmias. Postural hypotension and dizziness are most commonly associated with the use of chlorpromazine and thioridazine. These effects are presumably the result of phenothiazine-induced peripheral α-noradrenergic antagonism.[120,121] The more potent antipsychotics, particularly haloperidol, seem to be much less active in this regard.[121,167] Supraventricular and ventricular arrhythmias, conduction defects, and repolarization abnormalities have been associated with phenothiazine use.[87-91,117] Thioridazine is thought to be the most cardiotoxic drug of the antipsychotics.[87,89,117] Thioridazine also commonly produces electrocardiographic T-wave change which are thought to be reversible and benign in young patients. However, the severity of the T-wave changes appears to be related to chronological age.[88,92] The phenothiazines may produce a negative inotropic effect on the myocardium and papillary muscle. This can complicate the treatment of elderly patients with congestive heart failure or impaired left ventricular function.[93] The presence of concurrent heart disease or other illness, or use of other drugs affecting the cardiovascular system, all common occurrences in the elderly, place geriatric patients at increased risk of the adverse cardiovascular effects of antipsychotic drugs. Haloperidol appears to be the least toxic antipsychotic drug on the cardiovascular system.[167]

In summarizing the clinical use of antipsychotic agents in the elderly, these drugs appear to be therapeutically efficacious in treating the elderly chronic schizophrenic patient, the paranoid illnesses of late life, and to some degree the behavioral abnormalities associated with cognitive impairment in the elderly. Since these drugs possess no inherent differences in therapeutic efficacy, the selection of a particular agent should be determined on the basis of the potential adverse effects they may produce. If sedation is specifically indicated, chlorpromazine or thioridazine appear to be the drugs of choice. Otherwise, selecting one of the more potent antipsychotics and using low doses for the shortest duration possible would appear to be in the best interest of the elderly patient. Particularly in the elderly, the selection of an antipsychotic agent and the course of the treatment must be individualized, taking into consideration concomitant diseases, specific adverse effects of the antipsychotic agents, and potential for interaction with other drugs the patient may be using. As noted in Table 2, the "safe" range of the antipsychotics is significantly reduced in the elderly.

Antidepressant Drugs — Clinical Use

Although depression is common in the elderly, it is not frequently recognized as a clinical entity and remains undertreated.[94] Several obstacles may account for these difficulties.[95,96] Elderly patients infrequently present to the clinician with "depression" as a primary complaint. More commonly, depressed patients present complaining of multiple, vague somatic symptoms or pain, thereby often appearing hypochondriacal. Not infrequently the depressed elderly patient will deny or not experience a dysphoric mood when all other clinical findings suggest a significant depressive illness. In addition, the presence of serious medical disease and/or the use of various drugs, both more common in the aged, can produce depressive symptoms, thus confusing the clinical picture. If the clinician views depression as a normal consequence of aging, his/her ability to recognize a treatable, reversible illness is limited.

Table 2
COMMONLY PRESCRIBED ANTIPSYCHOTICS

Antipsychotic class Generic drug name	Trade name	Usual dose range (mg/day)		Sedation	Anticholinergic properties	Extrapyramidal symptoms
		Young adult	Elderly			
Phenothiazines						
Aliphatic						
Chlorpromazine	Thorazine®	50—800	10—100	+ + +	+ +	+
Piperidine						
Thioridazine	Mellaril®	50—800	10—100	+ + +	+ + +	+
Piperazine						
Perphenazine	Trilafon®	5—40	2—16	+	+	+ + +
Trifluoperazine	Stelazine®	8—64	2—15	+	+	+ + +
Fluphenazine	Prolixin®	2.5—20	1—10	+	+	+ + +
Butyrophenones						
Haloperidol	Haldol®	5—100	1—10	+ +	+	+ + +
Thioxanthines						
Thiothixene	Navane®	5—60	2—10	+	+	+ + +

Note: Degree of intensity: + = low; + + = moderate; and + + + = high.

Perhaps reflecting these difficulties are the reports of few clinical studies of antidepressant agents in the elderly.[64,176-198] Although the MAO inhibitors have been used to treat geriatric patients, adverse effects and dietary restrictions limit their use. The TCA receive wide clinical use and are the drugs of choice for the treatment of depression in the elderly. TCA have also been used to treat the emotional lability and pseudo-bulbar palsy secondary to organic brain damage, and to treat the incontinent and organically impaired elderly patient.[179,180] The double-blind, comparative or placebo-controlled trials of the antidepressant agents are presented in Table 3.

Although it has generally been accepted that TCA are equally efficacious in all patients, preliminary data suggesting the presence of subgroups of depressives, identified by pretreatment levels of MHPG and/or 5HIAA, may lead to a reappraisal of this assumption.[97] Presumably, patients could be preferentially treated by selecting a TCA according to its relative potency in blocking 5HT or NE reuptake. Although these findings await further validation, our growing knowledge of the relationship between plasma tricyclic antidepressant levels and therapeutic effect may be particularly relevant in the selection of a tricyclic antidepressant for the elderly. Nies et al.[184] have shown that older patients develop higher steady-state plasma levels of imipramine, desipramine, and amitriptyline. Plasma levels were correlated with age, and the disappearance half-lives of imipramine and desipramine were significantly longer in older patients than in younger. Although the literature on plasma TCA levels is still evolving and is controversial, there is growing evidence that the relationship between therapeutic effect and plasma levels for the tertiary amine TCA may be linear while that for the secondary amine TCA may be curvilinear.[98,99] These results are preliminary and need further support. If, however, high plasma levels of the secondary amine tricyclic antidepressants are associated with diminished efficacy, and since the pharmacokinetic changes associated with aging tend to produce higher steady-state plasma levels, then using a secondary amine tricyclic for an elderly patient may be more complicated than using a tertiary amine. Except for the report by Friedel and Raskind,[191] who found that depressed elderly

Table 3
DOUBLE BLIND TRIALS OF ANTIDEPRESSANT AGENTS IN THE ELDERLY

Drugs	Daily dose (mg)	Duration	N	Diagnosis	Results	Ref.
Nortriptyline Placebo	75	28 weeks	65	Anxiety, depression, chronic medical illness	Nortriptyline superior	188
Nortriptyline Placebo	25—100	12 weeks	92	Mixed[a]	Nortriptyline superior	187
Nortriptyline Desipramine	50—75 50—75	3 weeks	30	Depression	Equally effective	186
Trimipramine Placebo	50—100	6 weeks	12	Depression	Trimipramine superior	189
Doxepin Placebo	25—150	6—12 weeks	33	Memory impairment	No significant difference	192
Amitriptyline Imipramine	100—200	28 weeks	137	Depression	Amitriptyline superior in patients $\geq$ 50 years of age	183
Amitriptyline/ Chlordiazepoxide Amitriptyline	75/30—225/90 75—225	3 weeks	100	Depression	Combination superior	193
Amitriptyline/ Perphenazine Placebo	75/6—150/12	3 weeks	120	Depression	Combination superior	194
Amitriptyline/ Perphenazine Chlordiazepoxide	10/2—40/8 10—40	9 weeks	63	Anxiety, depression	Combination superior in depression, fewer adverse effects	195

[a] May include organic brain syndrome, schizophrenia, affective disease, alcoholism, and medical illness.

patients treated with doxepin to achieve plasma levels above 100 ng/mℓ responded better than those on doxepin with lower plasma levels, the relationship between efficacy and the plasma TCA levels has not been the subject of systematic studies exclusively in elderly patients.

The effectiveness of TCA alone in treating psychotic or delusional depression in younger patients is controversial.[100,101] Some authors suggest concomitant use of antipsychotic agents in these patients.[102] Combinations of TCA, MAOI, antipsychotics, and anxiolytic agents have also been investigated in elderly patients.[192-196] In two studies,[193,194] one comparing amitriptyline in combination with chlordiazepoxide vs. amitriptyline alone, the other comparing a combination of amitriptyline and perphenazine vs. placebo, Haider found the combinations to be more effective than one drug or placebo in the treatment of depression. Beber found a combination of amitriptyline and perphenazine more effective for depression than chlordiazepoxide alone in a crossover study of depressed and anxious older patients.[195]

The use of MAO inhibitors in treatment of depression in the elderly has received limited attention.[196-198] To the best of our knowledge, no controlled, double-blind trials of MAOI in the elderly have been reported. Renewed interest in the use of the MAOI has recently surfaced, particularly in treating atypical affective disorders.[103] Furthermore, there are reports that the hazards associated with MAOI use have been rather over-emphasized.[103-104] Recently, Robinson reported on an ongoing study of phenelzine which includes elderly subjects.[105]

Antidepressant Drugs — Adverse Effects

With the exception of EPS, the TCA produce adverse effects similar to those of the antipsychotics. Although the individual TCA have relatively different sedative and anticholinergic properties[75,107] (see Table 4), these properties markedly complicate TCA use in the elderly. Clinical evidence suggests that older patients are particularly sensitive to these adverse effects. Davies et al.[64] noted that the incidence of confusion in patients over 40 years of age was significantly higher then in patients under 40 years of age in a trial of imipramine and amitriptyline. Although confusion was thought by the investigators to be an idiosyncratic response, it is more likely that this symptom was related to higher steady-state plasma levels of the drugs and subsequent increased anticholinergic load.

The TCA can produce significant effects on the cardiovascular system. These include postural hypotension (possibly mediated through effects on central α-noradrenergic receptors),[108] sympathomimetic effects, anticholinergic effects, and quinidine-like effects. In a prospective and retrospective view of their patients treated with imipramine, Glassman et al.[109] found that orthostatic hypotension during treatment was best predicted by pretreatment orthostatic hypotension and was independent of age or plasma TCA concentration. Shader[185] noted cardiac changes in 4 of 9 patients over age 65 treated with imipramine. Cardiac effects included development of sinus tachycardia in two patients, nonspecific ST-T changes in one patient and development of left axis deviation and complete right bundle branch block in one patient. These effects are consistent with the TCA-induced electrocardiographic changes found in younger patients treated with TCA.[110] Although the cardiovascular effects of these drugs have not been systemically studied in the elderly, there is evidence supported by clinical lore, suggesting that doxepin causes fewer cardiovascular effects than the other TCA.[111,112,192] These empirical observations have yet to be confirmed in studies adequately controlled for plasma TCA concentration. The TCA routinely increase heart rate or produce tachycardia secondary to their anticholinergic effects.[110] In therapeutic doses, producing what are considered therapeutic plasma concentrations, the TCA appear to exert an antiarrhythmic effect as demonstrated by Bigger et al.[118] in two elderly patients. As plasma TCA concentrations approach toxic levels, progressive impairment of conduction through the His-Purkinje system and ventricle may occur.[112,119] In addition, animal data suggest that a direct myocardial depressant effect is exerted by the TCA in high concentration.[199,200] Since elderly patients have a higher incidence of cardiac disease, it is assumed that they are at higher risk for cardiac adverse effects of these drugs.

Table 4
COMMONLY PRESCRIBED TRICYCLIC ANTIDEPRESSANTS

Tricyclic antidepressant	Usual dose range (mg/day)		Sedative property	Anticholinergic property
	Young adult	Elderly		
Tertiary amines				
Amitriptyline (Elavil®)	100—300	25—150	+ + +	+ + + +
Imipramine (Tofranil®)	100—300	25—150	+ +	+ + +
Doxepin (Sinequan®)	100—300	25—150	+ + +	+ + + +
Secondary amines				
Nortriptyline (Pamelor®)	50—100	10—50	+	+ + +
Desipramine (Norpramin®)	100—300	25—150	0	+ +
Protriptyline (Vivactil®)	20—60	5—30	0	+ + +

Note: Degree of intensity: 0 = none; + = low; + + = moderate; + + + = high; and + + + + = very high.

The adverse effects associated with the MAOI have markedly limited their clinical usefulness in the elderly. Although the MAOI lack the anticholinergic properties which complicate TCA use, their tendency to produce postural hypotension in the elderly is a significant problem. They can also produce a clinical picture of CNS toxicity, which includes agitation, insomnia, and toxic psychosis. The most serious toxic effects of the MAOI stem from their ability to produce hypertensive crises associated with hyperpyrexia, intracranial bleeding, cardiovascular collapse, or seizures, if these drugs are used in conjunction with sympathomimetic drugs or tyramine-containing foods.

It is difficult to draw definitive conclusions on the appropriate use of the antidepressant agents in the elderly because of limited data. The TCA are effective in the treatment of depression and are the drugs of choice in the elderly. As noted with the antipsychotic agents, age-related pharmacokinetic changes require that these drugs be used in lower doses than in younger patients. For example, using imipramine to produce equivalent effects, the starting dose should be 10 to 50 mg/day, which can be increased in 25 mg increments at 3- to 4-day intervals, until a therapeutic effect, prohibitive adverse effects, or a maximum dose of 150 mg is achieved. Plasma TCA levels may be useful when patients fail to respond to a trial of adequate doses and duration, when a dose of 150 mg/day must be exceeded, when unusually prominent side effects occur at low doses, or when treating patients with heart disease or other high risk conditions. Antipsychotic agents may be useful as adjuncts to the TCA for treating markedly agitated or delusionally depressed elderly patients. The MAOI should play a secondary or tertiary role in the treatment of depression compared to the use of the TCA or electroconvulsive therapy.

Psychomotor Stimulants

The difficulties and imprecisions complicating the clinical trials of the antipsychotic agents and, to a lesser degree, the antidepressant drugs have been particularly troublesome in the stimulant drug literature. Most early reports described open, uncontrolled, usually promising trials whose results have not been supported by later controlled, double-blind investigations. Even the more rigorously designed trials present such variability in dose, duration of treatment, and clinical assessments that comparisons are difficult. The most glaring deficiency in many of these reports is the heterogeneity of study populations attributable to absence of diagnostic specificity in geropsychiatry.

Psychomotor stimulants have been used primarily to try to improve cognitive functioning in patients with irreversible organic brain syndromes or else to activate lethargic, unmotivated elderly patients with affective disease, schizophrenia, dementia, or chronic nonpsychiatric disease. These agents have been the subject of excellent reviews by Prien,[65] Lehmann and Ban,[67] and Ban.[70] As noted by Prien et al.[54] these drugs are used infrequently in clinical practice compared to the other psychotropic drugs. The most significant of these agents, pentylenetetrazol, pipradrol, methylphenidate, magnesium pemoline, and the amphetamines will be reviewed briefly. The results of the double-blind comparative or placebo-controlled studies are presented in Table 5.

Pentylenetetrazol has been the most widely studied of these drugs.[67,148,164,201-251,284] The majority of the early studies noted symptomatic and behavioral improvement in elderly patients. Several studies also reported intellectual improvement in cognitively impaired patients. As noted in Table 5, these claims have been unsupported by the more rigorously controlled trials of pentylenetetrazol alone or in combination with nicotinic acid. Although individual patients have occasionally responded remarkably well, in general it appears that this agent is of limited usefulness. It is generally well-tolerated but occasionally causes nausea, vomiting, headache, or dizziness.

As noted by Lehmann and Ban,[67] the evidence of therapeutic efficacy of pipradrol in geriatric patients is quite limited but generally positive. Improvement both in ward behavior and psychometric test performance have been noted.[252-256] In the only controlled study, Turek et al.[257] found 5 mg/day to be the most effective dose.

Clinical reports of methylphenidate use in geriatric patients have yielded contradictory results.[258-277] As noted in Table 5, 6 of 10 double-blind trials have reported improved mood or decreased fatigue in elderly patients receiving this agent.[266,270,271,276,277] Attempts to demonstrate beneficial effects on cognitive functioning or psychometric testing have been less convincing. Dube et al.[270] and Kaplitz[266] reported only global improvement on "mental status". In addition, a large comparative but not double-blind study by Lehmann and Ban[264] failed to demonstrate significant improvement in cognition or behavioral parameters. Although these studies are particularly complicated by differences in patient populations, it appears that some patients may respond to the stimulant effects of methylphenidate with improved energy or mood but that little benefit in cognitive functioning is likely to be produced.

Magnesium pemoline was actively investigated during the 1960s and early 1970s when initial reports suggested the drug had promise in reversing memory deficits in cognitively impaired elderly.[133] Initially thought to facilitate encoding of memory by increasing RNA synthesis, magnesium pemoline in subsequent investigations was not found to affect RNA synthesis, enzyme activity, or protein synthesis in rat brains.[114,115] Favorable therapeutic results were then attributed to its mild stimulating effect.[116] However, as noted in Table 5, 5 double-blind studies with elderly patients have failed to demonstrate any therapeutic effects.[276-281]

Although the amphetamines are used clinically, they have not been systematically evaluated in the elderly.[281-283] Dextroamphetamine sulfate, combined with meperidine hydrochloride, was evaluated by Lehmann et al.[283] in the treatment of 22 depressed patients, many of whom were elderly. In a pilot study and an uncontrolled trial they found the combination 10 mg d-amphetamine orally per 50 mg meperidine intramuscularly effective in the majority of patients. Clark and Mankikar used d-amphetamine,[282] 5 to 20 mg/day, to treat "poor motivation syndrome" in 88 elderly rehabilitation patients who were free of depression or dementia. They noted a positive response in more than half of the patients in an open trial, but the results appeared to be inversely related to age. Adverse effects, such as uncooperative behavior, confusion or delusions, hypomania, vomiting, and constipation resulted in 23 dropouts during the first 4 days of treatment.

In summary, recognizing the limitations and hazards in attempting to draw definitive

Table 5
DOUBLE-BLIND TRIALS OF STIMULANT DRUGS IN THE ELDERLY

Drugs	Daily dose (mg)	Duration	N	Diagnosis	Results	Ref.
(a) Pentylenetetrazol (b) Cytochrome C (c) Nicotinic acid (d) Placebo (e) a + b (f) a + b + c	600 300	20 weeks	30	Mixed[a]	Pentylenetetrazol/nicotinic acid superior for behavioral control	237
Pentylenetetrazol Placebo	800	4 weeks	24	Mixed	No significant difference	238
Pentylenetetrazol Placebo	300	30 days	50	Senile psychosis	No significant difference	239
Pentylenetetrazol Placebo	NR[b]	4 weeks	77	Mixed	Superior to placebo	240
Pentylenetetrazol i.v Pentylenetetrazol Placebo	100—500 300	12 weeks	41	Mixed	Oral pentylenetetrazol superior to i.v.; both superior to placebo globally	241
Pentylenetetrazol Placebo	300—1200	11—18 weeks	15	OBS[b]	No significant difference	242
Pentylenetetrazol Placebo	800	60 days	40	Mixed	No significant difference	243
Pentylenetetrazol Glutamic acid Placebo	600	8 weeks	48	OBS	Pentylenetetrazol superior	244
Pentylenetetrazol/ vitamins Vitamins	600—800	17 months	30	Senile psychosis	Combination superior on global clinical ratings	245
Pentylenetetrazol/nicotinic acid Pepsin-alcohol elixir Placebo	600/300	16 weeks	20	OBS	No significant difference	242
Pentylenetetrazol Placebo	400—800	Variable	131	"Epileptics" OBS "Little strokes"	Superior to placebo	247

	Dose	Duration	N	Diagnosis	Result	Ref.
Pentylenetetrazol Placebo	600—900	60 days	60	OBS	No significant difference	248
Pentylenetetrazol/ nicotinic acid Pentylenetetrazol Placebo	900/300 900	12 weeks	44	OBS	No significant difference	249
Pentylenetetrazol/ vitamins Placebo	600	8 weeks	100	"Mentally ill"	No significant difference	250
Pentylenetetrazol/ niacin Placebo	300	4 weeks	50	"Senility"	Combination superior	251
Pentylenetetrazol/ nicotinic acid Nicotinic acid Pentylenetetrazol	600—800 600—800	12 weeks	30	Chronic medical illness	No significant difference	236
Pentylenetetrazol Placebo	200—800	4 weeks	20	Mixed	Pentylenetetrazol superior	233
Pentylenetetrazol Papaverine Niacin	400—600 300—450 30—45	12 weeks	60	Memory impairment	No significant difference	234
Pentylenetetrazol/ thiamine Oxygen Placebo	800/8	NR[c]	92	OBS	No significant difference	284
Pentylenetetrazol Placebo	600	18 weeks	61	Mixed OBS	No significant difference	235
Pentylenetetrazol Placebo	300—600	9 weeks	50	Memory impairment	No significant difference	67
Pipradrol Placebo	2,5	6 weeks	68	OBS	Pipradrol 5 mg/day superior	257
Methylphenidate Reserpine Placebo	40 1	12 weeks	20	"Senility"	Methylphenidate superior	270
Methylphenidate/ placebo Methylphenidate/reserpine Reserpine/placebo	40 40/1 1	12 weeks	18	"Senility"	Methylphenidate/placebo combination superior	270

Table 5 (continued)
DOUBLE-BLIND TRIALS OF STIMULANT DRUGS IN THE ELDERLY

Drugs	Daily dose (mg)	Duration	N	Diagnosis	Results	Ref.
Methylphenidate Placebo	30	8 days	61	Medical illness Depression	Superior to placebo	271
Methylphenidate Placebo	10—60	8 weeks	70	OBS Senility	No significant difference	263
Methylphenidate Protriptyline Placebo	20 20	16 weeks	NR	Schizophrenia OBS	No significant difference	269
Methylphenidate Magnesium pemoline Placebo	15 75	4 weeks	55	Depression	Both superior to placebo in medical practice patients; placebo superior in psychiatric patients	276
Methylphenidate Magnesium pemoline Placebo	10—30 50—150	6 weeks	78	Normal	No significant memory improvement; methylphenidate reduced fatigue	277
Methylphenidate Diazepam Phenobarbital Placebo	15 6 45	1 week	100	Normal	No significant differences on psychometric tests; no antidepressant effect from methylphenidate	273
Methylphenidate Placebo	20	4—6 weeks	44	OBS "Senile apathy"	Superior to placebo	266
Methylphenidate Placebo	10—30	1 day	12	Memory deficits	No significant difference	265
Magnesium pemoline Methamphetamine Placebo	25—50 10	2—21 days	14	Korsakoff syndrome	No significant difference	281
Magnesium pemoline Placebo	25	4 weeks	29	OBS	No significant difference	278
Magnesium pemoline Placebo	50—150	6 weeks	26	Depression Anxiety "Apathy"	No significant difference	280

					279
Magnesium pemoline	75	24 weeks	42	Locomotor disabilities	No significant difference
Placebo					
No drug					

[a] May include organic brain syndrome, schizophrenia, affective disease, alcoholism, and medical illness.

[b] OBS = organic brain syndrome.

[c] NR = not reported.

conclusions from the clinical studies of the stimulant drugs, nevertheless some generalizations can be made. It appears that these agents have failed to a large extent to fulfill clinicians' hopes and expectations in offering symptomatic relief in the treatment of heterogeneous groups of elderly patients. Individual patients may derive such benefits as increased activity levels, improved alertness or attention, or a reduction in lethargy or depressed mood at least for brief periods. There is no compelling evidence that these drugs are generally effective in treating depression, in reducing behavioral problems, or in improving intellectual function in the elderly. Further research should explore the use of these agents in more specifically and homogeneously defined populations.

REFERENCES

1. **Barchas, J. D., Akil, H., Elliott, G. R., Holman, R. B., and Watson, S. J.,** Behavioral neurochemistry: neuroregulators and behavioral states, *Science,* 200, 964, 1978.
2. **Starke, K.,** Regulation of noradrenaline release by presynaptic receptor systems, *Rev. Physiol. Biochem. Pharmacol.,* 77, 1, 1977.
3. **Starke, K., Taube, H. D., and Borowski, E.,** Presynaptic receptor systems in catecholaminergic transmission, *Biochem. Pharmacol.,* 26, 259, 1977.
4. **Moore, R. Y. and Bloom, F. E.,** Central catecholamine neuron systems: anatomy and physiology of the dopamine system, *Ann. Rev. Neurosci.,* 1, 129, 1978.
5. **Lindvall, O. and Bjorklund, A.,** Anatomy of the dopaminergic neuron systems in the rat brain, *Adv. Biochem. Psychopharmacol.,* 19, 1, 1978.
6. **Maas, J. W.,** Biogenic amines and depression, *Arch. Gen. Psychiatry,* 32, 1357, 1975.
7. **Maas, J. W., Dekirmenjian, H., and Jones, F.,** The identification of depressed patients who have a disorder of norepinephrine metabolism and/or disposition, in *Frontiers of Catecholamine Research,* Usdin, E. and Snyder, S. H., Eds., Pergamon Press, New York, 1973, 1091.
8. **Schildkraut, J. J.** Norepinephrine metabolites as biochemical criteria for classifying depressive disorders and predicting responses to treatment: preliminary findings. *Am. J. Psychiatry,* 130, 695, 1973.
9. **Beckman, H. and Goodwin, E. K.,** Antidepressant response to tricyclics and urinary MHPG in unipolar patients, *Arch. Gen. Psychiatry,* 32, 17, 1975.
10. **Goodwin, F. K., Cowdry, R. W., and Webster, M. H.,** Predictors of drug response in the affective disorders: toward an integrated approach, in *Psychopharmacology: A Generation of Progress,* Lipton, M. A., DiMascio, A., and Killam, K. F., Eds., Raven Press, New York, 1978, 1277.
11. **Vetulani, J., Stawarz, R. J., Dingell, J. V., and Sulser, F.,** A possible common mechanism of action of antidepressant treatments, *Naunyn-Schmiedebergs Arch. Pharmacol.,* 293, 109, 1976.
12. **Vetalani, J., Stawarz, R. J., and Sulser, F.,** Adaptive mechanisms of the noradrenergic cyclic AMP generating system in the limbic forebrain of the rat: adaption to persistent changes in the availability of norepinephrine, *J. Neurochem.,* 27, 661, 1976.
13. **Sulser, F., Vetulani, J., and Mobley, P. L.,** Mode of action of antidepressant drugs, *Biochem. Pharmacol.,* 27, 257, 1978.
14. **Wolfe, B. B., Harden, T. K., Sporn, J. R., and Molinoff, P. B.,** Presynaptic modulation of beta adrenergic receptors in rat cerebral cortex after treatment with antidepressants, *J. Pharmacol. Exp. Ther.,* 207, 446, 1978.
15. **Whybrow, P. and Mendels, J.,** Toward a biology of depression: some suggestions from neurophysiology, *Am. J. Psychiatry,* 125, 45, 1969.
16. **Akiskal, H. S. and McKinney, W. T.,** Overview of recent research in depression, *Arch. Gen. Psychiatry,* 32, 285, 1975.
17. **Crews, F. T. and Smith, C. B.,** Presynaptic alpha-receptor subsensitivity after long term antidepressant treatment, *Science,* 202, 322, 1978.
18. **Svensson, T. H. and Usdin, T.,** Feedback inhibition of brain noradrenaline neurons by tricyclic antidepressants: alpha-receptor mediation, *Science,* 202, 1089, 1978.
19. **Matthysse, S.,** Dopamine and the pharmacology of schizophrenia; the state of the evidence, *J. Psychiatric Res.,* 11, 107, 1974.
20. **Carlsson, A.,** Antipsychotic drugs, neurotransmitters and schizophrenia, *Am. J. Psychiatry,* 135, 164, 1978.

21. **Carlsson, A.,** Does dopamine have a role in schizophrenia?, *Biol. Psychiatry,* 13, 3, 1978.
22. **Snyder, S. H.,** The dopamine hypothesis of schizophrenia: focus on the dopamine receptor, *Am. J. Psychiatry,* 133, 197, 1976.
23. **Creese, I., Burt, D. R., and Snyder, S. H.,** Biochemical actions of neuroleptic drugs: focus on the dopamine receptor, in *Handbook of Psychopharmacology,* Vol. 10, Iversen, L. L., Iversen, S. D., and Snyder, S. H., Eds., Plenum Press, New York, 1978, 37.
24. **Seeman, P., Tedesco, J. L., Lee, T., Chau-Wong, M., Muller, P., Bowles, J., Whitaker, P. M., McManus, C., Tittler, M., Weinreich, P., Friend, W. C., and Brown, G. M.,** Dopamine receptors in the central nervous system, *Fed. Proc., Fed. Am. Soc. Exp. Biol.,* 37, 130, 1978.
25. **McGeer, E. and McGeer, P. L.,** Neurotransmitter metabolism in the aging brain, in *Neurology of Aging,* Terry, R. D. and Gershon, S., Eds., Raven Press, New York, 1976, 389.
26. **McGeer, E. G.,** Aging and neurotransmitter metabolism in human brain, in *Alzheimer's Disease: Senile Dementia and Related Disorders,* Katzman, R., Terry, R. D., and Bick, K. L., Eds., Raven Press, New York, 1978, 427.
27. **Domino, E. F., Dren, A. T., and Giardina, W. J.,** Biochemical and neurotransmitter changes in the aging brain, in *Psychopharmacology: A Generation of Progress,* Lipton, M. A., Dimascio, A., and Killam, K. F., Eds., Raven Press, New York, 1978, 1507.
28. **McGeer, P. L., McGeer, E. G., and Suzuki, J. S.,** Aging and extrapyramidal function, *Arch. Neurol.,* 34, 33, 1977.
29. **Barbeau, A.,** Aging and the extrapyramidal system, *J. Am. Geriatr. Soc.,* 21, 145, 1973.
30. **Barbeau, A.,** Parkinson's disease: etiological considerations, in *The Basal Ganglia,* Yahr, M. D., Ed., Raven Press, New York, 1976, 281.
31. **Robinson, D. S., Davis, J. N., and Nies, A.,** Relation of sex and aging to monoamine oxidase activity of human brain, plasma end platelets, *Arch. Gen. Psychiatry,* 24, 536, 1971.
32. **Robinson, D. S.,** Changes in monoamine oxidase and monoamines with human development and aging, *Fed. Proc. Fed. Am. Soc. Exp. Biol.,* 34, 103, 1975.
33. **Nies, A., Robinson, D. S., Davis, J. M., and Ravaris, C. L.,** Changes in monoamine oxidase with aging, in *Psychopharmacology and Aging,* Eisdorfer, C. and Fann, W. E., Eds., Plenum Press, New York, 1974, 41.
34. **Gottfries, C. G., Gottfries, J., Johansson, B., Olsson, R., Persson, T., Roos, B. E., and Sjostrom, R.,** Acid monoamine metabolites in human cerebrospinal fluid and their relations to age and sex, *Neuropharmacology,* 10, 665, 1971.
35. **Adolfsson, R., Gottfries, C. G., Oreland, L., Roos, B. E., and Winblad, B.,** Reduced levels of catecholamines in the brain and increased activity of monoamine oxidase in platelets in Alzheimer's Disease: therapeutic implications, in *Alzheimer's Disease: Senile Dementia and Related Disorders,* Katzman, R., Terry, R. D., and Bick, K. L., Eds., Raven Press, New York, 1978, 441.
36. **McGeer, E. G., Fibiger, H. C., McGeer, P. L., and Wickson, V.,** Aging and brain enzymes, *Exp. Gerontol.,* 6, 391, 1971.
37. **Finch, C. E.,** Catecholamine metabolism in the brains of aging male mice, *Brain Res.,* 52, 261, 1976.
38. **Samorjaski, T. and Rolsten, C.,** Age and regional differences in the chemical composition of brains of mice, monkeys and humans, *Progr. Brain Res.,* 40, 253, 1973.
39. **Miller, A. E., Shaar, C. J., and Riegle, G. D.,** Aging effects on hypothalamic dopamine and norepinephrine content in the male rat, *Exp. Aging Res.,* 2, 475, 1976.
40. **Austin, J. H., Connole, E., Kett, D., and Collins, J.,** Studies in aging of the brain. V. Reduced norepinephrine, dopamine and cyclic AMP in rat brain with advancing age, *Age,* 1, 121, 1978.
41. **Ponzio, F., Brunello, N., and Algeri, S.,** Catecholamine synthesis in brain of aging rat, *J. Neurochem.,* 30, 1617, 1978.
42. **Joseph, J. A., Berger, R. E., Engel, B. T., and Roth, G. S.,** Age-related changes in the nigrostriatum: a behavioral and biochemical analysis, *J. Gerontol.,* 33, 643, 1978.
43. **Govoni, S., Spano, P. F., and Trabucchi, M.,** ^{3}H-Haloperidol and ^{3}H-spiroperidol binding in rat striatum during aging, *J. Pharm. Pharmacol.,* 30, 448, 1978.
44. **Saunders, D. R., Paolino, R. N., Bousquet, W. F., and Miya, T. S.,** Age-related responsiveness of the rat to drugs affecting the central nervous system, *Proc. Soc. Exp. Biol. Med.,* 147, 593, 1974.
45. **Weiss, B., Greenberg, L., and Cantor, E.,** Age-related alterations in the development of adrenergic denervation supersensitivity, *Fed. Proc., Fed. Am. Soc. Exp. Biol.,* 1915, 1979.
46. **Makman, M. H., Ahn, H. S., Thal, L. J., Sharpless, N. E., Dvorkin, B., Horowitz, S. G., and Rosenfeld, M.,** Aging and monoamine receptors in brain, *Fed. Proc., Fed. Am. Soc. Exp. Biol.,* 38, 1922, 1979.
47. **Puri, S. K. and Volicer, L.,** Effect of aging on cyclic AMP levels and adenylate cyclase and phosphodiesterase activities in the rat corpus striatum, *Mech. Aging Develop.,* 6, 53, 1977.
48. **Jonec, V. and Finch, C. E.,** Aging and dopamine uptake by subcellular fractions in the C57BL/6J male mouse brain, *Brain Res.,* 91, 197, 1975.

49. **Finch, C. E.,** The regulation of physiological changes during mammalian aging, *Q. Rev. Biol.,* 51, 49, 1976.

50. **Meek, J. L., Bertilsson, L., Cheney, D. L., Zsilla, G., and Costa, E.,** Aging-induced changes in acetylcholine and serotonin content of discrete nuclei, *J. Gerontol.,* 32, 129, 1977.

51. **Shih, J. C. and Young, H.,** The alteration of serotonin binding sites in aged human brain, *Life Sci.,* 23, 1441, 1978.

52. **Parish, P. A.,** The prescribing of psychotropic drugs in general practice, *J. R. Coll. Gen. Pract.,* 21 (Suppl. 4), 1, 1971.

53. **Rowe, I. L.,** Prescription of psychotropic drugs by general practitioners. I. General, *Med. J. Aust.,* 1, 589, 1973.

54. **Prien, R. F., Haber, P. A., and Caffey, E. M., Jr.,** Psychoactive drug use in elderly patients with psychiatric disorders: a survey of 12 Veterans Administration Hospitals, *J. Am. Geriatr Soc.,* 23, 104, 1975.

55. **Fracchia, J., Sheppard, C., and Merlis, S.,** Combination medications in psychiatric treatment: patterns in a group of elderly hospital patients, *J. Am. Geriatr. Soc.,* 19, 301, 1971.

56. **Learoyd, B. M.,** Psychotropic drugs and the elderly patients, *Med. J. Aust.,* 1, 1131, 1972.

57. **Greenblatt, D. J., Shader, R. I., and Koch-Weser, J.,** Psychotropic drug use in the Boston area: a report from the Boston Collaborative Drug Surveillance Program, *Arch. Gen. Psychiatry,* 32, 518, 1975.

58. **Parry, H. J., Balter, M. B., Mellinger, G. D., Cisin, I. H., and Manheimer, M. A.,** National patterns of psychotherapeutic drug use, *Arch. Gen. Psychiatry,* 28, 769, 1973.

59. **Greenblatt, D. J., Allen, M. D., and Shader, R. I.,** Toxicity of high-dose flurazepam in the elderly, *Clin. Pharmacol. Ther.,* 21, 355, 1977.

60. **Hurwitz, N.,** Predisposing factors in adverse reactions to drugs, *Br. Med. J.,* 1, 536, 1969.

61. **Smith, J. W., Seidl, L. G., and Cluff, L. E.,** Studies on the epidemiology of adverse drug reactions. V. Clinical factors influencing susceptibility, *Ann. Intern. Med.,* 65, 629, 1966.

62. **Ayd, F. J., Jr.,** Tranquilizers and the ambulatory geriatric patient, *J. Am. Geriatr. Soc.,* 8, 909, 1960.

63. **Siede, H. and Miller, H. F.,** Choreiform movements as side effects of phenothiazine medication in geriatric patients, *J. Am. Geriatr. Soc.,* 15, 517, 1967.

64. **Davies, R. K., Tucker, G. J., Hanow, M., and Detre, T. P.,** Confusional episodes and antidepressant medication, *Am. J. Psychiatry,* 128, 1971.

65. **Prien, R. F.,** Chemotherapy in chronic organic brain syndrome — a review of the literature, *Psychopharm. Bull.,* 9, 5, 1973.

66. **Stotsky, B. A.,** Psychoactive drugs for geriatric patients with psychiatric disorders, in *Aging,* Vol. 2, Gershon, S. and Raskin, A., Eds., Raven Press, New York, 1975, 229.

67. **Lehmann, H. E. and Ban, T. A.,** Central nervous system stimulants and anabolic substances in geropsychiatric therapy, in *Aging,* Vol. 2, Gershon, S. and Raskin, A., Eds., Raven Press, New York, 1975, 179.

68. **Friedel, R. O. and Raskind, M. A.,** Psychopharmacology of aging, in *Special Review of Experimental Aging Research: Progress in Biology,* Elias, M. F., Eleftheriou, B. E., and Elias, P. K., Eds., E. A. R., Inc., Bar Harbor, Maine, 1976, 105.

69. **Epstein, L. J.,** Anxiolytics, antidepressants, and neuroleptics in the treatment of geriatric patients, in *Psychopharmacology: A Generation of Progress,* Lipton, M. A., DiMascio, A., and Killam, K. F., Eds., Raven Press, New York, 1978, 1517.

70. **Ban, T. A.,** Vasodilators, stimulants, and anabolic agents in the treatment of geropsychiatric patients, in *Psychopharmacology: A Generation of Progress,* Lipton, M. A., DiMascio, A., and Killam, K. F., Raven Press, New York, 1978, 1525.

71. **Kay, D. W. K. and Roth, M.,** Environmental and hereditary factors in the schizophrenias of old age ("late paraphrenia") and their bearing on the general problem of causation in schizophrenia, *J. Ment. Sci.,* 107, 649, 1961.

72. **Post, F.,** Paranoid syndromes, in *The Clinical Psychiatry of Late Life,* Pergamon Press, Oxford, 1965, 106.

73. **Raskind, M. A., Alvarez, C., Pietrzyk, M., Westerlund, K., and Herlin, S.,** Helping the elderly psychiatric patient in crisis, *Geriatrics,* 31, 51, 1976.

74. **Synder, S. H., Banerjee, S. P., Yamamura, H. I., and Greenberg, D.,** Drugs, neurotransmitters and schizophrenia, *Science,* 184, 1243, 1974.

75. **Snyder, S. H., Greenberg, D., and Yamamura, H. I.,** Antischizophrenic drugs and brain cholinergic receptors: affinity for muscarinic sites predicts extrapyramidal effects, *Arch. Gen. Psychiatry,* 31, 58, 1974.

76. **Gershon, S., Holmberg, G., Mattson, E., Mattson, N., and Marshall, A.,** Imipramine hydrochloride. Its effects on clinical, autonomic, and psychological functions, *Arch. Gen. Psychiatry,* 6, 96, 1962.

77. **Klein, D. F. and Fink, M.,** Psychiatric reaction patterns to imipramine, *Am. J. Psychiatry,* 119, 432, 1962.

78. **Lehmann, H. E., Cahn, C. H., and DeVerteuil, E. L.,** Treatment of depressive conditions with imipramine (G 22355), *Can. Psychiatric Assoc. J.,* 3, 155, 1958.

79. **Baldessarini, R. J. and Wilmuth, R. L.,** Psychotic reactions during amitriptyline therapy, *Can. Psychiatric Assoc. J.,* 13, 571, 1968.
80. **Ayd, F. J., Jr.,** A survey of drug-induced extrapyramidal reactions, *J. Am. Med. Assoc.,* 175, 1054, 1961.
81. **Swett, C., Jr.,** Drug-induced dystonia, *Am. J. Psychiatry,* 132, 532, 1975.
82. **Kennedy, P. F., Hershon, H. I., and McGuire, R. J.,** Extrapyramidal disorders after prolonged phenothiazine therapy, *Br. J. Psychiatry,* 118, 509, 1971.
83. **Jus, A., Pineau, R., Lachance, R., Pelchat, G., Jus, K., Pires, P., and Villeneuve, R.,** Epidemiology of tardive dyskinesia, *Dis. Nerv. Syst.,* 37: Part I, 210, Part II, 257, 1976.
84. **Crane, G. E.,** High doses of trifluoperazine and tardive dyskinesia, *Arch. Neurol.,* 22, 176, 1970.
85. **Hershon, H. L., Kennedy, P. F., and McGuire, R. J.,** Persistence of extrapyramidal disorders and psychiatric relapse after long-term phenothiazine therapy, *Br. J. Psychiatry,* 120, 41, 1972.
86. **Brandon, S., McClelland, H. A., and Protheroe, C.,** A study of facial dyskinesia in a mental population, *Br. J. Psychiatry,* 118, 171, 1971.
87. **Huston, J. R. and Bell, G. E.,** The effect of thioridazine hydrochloride and chlorpromazine on the electrocardiogram, *J. Am. Med. Assoc.,* 198, 134, 1966.
88. **Wendkos, M. H.,** Cardiac changes related to phenothiazine therapy, with special reference to thioridazine, *J. Am. Geriatr. Soc.,* 15, 20, 1967.
89. **Alexander, C. S. and Nino, A.,** Cardiovascular complications in young patients taking psychotropic drugs, *Am. Heart J.,* 78, 757, 1969.
90. **Chouinard, G. and Annable, L.,** Phenothiazine-induced ECG abnormalities. Effect of a glucose load, *Arch. Gen. Psychiatry,* 34, 951, 1977.
91. **Hollister, L. E. and Kosek, J. C.,** Sudden death during treatment with phenothiazine derivatives, *J. Am. Med. Assoc.,* 192, 1034, 1965.
92. **Thorton, C. D. and Wendkos, M. H.,** EKG T-wave distortions among thioridazine treated psychiatric inpatients, *Dis. Nerv. Syst.,* 32, 320, 1971.
93. **Hollander, P. B. and Cain, R. M.,** Effects of thioridazine on transmembrane potential and contractile characteristics of guinea pig hearts, *Eur. J. Pharmacol.,* 16, 129, 1971.
94. **Epstein, L. J.,** Symposium on age differentiation in depressive illness. Depression in the elderly, *J. Gerontol.,* 31, 278, 1976.
95. **Salzman, C. and Shader, R. I.,** Depression in the elderly. I. Relationship between depression, psychologic defense mechanisms and physical illness, *J. Am. Geriatr. Soc.,* 26, 253, 1978.
96. **Salzman, C. and Shader, R. I.,** Depression in the elderly. II. Possible drug etiologies; differential diagnostic criteria, *J. Am. Geriatr. Soc.,* 26, 303, 1978.
97. **Maas, J. W.,** Clinical implications of pharmacological differences among antidepressants, in *Psychopharmacology: A Generation of Progress,* Lipton, M. A., DiMascio, A., and Killam, K. F., Eds., Raven Press, New York, 1978, 955.
98. **Glassman, A. H. and Perel, J. M.,** Tricyclic blood levels and clinical outcome: a review of the art, in *Psychopharmacology: A Generation of Progress,* Lipton, M. A., DiMascio, A., and Killam, K. F., Eds., Raven Press, New York, 1978, 917.
99. **Friedel, R. O., Veith, R. C., Bloom, V., and Bielski, R. J.,** Despiramine plasma levels and clinical response in depressed outpatients, *Comm. Psychopharm.,* 3, 81, 1979.
100. **Glassman, A., Perel, J., Shostak, M., Kantor, S. J., and Fleiss, J. L.,** Clinical implications of imipramine plasma levels for depressive illness, *Arch. Gen. Psychiatry,* 34, 197, 1977.
101. **Quitkin, F., Rifkin, A., and Klein, D. F.,** Imipramine response in deluded depressive patients, *Am. J. Psychiatry,* 135, 806, 1978.
102. **Nelson, J. C. and Bowers, M. B.,** Delusional unipolar depression. Description and drug response, *Arch. Gen. Psychiatry,* 35, 1321, 1978.
103. **Tyrer, P.,** Towards rational therapy with monoamine oxidase inhibitors, *Br. J. Psychiatry,* 128, 354, 1976.
104. **Schuckit, M., Robins, E., and Feighner, J.,** Tricyclic antidepressants and monoamine oxidase inhibitors, *Arch. Gen. Psychiatry,* 24, 509, 1971.
105. **Robinson, D. S.,** MAO inhibitors and the elderly, presented at Workshop on the Influences of Age on the Pharmacology of Psychoactive Drugs, Washington, D.C., April 16-17, 1979.
106. **Salzman, C., Shader, R. I. and Harmatz, J. S.,** Response of the elderly to psychotropic drugs: predictable or idiosyncratic?, in *Aging,* Vol. 2, Gershon, S. and Raskin, A., Eds., Raven Press, New York, 1975, 259.
107. **Snyder, S. and Yamamura, H. I.,** Antidepressants and the muscarinic acetylcholine receptor, *Arch. Gen. Psychiatry,* 34, 236, 1977.
108. **vanZwieten, P. A.,** Interaction between centrally acting hypotensive drugs and tricyclic antidepressants, *Arch. Int. Pharmacodyn.,* 214, 12, 1975.
109. **Glassman, A. H., Bigger, J. T., Giardina, E. V., Kantor, S. J., Perel, J. M., and Davies, M.,** Clinical characteristics of imipramine-induced orthostatic hypotension, *Lancet,* 1, 468, 1979.

110. **Bigger, J. T., Kantor, S. J., Glassman, A. H., and Perel, J. M.,** Cardiovascular effects of tricyclic antidepressant drugs, in *Psychopharmacology: A Generation of Progress,* Lipton, M. A., DiMascio, A., and Killam, K. F., Eds., Raven Press, New York, 1971, 1033.
111. **Pitts, N. E.** The clinical evaluation of doxepin, a new psychotherapeutic agent, *Psychosomatics,* 10, 164, 1969.
112. **Burrows, G. D., Vohra, J., Dumovic, P., Maguire, K., Scoggins, B. A., and Davies, B.,** Tricyclic antidepressant drugs and cardiac conduction, *Progr. Neuro-Psychopharm.,* 1, 329, 1977.
113. **Cameron, D. E.,** Memory drug tests are "encouraging," *J. Am. Med. Assoc.,* 196, 29, 1966.
114. **Morris, N. R., Agajanian, G. K., and Bloom, F. E.,** Magnesium pemoline: failure to affect *in vivo* synthesis of brain RNA, *Science,* 155, 1125, 1967.
115. **Yuwiler, A., Greenough, W., and Geller, E.** Biochemical and behavioral effect of magnesium pemoline, *Psychopharmacologica,* 13, 174, 1968.
116. **Jarvik, M. E., Gritz, E. R., and Schneider, N. G.,** Drugs and memory disorders in human aging, *Behav. Biol.,* 7, 643, 1972.
117. **Ban, T. A. and St. Jean, A.,** The effect of phenothiazines on the electrocardiogram, *Can. Med. Assoc. J.,* 91, 537, 1964.
118. **Bigger, J. T., Giardina, E. V., Perel, J. N., Kantor, S. J., and Glassman, A. H.,** Cardiac antiarrhythmic effect of imipramine hydrochloride, *N. Engl. J. Med.,* 296, 206, 1977.
119. **Burrows, G. D., Vohra, J., Hunt, D., Sloman, J. G., Scoggins, B. A., and Davies, B.,** Cardiac effects of different tricyclic antidepressant drugs, *Br. J. Psychiatry,* 129, 335, 1976.
120. **Snyder, S. H.,** Neuroleptic drugs and neurotransmitter receptors, *J. Continuing Educ. Psych.,* 39, 21, 1978.
121. **Peroutka, S. J., U'Prichard, D. C., Greenberg, D. A., and Snyder, S. H.,** Neuroleptic drug interactions with norepinephrine α-receptor binding sites in rat brain, *Neuropharmacology,* 16, 549, 1977.
122. **Judah, L., Murphree, O., and Seager, L.,** Psychiatric response of geriatric-psychiatric patients to Mellaril (TP-21 SANDOZ), *Am. J. Psychiatry,* 115, 1118, 1959.
123. **Ananth, J. V., Saxena, B. M., Lehmann, H. E., and Ban, T. A.,** Combined administration of thioridazine and nicotinic acid in treatment of geriatric patients, *Curr. Ther. Res.,* 13, 158, 1971.
124. **Barksdale, B.,** Behavior problems in nursing home patients: treatment with thioridazine, *Curr. Ther. Res.,* 13, 359, 1971.
125. **Boiullat, J. E., Saxena, B. M., Lehmann, H. E., and Ban, T. A.,** Combined administration of thioridazine, nicotinic acid, and fluoxymesterone in the treatment of geriatric patients, *Curr. Ther. Res.,* 13, 541, 1971.
126. **Cavero, C. V.,** Evaluation of thioridazine in the aged, *J. Am. Geriatr. Soc.,* 14, 617, 1966.
127. **Deutsch, M., Saxena, B. M., Lehmann, H. E., and Ban, T. A.,** Combined administration of thioridazine and fluoxymesterone in the treatment of geriatric patients, *Curr. Ther. Res.,* 12, 805, 1970.
128. **Felger, H.,** Thioridazine in the geriatric patient, *Dis. Nerv. Syst.,* 27, 537, 1966.
129. **Fleischl, H.,** Effects of thioridazine on chronically regressed patients, *J. Am. Geriatr. Soc.,* 15, 29, 1967.
130. **Fraiberg, P. L.,** Control of behavioral symptoms in patients with long-term illness, *Dis. Nerv. Syst.,* 33, 178, 1972.
131. **Hader, M.,** The use of selected phenothiazines in elderly patients: a review, *J. Mt. Sinai Hosp.,* 32, 622, 1965.
132. **Jackson, E. B.,** Mellaril in the treatment of the geriatric patient, *Am. J. Psychiatry,* 118, 543, 1961.
133. **Kral, V. A.,** The use of thioridazine in aged people, *Can. Med. Assoc. J.,* 84, 152, 1961.
134. **Kral, V. A. and Papetropoulos, D.,** Treatment of geriatric patients, in *Psychopharmacology,* Kline, N. S. and Lehmann, H. E., Eds., Little, Brown, Boston, 1965, 775.
135. **Lamberton, W. D.,** Mental illness, *Pa. Med.,* 70, 1967.
136. **Lehmann, H. E. and Ban, T. A.,** Comparative pharmacotherapy of the aging psychotic patients, *Laval Med.,* 38, 588, 1967.
137. **Lehmann, H. E., Ban, T. A., and Saxena, B. M.,** Nicotinic acid, thioridazine, fluoxymesterone and their combinations in hospitalized geriatric patients: a systematic clinical study, *Can. Psychiatric Assoc. J.,* 17, 315, 1972.
138. **Lifshitz, K. and Kline, N. S.,** Psychopharmacology in geriatrics, in *Principles of Psychopharmacology,* Clark, W. G. and Delguidice, J., Eds., Academic Press, New York, 1970, 695.
139. **Spencer, J.,** The management of behaviors in the geriatric patients, *Md. State Med. J.,* 18, 73, 1969.
140. **Wilson, J. D. and Mathis, E.,** Nursing home management of behavior problems in the geriatric patient, *J. Ark. Med. Soc.,* 65, 210, 1968.
141. **Altman, H., Mehta, D., Evenson, R. C., and Sletten, I. W.,** Behavioral effects of drug therapy on psychogeriatric inpatients. I. Chlorpromazine and thioridazine, *J. Am. Geriatr. Soc.,* 21, 241, 1973.
142. **Smith, G. R., Taylor, C. W., and Linkous, P.,** Haloperidol versus thioridazine for the treatment of psychogeriatric patients: a double-blind clinical trial, *Psychosomatics,* 15, 134, 1974.

143. **Tsuang, M. D., Lu, L. M., Stotsky, B. A., and Cole, J. O.,** Haloperidol versus thioridazine for hospitalized psychogeriatric patients: double-blind study, *J. Am. Geriatr. Soc.,* 19, 593, 1971.

144. **Goldstein, S. E. and Birnbom, F.,** Piperacetazine versus thioridazine in the treatment of organic brain disease: a controlled, double-blind study, *J. Am. Geriatr. Soc.,* 24, 355, 1976.

145. **Gallant, D. N. and Bishop, M. P.,** Quide vs. Mellaril in chronic schizophrenic patients, *Curr. Ther. Res.,* 14, 10, 1972.

146. **Tewfik, G. I., Jain, V. K., Harcup, M., and Magowan, S.,** Effectiveness of various tranquilizers in the management of senile restlessness, *Gerontol. Clin.,* 12, 351, 1970.

147. **Abse, W. and Dahlstrom, W. G.,** The value of chemotherapy in senile mental disturbance, *J. Am. Med. Assoc.,* 174, 2036, 1960.

148. **Robinson, D. B.,** Evaluation of certain drugs in geriatric patients, *Arch. Gen. Psychiatry,* 1, 41, 1959.

149. **Barton, R. and Hurst, L.,** Unnecessary use of tranquilizers in elderly patients, *Br. J. Psychiatry,* 112, 989, 1966.

150. **Seager, C. P.,** Chlorpromazine in treatment of elderly psychotic women, *Br. Med. J.,* 1, 882, 1955.

151. **Karland, A. A.,** Chlorpromazine in the management of the institutionalized aged psychiatric patient with organic brain syndrome, *Dis. Nerv. Syst.,* 16, 366, 1955.

152. **Pollack, B.,** The addition of chlorpromazine to the treatment program for emotional and behavior disorders in the aging, *Geriatrics,* 11, 253, 1956.

153. **Terman, L. A.,** Treatment of senile agitation with chlorpromazine, *Geriatrics,* 10, 520, 1955.

154. **Goldstein, B. J. and Dippy, W. E.,** A clinical evaluation of mesoridazine in geriatric patients, *Curr. Ther. Res.,* 9, 256, 1967.

155. **Goldstein, S. E.,** The use of mesoridazine in geriatrics, *Curr. Ther. Res.,* 16, 316, 1974.

156. **Hamilton, L. D. and Bennet, J. L.,** Acetophenazine for hyperactive geriatric patients, *Geriatrics,* 17, 596, 1962.

157. **Sheppard, C., Bhattacharyya, A., DiGiacomo, M., and Merlis, S.,** Effects of acetophenazine dimaleate on paranoid symptomatology in female geriatric patients: double-blind study, *J. Am. Geriatr. Soc.,* 12, 884, 1964.

158. **Honigfeld, G., Rosenblum, M. P., Blumenthal, I. J., Lambert, H. L., and Roberts, A. J.,** Behavioral improvement in the older schizophrenic patients: drug and social therapies, *J. Am. Geriatr. Soc.,* 13, 57, 1965.

159. **Witten, K. and Hermann, H. T.,** Clinical experience with acetophenazine in the elderly psychotic, *Dis. Nerv. Syst.,* 24, 314, 1962.

160. **Hader, M., Schulman, P. M., and Madonick, M. J.,** Paranoid conditions of late life treated with trifluoperazine, *Dis. Nerv. Syst.,* 27, 460, 1966.

161. **Hamilton, L. D. and Bennett, J. L.,** The use of trifluoperazine in geriatric patients with chronic brain syndrome, *J. Am. Geriatr. Soc.,* 10, 140, 1962.

162. **Kropach, K.** The treatment of acutely agitated senile patients with trifluoperazine (stelazine), *Br. J. Clin. Pract.,* 13, 859, 1959.

163. **Brooks, G. W. and MacDonald, M. G.,** Effects of trifluoperazine in aged depressed female patients, *Am. J. Psychiatry,* 117, 932, 1961.

164. **Danto, B. L.,** Triflupromazine versus pentylenetetrazol-nicotinic acid for treatment of chronic brain disease on a general-hospital psychiatric service, *J. Am. Geriatr. Soc.,* 17, 414, 1969.

165. **Sugarman, A. A., Williams, H., and Adlerstein, A. M.,** Haloperidol in the psychiatric disorders of old age, *Am. J. Psychiatry,* 120, 1190, 1964.

166. **Lapolla, A. and Nash, L. R.,** A butyrophenone (haloperidol) for the treatment of institutionalized patients, *Int. J. Neuropsychiatry,* 2, 129, 1966.

167. **Tobin, J. M., Brousseau, E. R., and Lorenz, A. A.,** Clinical evaluation of haloperidol in geriatric patients, *Geriatrics,* 25, 119, 1970.

168. **Kristjansen, P.,** Clinical evaluation of neuroleptic drug action, particularly considering butyrophenones, *Acta Psychiatr. Scand. (Suppl.),* 42, 171, 1966.

169. **Robbins, L. E. and Nagel, D. J.,** Haloperidol parenterally for treatment of vomiting and nausea from gastrointestinal disorders in a group of geriatric patients: double-blind placebo controlled, *J. Am. Geriatr. Soc.,* 23, 38, 1975.

170. **Post, F.,** The impact of modern drug treatment on old age schizophrenia, *Gerontol. Clin.,* 4, 137, 1962.

171. **Settle, E.,** The use of perphenazine (Trilafon) to control anxiety and agitation in aged patients, *J. Am. Geriatr. Soc.,* 5, 1003, 1957.

172. **Birkett, D. P., Hirschfield, W., and Simpson, G. M.,** Thiothixene in treatment of diseases of the senium, *Curr. Ther. Res.,* 14, 775, 1972.

173. **Rada, R. T. and Kellner, R.,** Thiothixene in the treatment of geriatric patients with chronic organic brain syndrome, *J. Am. Geriatr. Soc.,* 24, 105, 1976.

174. **Mohler, G.,** Clinical trial of thiothixene (Navane) in elderly chronic schizophrenics, *Curr. Ther. Res.,* 12, 377, 1970.

175. **Branchey, M. H., Lee, J. H., Simpson, G. M., Elgart, B., and Vincencio, A.,** Loxapine succinate as a neuroleptic agent: evaluation in two populations of elderly psychiatric patients, *J. Am. Geriatr. Soc.,* 26, 263, 1978.

176. **Cameron, D. E.,** The use of Tofranil in the aged, *Can. Psychiatr. Assoc. J., (Suppl),* 4, 160, 1959.

177. **Grauer, H. and Kral, V. A.,** The use of imipramine (Tofranil) in psychiatric patients of a geriatric outpatient clinic, *Can. Med. Assoc. J.,* 83, 1423, 1960.

178. **Delachaun, A. and Schwed, S.,** On the use of Tofranil in a geriatric rehabilitation clinic, *Praxis,* 23, 597, 1962.

179. **Aaronson, H. G. and Boger, W. P.,** Incontinence in the elderly: an attempt at control, *J. Am. Geriatr. Soc.,* 10, 626, 1962.

180. **Lawson, I. R. and MacLeod, R. D.,** The use of imipramine ("Tofranil") and other psychotropic drugs in organic emotionalism, *Br. J. Psychiatry,* 115, 281, 1969.

181. **Kendrick, D. C. and Post, F.,** Differences in cognitive status between healthy, psychiatrically ill, and diffusely brain-damaged elderly subjects, *Br. J. Psychiatry,* 113, 75, 1967.

182. **Nans, J., Cornil, J., and Allenberg, D.,** Therapeutic trials with G 22-355 (imipramine) in older patients in a psychiatric clinic, *Ann. Med. Psychol.,* 120, 57, 1962.

183. **Hordern, A. Burt, C. G., and Holt, N. F.,** *Depressive States: A Pharmacotherapeutic Study,* Charles C Thomas, Springfield, Ill., 1965.

184. **Nies, A., Robinson, D. S., Friedman, M. J., Green, R., Cooper, T. B., Ravaris, C. L., and Ives, J. O.,** Relationship between age and tricyclic antidepressant plasma levels, *Am. J. Psychiatry,* 134, 790, 1977.

185. **Shader, R.,** Cardiac effects of imipramine hydrochloride in the elderly, *Psychopharm. Bull.,* 11(1), 15, 1975.

186. **Haider, I.,** A comparative investigation of desipramine and nortriptyline in the treatment of depression, *Br. J. Psychiatry,* 114, 1293, 1968.

187. **Kernohan, W. J., Chambers, J. L., Wilson, W. T., and Daugherty, J. F.,** Effects of nortriptyline on mental and social adjustment of geriatric patients in a mental hospital, *J. Am. Geriatr. Soc.,* 15, 196, 1967.

188. **Chesrow, E. J., Kaplitz, S. E., Breme, J. T., Sabatini, T., Vetra, H., and Marquardt, G. H.,** Nortriptyline for the treatment of anxiety and depression in the chronically ill and geriatric patients, *J. Am. Geriatr. Soc.,* 12, 271, 1964.

189. **Kristoff, F. H., Lehmann, H. E., and Ban, T. A.,** Systematic studies with trimipramine — a new antidepressive drug, *Can. Psychiatr. Assoc. J.,* 12, 517, 1967.

190. **Ayd, F. J.,** Long term administration of doxepin (Sinequan), *Dis. Nerv. Sys.,* 32, 617, 1971.

191. **Friedel, R. O. and Raskind, M. A.,** Relationship of blood levels of Sinequan to clinical effects in the treatment of depression in aged patients, in *Sinequan, A Monograph of Recent Clinical Studies,* Mendels, J., Ed., Excerpta Medica, Princeton, 1975, 51.

192. **Goldberg, H. L., Finnerty, R. J., and Cole, J. O.,** The effects of doxepin in the aged: interim report on memory changes and electrocardiographic findings, in *Sinequan, A Monograph of Recent Clinical Studies,* Mendels, J., Ed., Excerpta Medica, Princeton, 1975, 65.

193. **Haider, I.,** A comparative-trial of RO 4-6270 and amitriptyline in depressive illness, *Br. J. Psychiatry,* 113, 933, 1967.

194. **Haider, I.,** Amitriptyline and perphenazine in depressive illness. A controlled trial, *Br. J. Psychiatry,* 113, 195, 1967.

195. **Beber, C. R.,** Treating anxiety and depression in the elderly: a double-blind crossover evaluation of two widely used tranquilizers, *J. Fla. Med. Assoc.,* 58, 35, 1971.

196. **Straker, N. and Brauer, H.,** Clinical study of a potent antidepressant, tranylcypramine with trifluoperazine (Parstelin) in the aged chronically ill, *Can. Med. Assoc. J.,* 85, 127, 1961.

197. **Wolff, K., Grasberger, J. C., and Kidorf, I. N.,** Nialamide in the treatment of schizophrenia in geriatric patients, *J. Am. Geriatr. Soc.,* 10, 148, 1962.

198. **Ayd, F. J., Jr.,** Nialamide therapy for the depressed geriatric patient, *J. Am. Geriatr. Soc.,* 10, 432, 1962.

199. **Langslet, A., Johansen, W. G., Ryg, M., and Skomedal, T.,** Effects of dibenzipine and imipramine on the isolated rat heart, *Eur. J. Pharmacol.,* 14, 333, 1971.

200. **Sigg, E. B., Osborn, M., and Korul, B.,** Cardiovascular effects of imipramine, *J. Pharmacol. Exp. Ther.,* 141, 237, 1963.

201. **Leake, C. D.,** Treating confused geriatric patients, *Geriatrics,* 19, 466, 1964.

202. **Andosca, J. B.,** Effects of pentylenetetrazol on senile patients, *N. Engl. J. Med.,* 250, 461, 1954.

203. **Aschenbach, E. H.,** The use of metrazol in non-institutionalized elderly patients, *Med. Ann. D. C.,* 25, 70, 1956.

204. **Bailey, K. G.,** Neuropsychiatric considerations peculiar to the aged, *J. Am. Osteopath. Assoc.,* Nov. 19, 1955.

205. **Butterworth, T. R., Jr.,** Some experiences with metrazol in geriatric practice, *Va. Med.,* 83, 540, 1956.

206. **Callan, J. R. and Starnes, W. L.,** Analeptic action of oral metrazol in geriatric practice (preliminary report), *Dis. Nerv. Syst.,* 15, 121, 1954.
207. **Cohn, A. G. and Cohn, W. M.,** Oral metrazol treatment of senile and arteriosclerotic psychoses, *N.Y. State J. Med.,* 55, 1324, 1955.
208. **Fong, T. C. C.,** Oral metrazol therapy in psychoses with cerebral arteriosclerosis, *J. Am. Geriatr. Soc.,* 1, 662, 1953.
209. **Jensen, E. and Leiser, R.,** The use of oral metrazol in psychosis with cerebral arteriosclerosis, *J. Mich. State Med. Soc.,* 52, 734, 1953.
210. **Kapernick, J. S.,** Metrazol for central nervous system arteriosclerosis in aging patients, *Geriatrics,* 12, 703, 1957.
211. **Kass, I. and Brown, E. C.,** The use of metrazol as a mood-conditioning drug: a discussion as to its mode of action (a preliminary report), *J. Nerv. Ment. Dis.,* 123, 57, 1956.
212. **Kolomeyer, N.,** A clinical evaluation of mephentermine sulfate and pentylenetetrazol as stimulant therapy for the geriatric patients, *J. Am. Geriatr. Soc.,* 6, 415, 1958.
213. **Levy, S.,** Drug therapy in the emotionally disturbed aged, *Northwest Med.,* 55, 298, 1956.
214. **Morrison, B. O.,** Oral metrazol in the care of the aged; a review of twenty-eight cases, *J. Am. Geriatr. Soc.,* 6, 895, 1958.
215. **Phipps, E. B. and Hogle, F. D.,** Clinical effects of the combined administration of nicotinamide and metrazol to a group of ten geriatric state hospital patients, *J. Ind. State M. Assoc.,* 51, 1661, 1958.
216. **Schall, E.,** Oral metrazol therapy in senile mental confusion and peripheral vascular spasm, *Clinical Med.,* 63, 859, 1956.
217. **Seidel, H., Silver, A., and Nagel, H.,** Effects of metrazol and nicotinamide on psychic and mental disorders in the geriatric patient: a preliminary report, *J. Am. Geriatr. Soc.,* 1, 280, 1953.
218. **Shapiro, R. P.,** A clinical evaluation of metrazol in senile women, *Clin. Med.,* 62, 29, 1955.
219. **Sluzynski, L.,** Experiences with metrazol therapy in senile individuals, *Ill. Med. J.,* 112, 65, 1957.
220. **Smigel, J. O., Serhus, L. N., and Barmak, S.,** Metrazol: its place in geriatric therapy, *J. Med. Soc. N.J.,* 50, 248, 1953.
221. **Smigel, J. O.,** Mood therapy in the aged, *Med. Times,* 85, 149, 1957.
222. **Sommer, R.,** Oral metrazol therapy in cerebral arteriosclerosis, *Ill. Med. J.,* 106, 323, 1954.
223. **Suter, W. B.,** Oral metrazol therapy in senility (a preliminary report), *Dis. Nerv. Syst.,* 16, 2, 1955.
224. **Thompson, L. J. and Procter, R. C.,** Effect of nicotinic acid and pentylenetetrazol in the therapy of psychiatric symptoms of cerebral arteriosclerosis, *N.C. Med. J.,* 15, 596, 1954.
225. **Travathan, R. D.,** Convulsive seizures during oral pentylenetetrazol therapy, *Geriatrics,* 9, 489, 1954.
226. **Tennent, H. J.,** Experiences with metrazol in psychosis with cerebral arteriosclerosis, *Psychiatr. Q.,* 30, 249, 1956.
227. **Wolff, K.,** Treatment of memory defects in geriatric patients, *Int. J. Neuropsychiatry,* 1, 216, 1965.
228. **Barrabee, P., Wingate, J. H., Phillips, B. D., and Greenblatt, M.,** Effects of L-Glutavite compared with metrazol and vitamins on aged female psychiatric patients, *Postgrad. Med.,* 19, 485, 1956.
229. **Williams, J. R., Csalany, L., and Misevic, G.,** Drug therapy with or without group discussion. Effects of various regimens on the behavior of geriatric patients in a mental hospital, *J. Am. Geriatr. Soc.,* 15, 34, 1967.
230. **Chesrow, E. J., Giacobe, A. J., and Wosika, P. H.,** Metrazol in arteriosclerosis associated with senility, *Geriatrics,* 6, 319, 1951.
231. **Detrick, R. E.,** Pentylenetetrazol with nicotinic acid in the management of chronic brain syndrome, *J. Am. Geriatr. Soc.,* 15, 191, 1967.
232. **Erwin, H. J.,** The geriatric patients; metalex in treatment, *Mo. Med.,* 56, 1971, 1956.
233. **Leckman, J., Ananth, J. V., and Goldberg, R. I.,** A double-blind study of pentylenetetrazol in the treatment of geriatric patients with disturbed memory function, *J. Clin. Pharmacol.,* 11, 301, 1971.
234. **Lu, L., Stotsky, B. A., and Cole, J. O.,** A controlled study of drugs in long-term geriatric psychiatric patients, *Arch. Gen. Psychiatry,* 25, 284, 1971.
235. **Stotsky, B. A., Cole, J. O., Lu, L., and Sniffin, C. M.,** A controlled study of the efficacy of pentylenetetrazol (Metrazol) with hard-core hospitalized psychogeriatric patients, *Am. J. Psychiatry,* 129, 387, 1971.
236. **Ananth, J. V., Deutsch, M., and Ban, T. A.,** Senilex in the treatment of geriatric patients, *Curr. Ther. Res.,* 13, 316, 1971.
237. **Levy, S.,** Pharmacological treatment of aged patients in a state mental hospital, *J. Am. Med. Assoc.,* 153, 1260, 1953.
238. **Mead, S., Mueller, E. E., Mason, E. P., Kheim, T., and Kountz, W. B.,** A study of the effects of oral administration of Metrazol in old individuals, *J. Gerontol.,* 8, 472, 1953.
239. **Swenson, W. M. and Grimes, B. P.,** Oral use of Metrazol in senile patients, *Geriatrics,* 8, 99, 1953.
240. **Kirkpatrick, W. L.,** The relationship between the state mental hospital and the general practitioner, *J. La. State Med. Soc.,* 106, 375, 1954.

241. **Lieberman, A. L., Schwartz, S. S., and Cooper, M.**, Evaluation of intravenous and oral use of Metrazol (pentylenetetrazol) on hospitalized psychiatric patients, *Geriatrics*, 9, 371, 1954.
242. **Gross, M. and Finn, M. H. P.**, Oral Metrazol® (pentylenetetrazol) therapy in psychotic patients, *J. Am. Geriatr. Soc.*, 2, 514, 1954.
243. **Hollister, L. end Fitzpatrick, W. F.**, Oral Metrazol® in the psychosis associated with old age, *J. Am. Geriatr. Soc.*, 3, 197, 1955.
244. **Lapinsohn, L. I.**, Metrazol® or glutamic acid in treating certain mental disorders, *Pa. Med. J.*, 58, 42, 1955.
245. **Linden, M. F., Courtney, E. D., and Howland, A. C.**, Interdisciplinary research in the use of oral pentylenetetrazol (Metrazol®) in the emotional disorders of the aged. Studies in gerontologic human relations, V., *J. Am. Geriatr. Soc.*, 4, 30, 1956.
246. **Johnson, F. G.**, Evaluation of Nicozol in the care of the senile psychotic, *Can. Psych. Assoc. J.*, 2, 132, 1957.
247. **Radich, B.**, Metrazol treatment of the geriatric patient, *Postgrad. Med.*, 22, 603, 1957.
248. **Swenson, W. M., Anderson, D. E., and Grimes, B. P.**, A re-evaluation of the oral use of Metrazol in senile patients, *J. Gerontol.*, 12, 401, 1957.
249. **Sheard, M. H., Coyne, E. P., and Hammons, P.**, A trial of oral Metrazol and nicotine acid in senile patients, *Geriatrics*, 13, 523, 1958.
250. **Haydu, G., Lange, H. S., and Whittier, J. R.**, Effects of Metrazol-vitamin administration in chronic psychoses, *Curr. Ther. Res.*, 3, 255, 1961.
251. **LaBrecque, D. C. and Goldberg, R. I.**, A double-blind study of pentylenetetrazol combined with niacin in senile patients, *Curr. Ther. Res.*, 9, 611, 1967.
252. **Pomeranze, J.**, A new antidepressant (MRD-108) in geriatrics, *J. Gerontol.*, 9, 486, 1954.
253. **Pomeranze, J. and Ladek, R. J.**, Clinical studies in geriatrics. III. The "tonic", *J. Am. Geriatr. Soc.*, 5, 997, 1957.
254. **LeHew, L. J.**, Pipradrol (Meratran) in institutionalized geriatric patients, *J. Am. Geriatr. Soc.*, 5, 534, 1957.
255. **Martin, K. E., Overly, G. H., and Krone, R. E.**, Pipradrol: combined therapy for geriatric and agitated patients, *Int. Record Med.*, 170, 33, 1957.
256. **Kleemeier, R. W., Rich, T. A., and Justiss, W. A.**, Effects of alpha-(2'-piperidyl) benzhydrol hydrochloride (Meratran) on psychomotor performance in group of aged males, *J. Gerontol.*, 11, 165, 1956.
257. **Turek, I., Kurland, A. A., Oya, K. Y., and Hanlon, R. E.**, Effects of pipradrol hydrochloride on geriatric patients, *J. Am. Geriatr. Soc.*, 17, 408, 1969.
258. **Zahn, L.**, Erfahrungen mit einem zentralen stimulans (Ritalin®) bei cerebralen Altersveranderungen, *Berl. Gesundheitsblatt*, 6, 419, 1955.
259. **Bare, W. W.**, A stimulant for the aged. Observations on a methyl-phenidate-vitamin-hormone combination (Ritonic), *J. Am. Geriatr. Soc.*, 8, 292, 1960.
260. **Jocobson, A.**, The use of Ritalin® in psychotherapy of depressions of the aged, *Psychiatr. Q.*, 32, 474, 1958.
261. **Bachrach, S.**, A new stimulant supplement for the geriatric patient, *J. Am. Geriatr. Soc.*, 7, 408, 1959.
262. **Bare, W. W. and Lin, D. Y.**, A stimulant for the aged. II. Long term observations with a methylphenidate-vitamin-hormone combination (Ritonic), *J. Am. Geriatr. Soc.*, 10, 539, 1962.
263. **Darvill, F. T., Jr.**, Double-blind evaluation of methylphenidate (Ritalin®) hydrochloride, *J. Am. Med. Assoc.*, 169, 1739, 1954.
264. **Lehmann, H. E. and Ban, T. A., II.**, Pharmacological load tests as predictors of pharmacotherapeutic response in geriatric patients, in *Psychopharmacology and the Individual Patient*, Wittenborn, J. R., Goldberg, S. C., and May, P. R. A., Eds., Raven Press, New York, 1975, 32.
265. **Crook, T., Ferris, S., Sathananthan, G. et al.**, The effect of methylphenidate on test performance in the cognitively impaired aged, *Psychopharm. Bull.*, 13(3), 46, 1977.
266. **Kaplitz, S. E.**, Withdrawn, apathetic geriatric patients responsive to methylphenidate, *J. Am. Geriatr. Soc.*, 23, 271, 1975.
267. **Sommerness, M. D. and Lucero, R. J.**, Pilot study of effects of stimulant drugs on regressed patients, *Minn. Med.*, 40, 831, 1957.
268. **Jaffe, G. V.**, Depression in general practice. A clinical trial of a new psychomotor stimulant, *Practitioner*, 186, 492, 1961.
269. **Holliday, A. R. and Joffe, J. R.**, A controlled evaluation of protriptyline compared to a placebo and to methylphenidate hydrochloride (abstract), *J. New Drugs*, 5, 257, 1965.
270. **Dube, A. H., Osgood, C. K., and Notkin, H.**, The effects of an analeptic (Ritalin®), an ataraxic (reserpine), and a placebo in senile states, *J. Chron. Dis.*, 5, 220, 1957.
271. **Landman, M. E., Preisig, R., and Perlman, M.**, A practical mood stimulant, *J. Med. Soc. N. J.*, 55, 55, 1958.

272. **Pritchard, J. G. and Mykyta, L. J.,** Use of a combination of methylphenidate and oxprenolol in the management of physically disabled, apathetic, elderly patients: a pilot study, *Curr. Med. Res. Opin.,* 3, 26, 1975.

273. **Salzman, C. and Shader, R. I.,** Responses to psychotropic drugs in the normal elderly, in *Psychopharmacology and Aging,* Eisdorfer, C. and Fann, W. E., Eds., Plenum Press, New York, 1973, 159.

274. **Ferguson, J. T. and Funderbeck, W. H.,** Improving senile behavior with reserpine and Ritalin®, *J. Am. Med. Assoc.,* 160, 259, 1956.

275. **Davidoff, E., Best, J. L., and McPheeters, H.,** Effect of Ritalin® (methylphenidylacetate-hydrochloride) on mildly-depressed ambulatory patients, *N.Y. State J. Med.,* 57, 1753, 1957.

276. **Rickels, K., Gordon, P. E., Gansman, D. H., Weise, C. C., Pereira-Ogan, J. A., and Hesbacher, M. A.,** Pemoline and methylphenidate in mildly depressed outpatients, *Clin. Pharmacol. Ther.,* 11, 698, 1970.

277. **Gilbert, J. G., Donnelly, M. A., Zimmer, L. E., and Kubis, J. F.,** Effect of magnesium pemoline and methylphenidate on memory improvement and mood in normal aging subjects, *Int. J. Aging Human Dev.,* 4, 35, 1973.

278. **Eisdorfer, C., Conner, J. F., and Wilkie, F. L.,** Effect of magnesium pemoline on cognition and behavior, *J. Gerontol.,* 23, 283, 1968.

279. **Droller, H., Bevans, H. G., and Jayaram, V. K.,** Problems of a drug trial (pemoline) on geriatric patients, *Gerontol. Clin.,* 13, 269, 1971.

280. **Goldstein, B. J. and Braunstein, J.,** Clinical evaluation of pemoline and magnesium hydroxide as a mild stimulant in geriatric patients, *Curr. Ther. Res.,* 10, 457, 1968.

281. **Talland, G. A., Hagen, D. Q., and James, R.,** Performance tests of amnesic patient with Cylert, *J. Nerv. Ment. Dis.,* 144, 421, 1967.

282. **Clark, A. N. G. and Mankikar, G. D.,** d-amphetamine in elderly patients refractory to rehabilitation procedures, *J. Am. Geriatr. Soc.,* 27, 174, 1979.

283. **Lehmann, H. E., Ananth, J. V., Geagea, K. C., and Ban, T. A.,** Treatment of depression with Dexadrine® and Demerol®, *Curr. Ther. Res.,* 13, 42, 1971.

284. **Gericke, O. L. and Lobb, L. G.,** Effect of Metrazol on the memory of the aged, *Psych. Studies Proj.,* 2, 2, 1964.

285. **Birkett, D. P. and Boltuch, B.,** Chlorpromazine in geriatric psychiatry, *J. Am. Geriatr. Soc.,* 20, 403, 1972.

NARCOTIC ANALGESICS

Frederick J. Goldstein

INTRODUCTION

Attenuation of pain in the elderly by administration of narcotic analgesics requires greater clinical assessment of the benefit-to-risk ratio than in younger individuals. Side effects related to opiate therapy include nausea, vomiting, constipation, urinary retention, sedation, and reduced respiratory function. These side effects tend to be more debilitating in the aged. A possible consequence of therapy with narcotic analgesics may be the conversion of an independent, ambulatory patient into one who is confined to bed, needing increased levels of attention from health personnel.

CODEINE

More than 30 years ago, Zelman cautioned that excessive use of codeine as an antitussive in geriatric patients could reduce the cough reflex and thereby cause atelectasis secondary to plugged bronchi.[1]

However, even in the course of normal use of codeine, the drug may exert adverse effects upon the respiratory system. In a healthy 75-year-old individual, only 1.5 ℓ of oxygen are extracted from the lung per minute, in comparison to 4 ℓ/min in an average 20-year-old.[2] This difference is probably due, in part, to reduced cardiac output and degenerative changes in lung tissue.[2] Respiratory efficiency is also affected by a decline in the breathing process. For example, maximum breathing capacity may decrease by 40% between 20 and 80 years of age. This change is related to progressive reductions in peripheral neuromuscular activity and associated central nervous system control.[2] The elderly patient may, therefore, be particularly susceptible to any further diminution in respiratory function, as can occur with use of codeine. The dose of codeine should be lowered accordingly.

As indicated above, constipation may result from administration of codeine for cough.[3] Since straining during defecation is undesirable, a modification of diet to include substances that produce a mild laxative effect will be of value in reversing codeine-induced intestinal atony.[3,4]

For low back pain and other types of chronic pain in the elderly, codeine has been recommended as the opiate analgesic.[4,5] For prolonged administration, advantages cited for codeine in comparison to other narcotics include lower toxicity, fewer adverse reactions, and minimal tendency to produce physical dependence.[4,5]

In contrast, when employed for analgesia in treatment of cancer pain in older patients (average age = 58 years), codeine, at 60 or 120 mg administered orally, was not superior to placebo administration.[6] Considering the ineffectiveness in cancer pain and an attendant constipating property, codeine therapy in such individuals seems unwarranted.[6]

MORPHINE

Administration of morphine for severe pain in the elderly is a preferred treatment modality. Extraordinary attention must be given to dosage regimens and patient selection.[7] In particular, patients presenting with deficiencies in respiratory reserve may be so sensitive to morphine that therapeutic doses could produce fatal respiratory depression.[7,8] To minimize the risk of respiratory depression, particularly during immediate postoperative periods, slow intravenous injection is recommended.[9]

An investigation by Bellville et al.[10] involving 712 patients with postoperative pain was designed to evaluate the relationship between narcotic analgesic activity and age. Morphine, 10 mg, was administered intramuscularly. Pain intensity was evaluated every 45 min for approximately 4.5 hr, at which time the antinociceptive activity of morphine was negligible. As patient mean age increased from 30 to 80 years, there was a corresponding elevation in morphine-induced analgesia. Similar relationships were not present with weight or body surface area. Sedation and other side effects were observed to occur with frequencies similar to those observed among subjects of all ages. This suggested that no difference occurred in absorption and distribution patterns of the drug in relation to age. From these data, Bellville et al.[10] concurred with others[11] that sensitivity to pain apparently decreases with age and this factor presumably accounted for the increased analgesic effectiveness of morphine reported by older individuals.

It is not clear whether the half-life of morphine in the circulation is influenced by aging. Stanski et al.,[12] upon injection of morphine (10 mg intravenously in young male volunteers), calculated an elimination half-life of 2.9 ± 0.5 hr. In aged patients who were anesthetized subsequent to morphine treatment, the half-life was 4.5 ± 0.3 hr. Although the dose was higher (45 to 80 mg) in the latter group, it was not regarded as a significant factor. The authors concluded that with advancing age, delayed elimination contributed, in part, to the longer half-life of morphine. In contrast, Berkowitz et al.,[13] after giving morphine (10 mg intravenously) to 31 surgical patients ranging in age from 23 to 75 years, found no difference in serum half-lives. However, morphine serum levels at 2 and 5 min post-injection were significantly higher in the older group (subjects older than 50 years). Reduced cardiac output in the elderly may be responsible for altered distribution of morphine[14] and thus account for the elevated concentrations shortly after injection.[13]

Orally administered morphine is less effective in producing analgesia than parenterally injected morphine. Brompton's mixture is used as the oral form of morphine. It finds its major use in treatment of chronic pain of carcinoma. While the usual oral dose of morphine varies from 5 to 20 mg, elderly patients may experience antinociceptive activity at 2.5 mg.[15]

MEPERIDINE

To provide sedation and analgesia in aged patients being prepared for extensive dental procedures, meperidine, in doses not greater than 25 mg intravenously, has been given safely in combination with other central nervous system depressants and local anesthetics.[16] Prior to elective surgery, 25 to 100 mg were administered subcutaneously without adverse incidence in patients 60 years of age; there was minimal alteration of pO_2 and pCO_2.[17] In both investigations, extreme caution was urged during injection due to the possibility of respiratory depression and hypotension.

A retrospective study of meperidine in 3263 hospitalized patients (mean age = 53 years) revealed that frequency of parenteral administration of 100 mg unit doses decreased from 13.8% in those 20 to 29 years old to 6.2% in subjects 70 and older; age was not a factor in the occurrence of adverse reactions.[18]

Effectiveness of lower doses of meperidine in the elderly may be linked to elevated levels of unbound drug. Following intravenous injection of 50 mg, Mather et al.[19] reported significantly higher fractions of free meperidine in patients over 45 years old than in younger subjects. Circulating half-life of meperidine appears to be unrelated to age. Chan et al.[20] administered meperidine, 1.5 mg/kg intramuscularly, to anesthetized patients under 30 and over 70 years of age. Mean plasma meperidine concentrations at 30 min were much greater in the elderly group; the difference was smaller but remained significant at 8 hr. There were no apparent differences in rate of biotransformation, packed cell volume, or protein binding. However, older patients exhibited a substantially lower percentage binding of meperidine to red blood cells, which may account for the higher free meperidine plasma levels. Elderly subjects also excreted more of the metabolite, normeperidine, probably because of greater entrance of unbound meperidine into hepatic sites of inactivation.[20]

PENTAZOCINE

To alleviate postoperative pain, pentazocine was given in a standardized dose of 20 mg, intramuscularly, to groups of patients ranging in mean age from 30 to 80 years.[10] Generally, pain relief became greater as patient age increased. Similar results were observed with morphine as discussed earlier.

In young (age unspecified) volunteers, pentazocine, 0.2 mg/kg, was injected intravenously during halothane anesthesia.[21] As a result, it was possible to lower the minimum alveolar anesthetic concentration. Pentazocine was, therefore, recommended as an adjunct to halothane use in elderly patients. In contrast to the results obtained in the young group, in a group of 25 males age 60 to 69 years, pentazocine (0.8, 1.3, or 1.8 mg/kg), administered intravenously; it lowered pO_2 and elevated pCO_2 in arterial blood.[22] Thus, if pentazocine is administered to the aged, there may be adverse effects upon the respiratory system.

FENTANYL

As a component of Innovar®, fentanyl provides analgesia during various types of operations. When employed in 35 surgical patients (age range = 18 to 78 years) receiving regional anesthesia, Innovar® reduced the ventilatory response to CO_2.[23] Although this effect was minor and unrelated to age, depression of central sensitivity to CO_2 by Innovar® may be more significant in elderly subjects with preexisting deficiencies in respiratory function.

In 9 patients, 85 to 96 years, fentanyl was administered as an adjunct to flunitrazepam anesthesia.[24] A severe reduction in blood pressure, due to a decline in total peripheral resistance, occurred in four patients. The authors concluded that fentanyl could be utilized in the elderly provided there is adequate preparation to reverse drug-induced hypotensive events.

REFERENCES

1. **Zelman, F. D.,** Infectious diseases in old age, *Clinics,* 4, 1157, 1946.
2. **Timiras, P. S.,** Biological perspectives on aging, *Am. Sci.,* 66, 605, 1978.
3. **Friend, D. G.,** Drug therapy and the geriatric patient, *Clin. Pharmacol. Ther.,* 2, 832, 1961.
4. **Hunt, T. E.,** Management of chronic non-rheumatic pain in the elderly, *J. Am. Geriatr. Soc.,* 24, 402, 1976.
5. **Burton, C., Nida, G., Ray, C., and Heithoff, K.,** Treating low back pain in the elderly, *Geriatrics,* 33, 61, 1978.
6. **Jochimsen, P. R. and Noyes, R.,** Appraisal of codeine as an analgesic in older patients, *J. Am. Geriatr. Soc.,* 26, 521, 1978.
7. **Judge, T. G. and Caird, F. I.,** *Drug Treatment of the Elderly Patient,* Pitman Medical, Kent, England, 1978, 54.
8. **Jaffe, J. H. and Martin, W. R.,** Narcotic analgesics and antagonists, in *The Pharmacological Basis of Therapeutics,* Goodman, L. S. and Gilman, A., Eds., Macmillan, New York, 1975, 245.
9. **Inglis, J. M.,** Premedication in the geriatric patient, *Geriatrics,* 22, 115, 1967.
10. **Bellville, J. W., Forrest, W. H., Jr., Miller, E., and Brown, B. W.,** Influence of age on pain relief from analgesics: a study of postoperative patients, *J. Am. Med. Assoc.,* 217, 1835, 1971.
11. **Sherman, E. D. and Robillard, E.,** Sensitivity to pain in the aged, *Can. Med. Assoc. J.,* 83, 944, 1960.
12. **Stanski, D. R., Greenblatt, D. J., and Lowenstein, E.,** Kinetics of intravenous and intramuscular morphine, *Clin. Pharmacol. Ther.,* 24, 52, 1978.
13. **Berkowitz, B. A., Ngai, S. H., Yang, J. C., Hempstead, B. S., and Spector, S.,** The disposition of morphine in surgical patients, *Clin. Pharmacol. Ther.,* 17, 629, 1975.

14. **Brandfonbrener, M., Landowne, M., and Shock, N.,** Changes in cardiac output with age, *Circulation,* 12, 557, 1955.
15. **Mount, B. M., Ajemian, I., and Scott, J. F.,** Use of the Brompton mixture in treating the chronic pain of malignant disease, *Can. Med. Assoc. J.,* 115, 122, 1976.
16. **Stacy, G. C.,** Methods of attaining sedation for dental procedures, *Aust. Dent. J.,* 19, 100, 1974.
17. **Dobkin, A. B., Su, J. P. G., and Byles, P. H.,** ''Normal'' PaO_2 and SaO_2 in elderly patients and the effect of premedication with atropine and meperidine, *Acta Anaesthesiol. Scand. Suppl.,* 23, 542, 1966.
18. **Miller, R. R. and Jick, H. J.,** Clinical effects of meperidine in hospitalized medical patients, *J. Clin. Pharmacol.,* 18, 180, 1978.
19. **Mather, L. E., Tucker, G. T., Pflug, A. E., and Lindop, M. J.,** Meperidine kinetics in man: intravenous injections in surgical patients and volunteers, *Clin. Pharmacol. Ther.,* 17, 21, 1975.
20. **Chan, K., Kendall, M. J., Mitchard, M., and Wells, W. D. E.,** Proceedings: the effect of ageing on plasma pethidine concentrations, *Br. J. Clin. Pharmacol.,* 2, 297, 1975.
21. **Tsunodo, Y., Hattori, Y., Takatsuka, E., Suwa, T., Hori, T., and Ikezono, E.,** Effects of hydroxyzine, diazepam, and pentazocine on halothane minimum alveolar anesthetic concentration, *Anesth. Analg.,* 52, 390, 1973.
22. **Siemoneit, K. D., Stojilikovic, D., Marquardt, B., Strunz, E., Eberlein, H. J., and Reinhardt, H. W.,** Effects of pentazocine upon arterial blood gases. A study in elderly subjects, *Arzneim Forsch.,* 24, 1835, 1974.
23. **Mulroy, M. F., Coombs, J. H. B., Isenberg, M. D., and Fairley, H. B.,** Age, chronic obstrucive pulmonary disease, and Innovar®-induced ventilatory depression during regional anesthesia, *Anesth. Analg.,* 56, 826, 1977.
24. **Haldemann, G., Hossli, G., and Schaer, H.,** Die anaesthesie mit rohypnol (fluritrazepam) und fentanyl beim geriatrischen patienten, *Anaesthesist,* 26, 168, 1977.

AGE-ASSOCIATED CHANGES OF NONNARCOTIC ANALGESICS

Steven I. Baskin and Allan H. Goldfarb

INTRODUCTION

Aspirin and nonnarcotic analgesics can be effective antipyretic, analgesic, and anti-inflammatory agents, but their use in the elderly is often excessive.[1] In a survey by Gillies and Skyring,[2] the overall prevalence of daily aspirin intake was greater in middle- and older-age groups than in persons less than 40 years of age. Age-related physiological changes modify the response to aspirin in the elderly. The cases cited throughout this report substantiate the need for caution on the part of the geriatric patient and the patient's physician when considering analgesic therapy.

Additional investigations are needed to determine the full range of side effects and their seriousness for the nonnarcotic analgesics often prescribed for elderly patients. It is also important to discover more about the mechanism of these side effects and to better understand the pharmacologic interactions of drugs in the elderly.

The easy availability and the numerous therapeutic applications of nonnarcotic analgesic compounds make them one of the most commonly used groups of agents worldwide. Aspirin, the best known nonnarcotic analgesic, is used variously as an analgesic and an anti-inflammatory agent. Significant age-related differences in both therapeutic and toxic effects of aspirin and aspirin-related compounds have been observed in a number of recent studies. As will be detailed in what follows, these will be drawn upon in determining what the age-related effects of nonnarcotic analgesics are as a whole. This review evaluates the clinical and pharmacological studies which do exist.

ASPIRIN

Intolerance to aspirin has been documented during almost the entire history of its clinical use. Reports of death resulting from aspirin overdose are scattered throughout the literature. Angioedema and rhinitis, nasal polyposis, bronchial asthma, and the development of gastric complications (i.e., gastrointestinal upset, gastric ulcer, and gastric and duodenal bleeding) are commonly cited toxic reactions to aspirin.[1] Abdominal pain, nausea, tinnitus, shock, and unconsciousness are additional possible manifestations of aspirin toxicity.[3,4] Disturbances of acid-base balance have been attributed to aspirin.[3,4] Respiratory alkalosis resulting from altered respiratory stimulation has also been documented.[3,4] Approximately 10% of all adverse drug reactions that have been reported in American hospitals appear to be aspirin related. Stanford University Hospital reports that of the cases of toxicity it encountered from August 1974 to March 1975, the third highest number were related to salicylates.[5] These statistics indicate the necessity for a greater understanding of the toxic mechanisms of salicylates and nonnarcotic analgesics.

A documented composite of the dangerous side effects associated with nonnarcotic analgesics, particularly as a function of age, is necessary to aid the practicing physician.[6] Given common prescription patterns of physicians, an increase in immune response in elderly patients and an increase in arthritic types of diseases often results in elderly patients taking increasing amounts of aspirin or other nonnarcotic analgesic compounds.[7] Also, because of the increased incidence of pain due to diseases particularly prevalent in the elderly,[8] not only may the frequency of usage increase, but there may also be an increased dosage of aspirin. The normal adult dose range for aspirin as an analgesic is 300 to 1000 mg 4 times per day.[9] Toxicity, which is variable, can result from doses of aspirin as low as 5 g/day, but usually occurs between 10 to 15 g.[4,9]

Table 1
PHARMACOKINETICS OF NONNARCOTIC ANALGESICS

Drug	Time to peak absorption (hr)	Plasma half-life (hr)	Plasma protein binding (%)	Biotransformation	Dosage
Salicylates	2	3—6 (low dose)[a] 15—30 (high dose)[b]	50—90	Hepatic microsomal and mitochondrial systems	325 mg to 1.0 gm every 4 hr not to exceed 3.6 g/day
Aspirin	2	0.33			
Phenylbutazone	2	50—100	90—98	Hepatic microsomal system	400—600 mg/day
Indomethacin	3	2	90	Hepatic microsomal and mitochondrial systems	25—50 mg twice daily
Acetaminophen	1/2—1	1— 3	25—50	Hepatic microsomal system	325—650 mg every 4 hr not to exceed 2.6 g/day
Antipyrine[c]	1—2	7—20	<10	Hepatic microsomal system	300—600 mg every 4 hr not to exceed 4.0 g/day

[a] A low dose is represented by 1 gm or less per day.
[b] A high dose is represented by 3 gm or more per day.
[c] Sales prohibited in the U.S.

Absorption of aspirin is rapid, partly from the stomach, but mostly from the upper small intestine. Absorption occurs by passive diffusion and is affected by pH and the presence of food. Once absorbed into the circulation, salicylates are rapidly distributed throughout the body by pH-dependent passive processes. Plasma concentrations of aspirin are usually low and rarely exceed 20 µg/mℓ at ordinary therapeutic doses. Salicylates are bound to plasma protein to the extent of 50 to 90%, principally to albumin.

The major sites for biotransformation of salicylates are the microsomal and mitochondrial enzyme systems of the liver. Salicylates and metabolites are eventually excreted primarily by the kidney. The plasma half-life for aspirin is approximately 20 min; for salicylate it depends on the dosage. At low doses, plasma half-life is dependent on the ability of the liver to transform salicylate to its metabolites.

With decreased renal and liver function (see chapter by Dr. Richey), the elderly patient may not be sufficiently equipped to handle increasing loads of nonnarcotic analgesic agents and drugs in general.[10] Table 1 illustrates some differences and similarities in the pharmacokinetic profiles of nonnarcotic analgesics. The time to peak absorption of drug, the plasma half-life, the percent of drug bound to plasma proteins, and the dosage of drug are factors which should be considered when administering these agents. The comparison of data in Tables 1 and 2 should provide insight into how a knowledge of the pharmacokinetics of nonnarcotic analgesics can enable a more rational use of these drugs in the geriatric patient.

PROPOSED MECHANISM OF NONNARCOTIC ANALGESICS

Acetylsalicylic acid (aspirin) was first used for medicinal purposes some 75 years ago.[9] Despite the long and widespread use of salicylates in medicine, it was not until recently that the mechanism for their mode of action was discovered.[11] Vane found that aspirin inhibited prostaglandin biosynthesis in various species of animals, including man.[12] In man, this inhibition is achieved with ordinary therapeutic doses.[13]

It is helpful to look at the biosynthetic pathway of prostaglandins (PG) in order to understand the step at which aspirin influences the process.

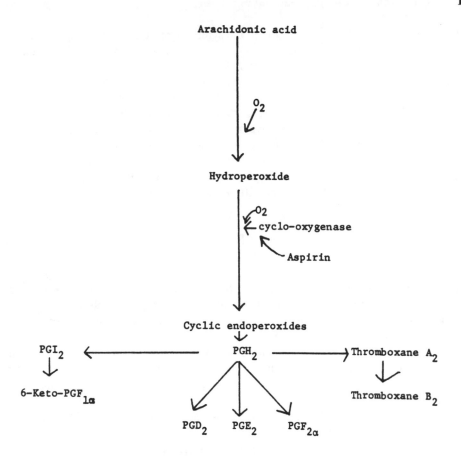

The cyclo-oxygenase enzyme system is necessary to generate cyclic endoperoxides from the precursor arachidonic acid, an essential fatty acid.[11] It is at this point in the synthetic chain that aspirin exerts its inhibitory effect by acetylating the active site of the cyclo-oxygenase enzyme protein.[12]

Endoperoxidases participate in various physiological as well as pathological processes in the body, such as anaphylaxis and thrombosis.[11,13] PGE_1, PGE_2, and Thromboxane A_2 can cause edema.[14] The pathology of fever may be due to the effects of PGE_1 and PGE_2 on the central nervous system (CNS).[15] PGE_1 and PGE_2 have been implicated in the production of fever systemically by actions in the anterior hypothalamic preoptic region.[16] Aspirin can also inhibit PG synthesis in the CNS.[17] The ability of aspirin to inhibit PG synthesis in the CNS, together with the action of PG in the CNS, does not negate a peripheral site of action for aspirin, as has been held for some time.

It has been demonstrated that PGs produce pain along the veins into which they are infused, and headache may also result.[18,19]

Prostaglandins protect the stomach lining by promoting mucus production, decreasing acid production, and increasing the blood supply to the mucosa.[20] Aspirin inhibition of PG synthesis in the stomach causes a decrease in mucin, an increased acid level, and a decrease in blood supply to the gastric lining.[20] This condition may lead to gastric problems such as gastric ulceration.

Asthma attacks in patients sensitive to aspirin have also been related to the ability of the drug to inhibit PG synthesis. Two PGs have been identified in the lung: PGE_1, a bronchodilator found primarily in the airways; and $PGF_{2\alpha}$, a bronchoconstrictor found primarily in the parenchyma. Szczeklik et al.[21] proposed that asthma attacks may be related to an imbalance of the two different groups of PG. The bronchoconstrictor, $PGE_{2\alpha}$, is balanced by the bronchodilator, PGE_1. Inhibition of the synthesis of PGE_1, for example, would result in bronchoconstriction via the action of $PGF_{2\alpha}$, as well as histamine (a bronchoconstrictor) which is also physiologically balanced by PGE_1.

Vane proposed that any biological reaction which is in some way changed or prevented by non-narcotic analgesics is probably a result of the inhibition of PG synthesis.[11] The inhibitory effects of nonnarcotic analgesics on PG synthesis in the elderly should be investigated to determine if these agents have similar actions as in younger populations. Such studies would help to clarify some of the toxic side effects observed in the elderly (e.g., acid-base imbalance, nasal polyposis, and bronchial asthma). To date, no such studies have been performed. Based on actions of aspirin in elderly (e.g., analgesic, anti-inflammatory, and antipyretic), one would expect the differences (inability to inhibit PG synthesis) to be quantitative and not qualitative.

AGE-ASSOCIATED CONSIDERATIONS IN PHARMACOKINETICS AND SIDE EFFECTS

Most of the work on the pharmacology of nonnarcotic analgesics in relation to age has been in the area of pharmacokinetics. Thus, for several drugs, the plasma half-life (t1/2), volume of distribution (V≡) and clearance (C) have been determined in young and old humans. These data are given in Table 2.

Two case reports point to serious consequences in elderly patients undergoing therapy of glaucoma with carbonic anhydrase inhibitor in combination with therapy of chronic arthritis with aspirin.[41] Systemic acidosis, an inevitable concern in therapy with carbonic anhydrase inhibitors, enhances the transport of salicylates into the CNS. High doses of salicylates can cause CNS dysfunction (e.g., acid-base imbalance). It has been postulated that in the elderly trying to compensate for decreased blood flow, more blood is sent to the brain, muscles, and heart. If this is true, increased blood volume might cause higher amounts of aspirin to be available to the CNS.[42]

The absorption of acidic drugs is not significantly impaired in the elderly.[43] However, other factors involved in drug disposition are altered, e.g., renal function is diminished.[22,44,45] With increasing age, there is a progressive loss of nephrons, together with a decrease in renal blood flow, glomerular filtration rate, and renal tubular secretion. The accumulation of these factors can result in higher, perhaps toxic, levels of salicylates being retained in the body.[17] Diminished glomerular filtration rate appears to be correlated with severity of rheumatoid disease.[46,47] Nonnarcotic analgesics may exacerbate this already diminished renal function by causing further renal impairment.[47]

Slight changes in urine pH alter renal capacity for aspirin excretion. Acidic urine favors reabsorption of salicylates by the renal tubules, while alkaline urine brings about excretion of salicylates from the body. Alkalinizing and acidifying agents can, therefore, interact with salicylates by altering urine pH.[44]

Murray et al.[48] conducted a 5-year study of patients who misused analgesics. These patients were admitted initially with a raised blood urea but with no other obvious cause of renal damage except analgesic abuse. All of the patients were warned of the dangers of continued analgesic abuse. Renal function deteriorated in 23 of 28 patients who persisted in abuse. Of these 28 patients, 11 died of renal failure. Of the 26 patients who ceased abuse, renal function remained static in 6, was improved in 17, and failed in 3, resulting in death.

Russel et al.[49] found raised serum transaminase levels correlated with high levels of salicylates. Pronounced transaminase levels per se are often indicative of significant liver damage. Aspirin alone does not appear to cause liver damage in the healthy adult. It may, however, exacerbate preexisting liver diseases.[20]

Toxicity seems to be related to tissue, rather than blood levels of salicylates.[41] The

Table 2
PHARMACOKINETICS OF NONNARCOTIC ANALGESICS IN THE YOUNG AND ELDERLY

Drug	Ages	Half-life (hr)	Volume of distribution	Clearance rate	Ref.
Acetaminophen	22—27	1.82	1.03	477mℓ/min/1.73M²	22
	73—91	2.18	1.05	379mℓ/min/1.72M²	
	20—40	1.79	—	—	23
	Over 65	2.27	—	—	
	23.9	—	0.62	21.8 ℓ/hr	24
	75.8	—	0.48	14.4 ℓ/hr	
	20—40	1.75	0.863	0.340 ℓ/kg/hr	25
	Over 65	2.17	0.771	0.254 ℓ/kg/hr	
Aminopyrine	25—30	3.3	—	—	26
	65—80	8.1	—	—	
Antipyrine	20—50	12.0	40.6	2.4 ℓ/hr	27
	70—100	17.4	31.2	1.5 ℓ/hr	28
	18—39	12.7	0.57	0.34⁶ ℓ/kg/hr	29
	60—92	14.8	0.54	0.0282 ℓ/kg/hr	
	20—40	12.5	—	—	23
	Over 65	16.8	—	—	
	20—40	12.5	0.60	—	30
	Over 65	16.8	0.56	—	
	22—72	—	—	↓	31
	Old	—	—	↓	
		11.8	41.6	41.8 ℓ	36
		16.7 N[a]	32.8 N[a]	24.1 N[a]	
		10.4 H[b]	28.0 H[b]	33.7 H[b]	
Indomethacin	20—50	1.53	—	—	32
	71—83	1.73	—	—	
	22—59	2.06	47.52	7.79	33
	Old	—	—	—	
Phenylbutazone	20—50	81.2	9.6	0.086 ℓ/hr	27
	70—100	104.6	0.2	0.065 ℓ/hr	28
	22—30	110	0.172	—	22
	73—91	87	0.165	—	
		—	0.172	—	34
		—	0.165	—	
	Offspring	110	—	—	35
	Parents	109	—	—	
Salicylates		3—6[c]	0.150	—	9
		15—30[d]	—	—	37
		10.0	—	—	38
		—	—	—	
(Aspirin)		0.33	—	—	9
		—	—	—	
(Aspirin)		0.29	—	—	39
		—	—	—	
(Aspirin)		—	0.08	0.02 ℓ/kg/hr	40
		—	0.11	0.017 ℓ/kg/hr	

[a] N = normal.
[b] H = hospitalized.
[c] 3 to 6 hr in low doses (less than 1 gm).
[d] 15 to 30 hr in high doses (3 gm or greater).

therapeutic ratio, [ED_{50}(ulcerogenic action)/$ED_{20\text{-}30}$ (anti-inflammatory action)] is relatively high compared to other nonsteroidal anti-inflammatory drugs.[50] The required therapeutic dosage in the elderly is often high (greater than 1.0 g/day) for the treatment of rheumatoid arthritis and other chronic pain. At the same time, toxic salicylate levels are reached at lower dosages in the elderly.[7] Thus, the safety margin between therapeutic and toxic doses is narrowed.

Several problems arise with the aged when diagnosing the etiology of chronic pain other than pain associated with rheumatism.[7] Attention span is limited and many problems stem from difficulty in communication.[1] Minor incidents (e.g., falling against a piece of furniture) which serve as precipitating agents at the onset of pain may be forgotten soon afterwards.[7,51] Thus, inaccurate data concerning the onset of pain results in the overlooking of clues helpful in diagnosis of dosage. "Aches and pains," especially of the rheumatoid variety, are common in the elderly. Elderly patients may often have trouble describing general aches in an accurate fashion, since referred pain tends to dominate over local pain at the site of origin.[7] As a result of the process of aging, perception and recognition of pain may be irregularly altered.[7]

Self-medication errors can occur more easily in elderly patients because of failing vision and decreased mental activity, especially if tablets or capsules of various sizes, shapes, and colors are prescribed concurrently.[15] A survey by Achong et al.[15] revealed that approximately two thirds of the patients undergoing long-term institutionalization had either physical or mental impairment, or both, causing an inability to self-administer medication.[15] A review of elderly patients living at home disclosed that not less than 25% made errors in self-administration of medication.[5]

In general, drug interactions occur more frequently in the elderly and their consequences can be hazardous.[52] Due to multiple health problems among the elderly, several different drug therapies may be administered simultaneously along with aspirin. Drug interactions may occur by the mechanism of displacement of one drug by another at the protein-binding sites. This displacement creates higher than expected levels of the displaced drug in the free state. Salicylates have been shown to exhibit this mechanism of drug interaction.[9,53] Displacement effects are more likely to occur in the elderly than in other age groups as a result of a decrease in serum albumin levels.[1]

Clinically significant interactions can occur between aspirin and oral hypoglycemic agents, methotrexate, uricosuric agents, spironolactone, corticosteroids, and nonsteroidal anti-inflammatory agents.[20] Gokal and Matthews showed evidence linking a nonsteroidal compound (alclofenac) in combination with aspirin to the development of renal papillary necrosis.[54] Aspirin increases prothrombin time and inhibits the second phase of platelet aggregation. Aspirin used concurrently with an anticoagulant may cause severe hemorrhage.[1]

In regulating aspirin dosage for intensive salicylate therapy, the clinical precept often is to increase the dose until tinnitus is observed, then decrease dosage slightly to a subtinnitus level.[55] However, in the elderly, tinnitus is not always a reliable clinical guide for salicylate toxicity. Monitoring of serum salicylate levels provides a more reliable guide for dose determination in the elderly. Experiments have shown that salicylates can cause pathological cochlear changes and deafness.[56,57] In a study of salicylate ototoxicity, a 76-year-old woman receiving approximately 4.0 g/day of aspirin as therapy for rheumatoid arthritis complained of decreased bilateral hearing but had no complaint of tinnitus.[56] She had no previous history of ear disease. Within 3 days after cessation of salicylate therapy, her hearing improved significantly. It was concluded that salicylate ototoxicity is reversible. Experimental evidence suggests that aspirin-induced deafness correlates with the unit dose of aspirin.[57]

Sahud and Cohen suggested that patients receiving high-dose aspirin therapy for rheumatoid arthritis take vitamin C supplements.[58] Their investigation showed that rheumatoid patients receiving constant large doses of aspirin had drastically reduced platelet and plasma levels of ascorbic acid.

Aspirin has been known to induce asthmatic episodes.[59] The triad of symptoms, skin reactions, nasal polyposis, and bronchial asthma, are characteristic of aspirin intolerance, a disease entity in itself.[3,59] Although not every patient experiences every aspect of the aspirin intolerance syndrome, the onset and progression of the changes occurring in the skin and respiratory tract usually demonstrate the following pattern: (1) vasomotor rhinitis, developing in the second or third decade; (2) bilateral nasal and paranasal polyps; (3) bronchial asthma occurring as a rule, in middle age. The severity of the reactions is largely an idiosyncratic function of the individual patient and tends to remain the same regardless of the frequency with which patients have taken aspirin in the past.[3]

Gastrointestinal irritation is experienced by 2 to 10% of the people who take aspirin occasionally. Among rheumatoid patients on high-dose aspirin therapy, about 30 to 50% experience disturbing gastrointestinal distress and about 25% of these patients have to discontinue the drug.[20] Gastric damage is thought to be the most serious adverse effect of aspirin ingestion.[60] A histological study of 51 patients with chronic gastric ulcers indicated an association between habitual use of aspirin-containing preparations and ulceration of the mucosa.[61] A study by Duggan and Chapman supported the hypothesis that aspirin ingestion is a cause of gastric ulcer.[62] However, their study suggested that there is no association between aspirin and duodenal ulcer. Jabbari and Valberg found that the gastric mucosa of achlorhydria patients is less susceptible to aspirin-induced gastric mucosal injury than that of subjects with normal gastric acid levels.[63] Hydrochloric acid is not essential for the occurrence of aspirin-induced occult gastrointestinal blood loss. This blood loss is significantly increased in patients with pernicious anemia and/or achlorhydria.[64]

It has been claimed that gastrointestinal blood loss is clinically insignificant in almost all patients taking moderate-to-high doses of aspirin. Hemorrhage of any other origin in the gastrointestinal tract may be a more serious and life-threatening type of blood loss than that induced by aspirin. A study by Duggan suggested that a significant relationship between aspirin and acute hemorrhage exists and depends on the repeated use of aspirin rather than on its isolated administration.[65] A report by Valman and associates,[66] on the other hand, confirmed that aspirin is a precipitating factor in overt hemorrhage in acute and chronic peptic ulcers, and that it is a significant cause of gastric and/or duodenal bleeding in absence of a chronic peptic ulcer.

It has been suggested that aspirin may be a causal factor in iron deficiency anemia observed in the elderly.[53] Aspirin has also been found to be a causative agent of aplastic anemia.[67]

Venous and arterial thrombosis are problems among the elderly which may create complications during surgery and postoperatively.[68-70] On the basis that aspirin inhibits the second phase of platelet aggregation in vitro, it was proposed in several studies that aspirin may exert an antithrombotic effect in vivo.[68-70] However, the results of these studies indicate that aspirin does not exhibit an antithrombotic effect.

Two independent studies propose that aspirin protects against nonfatal myocardial infarction.[71,72] The results of one study were inconclusive,[71] while the data of the second study were consistent with the hypothesis that aspirin reduces myocardial infarction.[72] Results inconsistent with this hypothesis were reported in a similar study by Hammond and Garfinkel.[73] Additional studies are necessary to provide further information concerning the relationship between aspirin and acute myocardial infarction.

Since 1966, studies have reported that acetaminophen (paracetamol) is potentially fatal.[74-78] Acetaminophen can cause centrilobular hepatic necrosis and hepatic failure.[79] The mechanism for acetaminophen hepatoxicity has been elucidated by Mitchell et al.[75,80-82] Normally, only a small proportion of acetaminophen is metabolized to a toxic metabolite by the hepatic cytochrome P-450 mixed-function oxidase system.[75,80] Detoxification of this metabolite occurs by conjugation with glutathione and excretion in this form.[81] In cases of acetaminophen overdose, when a relatively greater amount of the toxic metabolite is formed, there is insufficient glutathione to combine with all of the metabolite, enabling the excess to bind with other components of the cell to produce necrosis. This problem may be more severe in the elderly as a result of their decreased ability to metabolize and detoxify certain substances in the body. For example, Kato and Takanaka have reported a decreased ability to metabolize a number of related drugs in old (600 day) rats.[83] These in vitro studies demonstrated hepatic cytochrome P-450 mixed-function oxidase system activity was decreased in both male and female old (600 day) rats. In a follow-up investigation, Kato and Takanaka compared the ability of young (40, 100, and 300 days) and old (600 days) rats to metabolize drugs in vivo.[84] They reported a decreased ability to metabolize carisoprodol and pentobarbital by the old (600 days) rats. The decreased biotransformation was attributed to a decrease in hepatic microsomal enzyme activity. This study did not consider changes in blood flow with aging, which might have contributed to the altered metabolism in the older animals. Fulton et al.[24] compared the pharmacokinetics of acetaminophen in the elderly. The elderly group (mean age, 75.8 years) demonstrated an increase in plasma acetaminophen and a decrease in clearance compared to a young group (mean age, 23.9 years). It was suggested that the bioavailability of acetaminophen was normal in the elderly, but its conjugation was impaired. These investigators did not measure the conjugated metabolite of acetaminophen to determine if the elderly demonstrated impaired hepatic microsomal enzyme activity. Triggs et al.[22] determined the pharmacokinetics of acetaminophen in the elderly (mean age 80.9 years). The results suggest impaired metabolism of acetaminophen. They measured unconjugated and conjugated metabolites excreted in the urine after 24 hr. The elderly group (age 73 to 91 years) demonstrated a wide range (1.7 to 51.7%) in percentage of total unconjugated drug excretion; whereas, the young group demonstrated a narrow range. Unfortunately, three of the geriatric subjects were receiving other drugs which might have influenced the results. It is recommended, therefore, that in further studies of acetaminophen conjugation in the elderly, the results be adjusted to blood flow rates or else be expressed as percentage of total drug conjugated, to determine whether hepatic microsomal enzyme activity in vivo is impaired. Swift et al.[36] studied the disposition of antipyrine in relation to liver size in the elderly (age 70 to 89 years). They found the liver volume to be decreased. Antipyrine plasma half-life was prolonged and its clearance was reduced in normal, nonhospitalized elderly individuals. There was no difference of antipyrine elimination in an elderly hospitalized group compared to a young group. It was concluded that both decreased liver mass and decreased hepatic enzyme activity contributed to the impairment of drug biotransformation in the elderly. Unfortunately, these investigators did not measure hepatic enzyme activity or the conjugated and nonconjugated metabolites of this drug to confirm their conclusions. To understand the changes in drug metabolism that might occur in the elderly, Jori et al.[26] investigated the metabolites of aminopyrine in persons aged 65 to 86 years. They reported a decrease with increasing age in the hydroxylation of aminopyrine. Wallace and Whiting explored some of the factors that might affect the binding of nonnarcotic analgesics in plasma.[85] They concluded that higher concentrations of free-drug occur in the elderly (mean age 81.5 years) partly as a result of decreased concentrations of plasma albumin. They also stressed that with multiple drug therapy elderly patients are more susceptible to side effects resulting from the decreased availability of drug-binding sites.

Progeria (a disorder of premature aging) has been utilized as a model for aging, for example, in a study by Caldwell and co-workers.[87] The metabolism of acetaminophen in a child with progeria was investigated and compared to its metabolism in both a normal child and in an adult. The comparison indicated that acetaminophen was biotransformed differently by the progeria subject than by either the normal child or the adult. Most of the conjugated acetaminophen in the progeria subject was in the sulphate form, whereas in both the normal child and the adult, most of the conjugate was in the glucuronide form. Therefore, it appears that progeria is not a good model for studying drug biotransformation in relation to aging.

Side effects of nonnarcotic analgesics may occur more frequently in the elderly than in the young for several reasons. The aged are more likely to have multiple diseases which can alter the body's ability to handle drugs. They utilize a greater number of different drugs, which increases the likelihood for drug interaction. Their homeostatic mechanisms could be less adaptable to drug side effects than those of younger persons. Unfortunately, there are still too few studies which have addressed the issue of side effects resulting from nonnarcotic analgesics in the elderly.

McMahon et al.[88] investigated the effects of fenoprofen in 24 female geriatric patients (48 to 75 years) with osteoarthritis. Fenoprofen was compared with aspirin and a placebo for ability to relieve pain. The results showed fenoprofen and aspirin equal in effectiveness and both provided significantly greater relief of osteoarthritis symptoms than the placebo. This study also demonstrated a broad spectrum of side effects for both aspirin and fenoprofen: these included nausea, vomiting, dyspepsia, tinnitus, blurred vision, dizziness, nervousness, headache, and skin rash. Unfortunately, all of the patients in this study had at least one other concomitant illness, thus making it difficult to interpret the findings.

Inman investigated the cause of fatal bone marrow depression in relation to age in 269 patients whose death certificate did not mention a drug as the possible cause of aplastic anemia or agranulocytosis.[89] It was concluded that 83 deaths were probably attributable to drugs, the most common being phenylbutazone (28 cases) and oxyphenbutazone (11 cases). The probability of death due to phenylbutazone has been estimated as 0.5 per 100,000 for men under age 65, and 1.3 per 100,000 for men aged 65 or older. For women, it is 1.2 per 100,000 at ages under 65 and 6.5 per 100,000 for ages 65 or older. The dosage used by these patients was not abnormally high; usually 100 mg, 3 times daily.

Larsen and Moller have reported that prolonged misuse of phenacetin reduces the concentrating ability of the kidneys, resulting in uremia.[90] Kasanen and Salmi found that of 800 patients studied, 21% were daily users of phenacetin.[91] They reported a positive relationship of renal disease with the use of phenacetin, i.e., the more prevalent the use of phenacetin, the more common the renal disease. Ruikka and Sourander investigated the occurrence of urinary tract infection in relation to phenacetin consumption in geriatric hospital patients.[92] They reported no difference in the percentage of cases demonstrating urinary tract infection in users compared with nonusers of phenacetin, and there was no difference in this relationship with respect to age.

Triggs et al.[22] reported no difference in the rate of gastrointestinal absorption of acetaminophen and phenylbutazone in the elderly (mean age 80.9 years). Unfortunately, three of the seven geriatric subjects received other drugs during the study, so the findings lost some of their significance. Salem and Stevenson investigated the absorption kinetics of aspirin in the elderly (age greater than 65) and reported no significant difference in the absorption rate compared to the rate in younger individuals.[40] Melander and associates studied the absorption of a single dose of a combination tablet containing acetylsalicylic acid, antipyrine, and d-propoxyphene.[93] They reported no significant differences in the absorption of the different drugs in the elderly. The problems with this investigation were the small number of subjects (six) and the wide interindividual variation within the groups, i.e., the time range of drug absorption was from 20 to 125 min. Crooks et al.[94] reported no major change attributable to age in absorption of drugs they examined. Castelden and co-workers[95] determined the absorption rate of a single dose of aspirin in young and old subjects. They found no drug- or age-related differences. It is suggested that this area be further investigated to obtain a clearer understanding of absorption kinetics as they relate to age.

O'Malley et al.[28] have reported that the apparent volume of distribution of phenylbutazone was significantly increased in their geriatric group. In the same investigation, antipyrine demonstrated a similar volume of distribution for the two age groups. Triggs reported no significant difference between young and aged groups in the apparent volume of distribution of acetaminophen and phenylbutazone.[22] Liddell et al.[30] also reported no significant differences in the volume of distribution of antipyrine in a geriatric group compared to a young group. Salem and Stevenson have also found similar volumes of distribution of aspirin in the elderly and young subjects.[40] Fulton et al.[24] reported, however, a significant reduction in the volume of distribution for acetaminophen in the aged. Further investigations are recommended to determine if the volume of distribution for all drugs is altered in the elderly.

The plasma half-lives of antipyrine and phenylbutazone were studied in the elderly (65 to 85 years) by O'Malley.[28] The mean plasma half-life of antipyrine in this geriatric group was significantly longer than in a control group of younger persons (ages 20 to 50 years). O'Malley et al.[27] found the half-lives of antipyrine and phenylbutazone to be prolonged in a group of geriatric patients. For phenylbutazone, a longer half-life was found in the control group, but the difference between the control and old groups was not significant. Liddell et al.[30] reported results which concur with those of O'Malley. They found an increased plasma half-life of antipyrine in a geriatric group (mean age 78.9 years). Triggs et al.[22] reported significant increases in plasma half-life for acetaminophen in the elderly. Phenylbutazone half-life was not significantly diffferent in the elderly group in this investigation. Vestal et al.[29] have reported an increase in plasma half-life for antipyrine in the aged. It appears that antipyrine has an increased half-life in the elderly; whereas, results with phenylbutazone do not always demonstrate this effect in the elderly.

Fulton et al.[24] reported that acetaminophen clearance was significantly reduced in the aged as compared with the young. Vestal et al.[29] found a decreased clearance of antipyrine in the elderly. It was indicated that clearance rates were widely scattered for all ages. Wood et al.[31] demonstrated a reduction in the clearance of antipyrine in the aged. It was also reported that smoking decreases clearance more drastically in the elderly than in younger subjects. Salem and Stevenson have reported no difference between young and old persons in the clearance of aspirin.[40] Triggs et al.[22] found acetaminophen plasma clearance was not significantly different between young and geriatric subjects. Clearance studies indicate differences among the nonnarcotic analgesics, but there are insufficient data as yet for making definitive statements regarding the nature of the differences.

CONCLUSION

In conclusion, the pharmacological processes which are responsible for determining the capacity and frequency of drugs to interact with biological receptors most certainly appear to be affected by the process which we call aging. For nonnarcotic analgesics, as well as other drugs to be used properly in the treatment or diagnosis of disease in the elderly, the pharmacology of drugs must be utilized.

REFERENCES

1. **Ward, M. and Blatman, M.,** Drug therapy in the elderly, *Am. Family Physician*, 19(2), 143, 1979.
2. **Gillies, M. A. and Skyring, A. P.,** The pattern and prevalence of aspirin ingestion as determined by interview of 2,921 inhabitants of Sydney, *Med. J. Aust.*, 1, 974, 1972.
3. **Samter, M. and Beers, R. F.,** Intolerance to aspirin, clinical studies and consideration of its pathogenesis, *Ann Intern. Med.*, 68, 975, 1968.
4. **Ali Abrishami, M. and Thomas, J.,** Aspirin intolerance, a review, *An. Allergy*, 39, 28, 1977.
5. **Stewart, R. B. and Cluff, L. E.,** A review of medication errors and compliance in ambulent patients, *Clin. Pharmacol. Ther.*, 13, 463, 1972.
6. **Mendelson, J. and Grisolia, S.,** Age-dependent sensitivity to salicylate, *Lancet*, 2, 974, 1975.

7. **Hunt, T. E.,** Management of chronic non-rheumatic pain in the elderly, *J. Am. Geriatr. Soc.,* 24, 402, 1979.
8. **Reichel, W.,** *Clinical Aspects of Aging,* Williams & Wilkins, Baltimore, 1978, 3.
9. **Goodman, L. S. and Gilman, A.,** *The Pharmacological Basis of Therapeutics,* 5th ed., Macmillan, New York, 1975.
10. **Birnbaum, L. S. and Malcolm, B. B.,** Induction of hepatic mixed function oxidases in senescent rodents, *Exp. Gerontol.,* 13, 229, 1978.
11. **Vane, J. R.,** The mode of action of aspirin and similar compounds, *Hosp. Form.,* 10-11, 618, 1976.
12. **Vane, J. R.,** Inhibition of prostaglandin synthesis as a mechanism of action for aspirin-like drugs, *Nature (London), New Biol.,* 231, 232, 1971.
13. **Roth, G. J., Stanford, N., and Majerus, P. W.,** Acetylation of prostaglandin synthetase by aspirin, *Proc. Natl. Acad. Sci., U.S.A.,* 72, 3073, 1975.
14. **Glenn, E. M., Bowman, B. J., and Rohloff, N. A.,** Proinflammatory effects of certain prostaglandins, in *Prostaglandins in Cellular Biology,* Ramwell, P. W. and Pharris, B. B., Eds., Plenum Press, New York, 1972, 329.
15. **Achong, M. R., Bayne, J. R. D., Gerson, L. W., and Golshani, W.,** Prescribing of psychoactive drugs for chronically ill elderly patients, *Can. Med. Assoc. J.,* 188, 1503, 1978.
16. **Wolfe, L. S. and Coceani, F.,** The role of prostaglandins in the central nervous system, *Ann. Rev. Physiol.,* 41, 669, 1979.
17. **Anon.,** Drugs and the elderly, *Lancet,* 2, 693, 1977.
18. **Bergstrom, S., Duner, H., von Euler, U. S., Pernow, B. J., and Sjovall, J.,** Observations on the effects of infusion of prostaglandin E in man, *Acta Physiol. Scand.,* 45, 145, 1959.
19. **Collier, J. G., Karim, S. M. M., Robinson, B., and Somers, K.,** Action of prostaglandins A_2, B_1, E_2 and F_2 on superficial hand veins of man, *Br. J. Pharmacol.,* 44, 374, 1972.
20. **Beaver, W. T., Kantor, T. G., and Levy, G.,** On guard for aspirin's harmful effects, *Patient Care,* 13, 16, 1979.
21. **Szczeklik, A., Gryglewski, R. J., and Czerniawska-Mysik, G.,** Relationship of inhibition of prostaglandin biosynthesis by analgesics to asthma attacks in aspirin-sensitive patients, *Br. Med. J.,* 1, 67, 1975.
22. **Triggs, E. J., Nation, R. L., Long, A., and Ashly, J. J.,** Pharmacokinetics in the elderly, *Eur. J. Clin. Pharmacol.,* 8, 55, 1975.
23. **Briant, R. H., Dorrington, R. E., Cleal, J., and Williams, F. M.,** The rate of acetaminophen metabolism in the elderly and the young, *J. Am. Geriatr. Soc.,* 24, 359, 1976.
24. **Fulton, B., James, O., and Rawlins, M. D.,** The influence of age on the pharmacokinetics of paracetamol, *Br. J. Clin. Pharmacol.,* 7, 418, 1979.
25. **Briant, R. H., Liddell, D. E., Dorrington, R., and Williams, F. M.,** Plasma half-life of two analgesic drugs in young and elderly adults, *N.Z. Med. J.,* 82, 136, 1975.
26. **Jori, A., DiSalle, E., and Quadri, A.,** Rate of aminopyrine disappearance from plasma in young and aged humans, *Pharmacology,* 8, 273, 1972.
27. **O'Malley, K., Crooks, J., Duke, E., and Stevenson, I. H.,** Effect of age and sex on human drug metabolism, *Br. Med. J.,* 3, 607, 1971.
28. **O'Malley, K., Stevenson, I. H., and Crooks, J.,** Drug metabolism in a geriatric population, *Clin. Sci.,* 41, 6P, 1971.
29. **Vestal, R. E., Norris, A. H., Tobin, J. D., Cohen, B. H., Shock, N. W., and Andres, R.,** Antipyrine metabolism in man: influence of age, alcohol, caffeine and smoking, *Clin. Pharmacol. Ther.,* 18, 425, 1975.
30. **Liddell, D. E., Williams, F. M., and Briant, R. H.,** Phenazone (antipyrine) metabolism and distribution in young and elderly adults, *Clin. Exp. Pharmacol. Physiol.,* 2, 481, 1975.
31. **Wood, A. J. J., Vestal, R. E., Wilkinson, G. R., Branch, R. A., and Shand, O. G.,** Effect of aging and cigarette smoking on antipyrine and indocyanine green elimination, *Clin. Pharmacol. Ther.,* 26, 16, 1979.
32. **Traeger, A., Kunze, M., Stein, G., and Ankerman, H.,** Zur pharmakokinetik von indomethazin bei alten menschen, *Z. Alternsforsch,* 27, 151, 1973.
33. **Duggan, D. E., Hogans, A. F., Kwan, K. C., and McMahon, F. G.,** The metabolism of indomethacin in man, *J. Pharmacol. Exp. Ther.,* 181, 563, 1972.
34. **Gibaldi, M., Nagashima, R., and Levy, G.,** Relationship between drug concentration in plasma or serum and amount of drug in the body, *J. Pharm. Sci.,* 58, 193, 1969.
35. **Whittaker, J. A. and Price Evans, D. A.,** Genetic control of phenylbutazone metabolism in man, *Br. Med. J.,* 4, 323, 1970.
36. **Swift, C. G., Homeida, M., Halliwell, M., and Roberts, C. J.,** Antipyrine disposition and liver size in the elderly, *Eur. J. Clin. Pharmacol.,* 14, 149, 1978.
37. **Levy, G., Tsuchiya, T., and Amsel, L. P.,** Limited capacity for salicyl phenolic glucuronide formation and its effect on the kinetics of salicylate elimination in man, *Clin. Pharmacol. Ther.,* 13, 258, 1972.

38. **Davison, C.,** Salicylate metabolism in man, *Ann. N.Y. Acad. Sci.,* 179, 249, 1971.
39. **Sholkoff, S. D., Rowland, M., Eyring, E. J., and Riegelman, S.,** Pharmacokinetic studies of acetylsalicylic acid in patients with rheumatoid arthritis, *Arthritis Rheum.,* 10, 312, 1967.
40. **Salem, S. A. M. and Stevenson, I. H.,** Absorption kinetics of aspirin and quinine in elderly subjects, *Br. J. Clin. Pharmacol.,* 4, 397P, 1977.
41. **Anderson, C. J., Kaufman, P. L., and Sturm, R. J.,** Toxicity of combined therapy with carbonic anhydrase inhibitors and aspirin, *Am. J. Ophthalmol.,* 86, 516, 1978.
42. **Vancura, E. J.,** Guard against unpredictable drug responses in the aging, *Geriatrics,* 34, 63, 1979.
43. **Thompson, J. F. and Floyd, R. A.,** Effect of aging on pharmecokinetics, in *Drugs and the Elderly,* R. C. Kayne, Ed., University of Southern California Press, 1978, 143.
44. **Krupka, L. R. and Vener, A. M.,** Hazards of drug use among the elderly, *Gerontologist,* 19(1), 90, 1979.
45. **Weg, R. B.,** Drug interaction with the changing physiology of the aged, practive and potential, in *Drugs and the Elderly,* R. C. Kayne, Ed., University of Southern California Press, 1978, 103.
46. **Sorensen, A. W. S.,** Investigation of kidney function in rheumatoid arthritis, *Acta Rheum. Scand.,* 6, 115, 1960.
47. **Burry, H. C.,** Reduced glomerular function in rheumatoid arthritis, *Ann. Rheum. Dis.,* 31, 65, 1972.
48. **Murray, R. M., Lawson, D. H., and Linton, A. L.,** Analgesic nephropathy, clinical syndrome and prognosis, *Br. Med. J.,* 1, 479, 1971.
49. **Russell, A. S., Sturge, R. A., and Smith, M. A.,** Serum transaminases during salicylate therapy, *Br. Med. J.,* 2, 428, 1971.
50. **Rainsford, K. D.,** The biochemical pathology of aspirin-induced gastric damage, *Agents Actions,* 5(4), 326, 1975.
51. **van Praag, H. M.,** Psychotropic drugs in the aged, *Compr. Psychiatry,* 18(5), 429, 1977.
52. **Brady, E. S.,** Drugs and the elderly, in *Drugs and the Elderly,* R. C. Kayne, Ed., University of Southern California Press, 1978, 1.
53. **Riley, G. A.,** How aging influences drug therapy, *U.S. Pharm.,* 2, 28, 1977.
54. **Gokal, R. and Matthews, D. R.,** Renal papillary necrosis after aspirin and alclofenac, *Br. Med. J.,* 2, 1517, 1977.
55. **Mongan, E., Kelly, P., Nies, K., Porter, W. W., and Paulus, H. E.,** Tinnitus as an indication of therapeutic serum salicylate levels, *J. Am. Med. Assoc.,* 226(2), 142, 1973.
56. **Perez De Moura, L. F. and Hayden, R. C., Jr.,** Salicylate ototoxicity. I. Human temporal bone report, *Arch. Otolaryngol.,* 87, 60, 1968.
57. **Miller, R. R.,** Deafness due to plain and long-acting aspirin tablets, *J. Clin. Pharmacol.,* 18, 468, 1978.
58. **Sahud, M. A. and Cohen, R. J.,** Effect of aspirin ingestion on ascorbic acid levels in rheumatoid arthritis, *Lancet,* 1, 937, 1971.
59. **Mielens, Z. E. and Rosenberg, F. J.,** Dual effects of aspirin in guinea-pig lungs, *Br. J. Pharmacol.,* 57, 495, 1976.
60. **Rainsford, K. D.,** Aspirin: actions and uses, *Aust. J. Pharmacol.,* 56, 373, 1975.
61. **MacDonald, W. C.,** Correlation of mucosal histology and aspirin intake in chronic gastric ulcer, *Gastroenterology,* 65(1), 381, 1973.
62. **Duggan, J. M. and Chapman, B. L.,** The incidence of aspirin ingestion in patients with peptic ulcer, *Med. J. Aust.,* 1(16), 797, 1970.
63. **Jabbari, M. and Valberg, L. S.,** Role of acid secretion in aspirin-induced gastric mucosal injury, *Can. Med. Assoc. J.,* 102, 178, 1970.
64. **St. John, D. J. B. and McDermott, F. T.,** Influence of achlorhydria on aspirin-induced occult gastrointestinal blood loss: studies in Addisonian pernicious anaemia, *Br. Med. J.,* 2, 450, 1970.
65. **Duggan, J. M.,** Gastrointestinal haemorrhage, gastric ulcer and aspirin, *Aust. An. Med.,* 2, 135, 1970.
66. **Valman, H. B., Parry, D. J., and Coghill, N. F.,** Lesions associated with gastroduodenal haemorrhage, in relation to aspirin intake, *Br. Med. J.,* 4, 661, 1968.
67. **Eldar, M., Aderka, D., Shoenfeld, Y., Livini, E., and Pinkhas, J.,** Aspirin-induced aplastic anaemia, *S. Afr. Med. J.,* 55(9), 318, 1979.
68. **Morris, G. K. and Mitchell, J. R. A.,** Preventing venous thromboembolism in elderly patients with hip fractures, studies of low-dose heparin, dipyridamole, aspirin and flurbiprofen, *Br. Med. J.,* 1, 535, 1977.
69. **Butterfield, W. J. H.,** Effect of aspirin on postoperative venous thrombosis, *Lancet,* 2, 441, 1972.
70. **Freed, M. D., Rosenthal, A., and Fyler, D.,** Attempts to reduce arterial thrombosis after cardiac catheterization in children, use of percutaneous techniques and aspirin, *Am. Heart J.,* 87(3), 293, 1974.
71. **Elwood, P. C., Cochrane, A. L., Burr, M. L., Sweetnam, P. M., Williams, G., Welsby, E., Hughes, S. J., and Renton, R.,** A randomized controlled trial of acetylsalicylic acid in the secondary prevention of mortality from myocardial infarction, *Br. Med. J.,* 1, 436, 1974.
72. Boston Collaborative Drug Surveillance Group, Regular aspirin intake and acute myocardial infarction, *Br. Med. J.,* 1, 440, 1974.

73. **Hammond, E. C. and Garfinkel, L.,** Aspirin and coronary heart disease: findings of a prospective study, *Br. Med. J.,* 2, 269, 1975.

74. **Davidson, D. G. D. and Eastham, W. N.,** Acute liver necrosis following overdose of paracetamol, *Br. Med. J.,* 2, 497, 1966.

75. **Mitchell, J. R., Jollow, D. J., Potter, W. Z., Davis, D. C., Gillette, J. R., and Brodie, B. B.,** Acetaminophen induced hapatic necrosis I: role of drug metabolism, *J. Pharmacol. Exp. Ther.,* 187, 185, 1973.

76. **Proudfoot, A. T. and Wright, N.,** Acute paracetamol poisoning, *Br. Med. J.,* 3, 557, 1970.

77. **Rumack, B. H. and Matthew, H.,** Acetaminophen poisoning and toxicity, *Pediatrics,* 55, 871, 1975.

78. **Thomson, J. S. and Prescott, L. F.,** Liver damage and impaired glucose tolerance after paracetamol overdosage, *Br. Med. J.,* 2, 506, 1966.

79. **James, O., Lesna, M., Roberts, S. M., Pulman, L., Douglas, A. P., Smith, P. A., and Watson, A. J.,** Liver damage after paracetamol overdose, *Lancet,* 2, 579, 1975.

80. **Jollow, D. J., Mitchell, J. R., Potter, W. Z., Davis, D. C., Gillette, J. R., and Brodie, B. B.,** Acetaminophen induced hepatic necrosis. II. Role of covalent binding *in vivo, J. Pharmacol. Exp. Ther.,* 187, 195, 1973.

81. **Mitchell, J. R., Jollow, D. J., Potter, W. Z., Gillette, J. R., and Bordie, B. B.,** Acetaminophen induced hepatic necrosis. IV. Protective role of glutathione, *J. Pharmacol. Exp. Ther.,* 187, 211, 1973.

82. **Potter, W. Z., Davis, D. C., Mitchell, J. R., Jollow, D. J., Gillette, J. R., and Brodie, B. B.,** Acetaminophen binding *in vitro, J. Pharmacol. Exp. Ther.,* 187, 203, 1973.

83. **Kato, R. and Takanaka, A.,** Metabolism of drugs in old rats. I. Activities of NADPH-linked electron transport and drug-metabolizing enzyme systems in liver microsomes of old rats, *Jpn. J. Pharmacol.,* 18, 381, 1968.

84. **Kato, R. and Takanaka, A.,** Metabolism of drugs in old rats. II. Metabolism *in vivo* and effect of drugs in old rats, *Jpn. J. Pharmacol.,* 18, 389, 1968.

85. **Wallace, S. and Whiting, B.,** Factors affecting drug binding in plasma of elderly patients, *Br. J. Clin. Pharmacology.,* 3, 327, 1976.

86. **Larking, P. W.,** Salicylate binding, effect of age and regular aspirin ingestion, *Aust. J. Pharm. Sci.,* 8, 123, 1979.

87. **Caldwell, J., Smith, R. L., and Davies, S. A.,** Drug metabolism in a case of Progeria, *Gerontology,* 24(5), 373, 1978.

88. **McMahon, F. G., Jain, A., and Onel, A.,** Controlled evaluation of fenoprofen in geriatric patients with osteoarthritis, *J. Rheumatol.,* 3(Supp. 2), 76, 1976.

89. **Inman, W. H. W.,** Study of fatal bone marrow depression with special reference to phenylbutazone and oxyphenbutazone, *Br. Med. J.,* 1, 1500, 1977.

90. **Larsen, K. and Moller, C. E.,** A renal lesion caused by abuse of phenacetin, *Acta Med. Scand.,* 165, 321, 1979.

91. **Kasanen, A. and Salmi, H.,** The use of phenacetin by and its detrimental effects on a series of hospital patients, *Ann. Med. Intern. Fenn.,* 50, 195, 1961.

92. **Ruikka, I. and Sourander, L. B.,** Phenacetin consumption, occurrence of urinary tract infection and renal function in a series of aged hospital patients, *Gerontol. Clin. (Basel),* 9, 99, 1967.

93. **Melander, A., Bodin, N. O., Danielson, K., Gustafsson, B., Haylund, G., and Westerlund, D.,** Absorption and elimination of D-propoxyphene, acetylsalicylic acid, and phenazone in a combination tablet (Doleron®), comparison between young and elderly subjects, *Acta Med. Scand.,* 203, 121, 1978.

94. **Crooks, J., O'Malley, K., and Stevenson, I. H.,** Pharmacokinetics in the elderly, *Clin. Pharmacokinet.,* 1, 280, 1976.

95. **Castelden, C. M., Volans, C. N., and Raymond, K.,** The effect of aging on drug absorption from the gut, *Age Aging,* 6, 138, 1977.

LOCAL ANESTHETICS

N. Lakshminarayanaiah and C. Paul Bianchi

INTRODUCTION

Local anesthetics are drugs that reversibly block impulse conduction in nerve. Because the ionic mechanism of excitability (i.e., production of action potential) is similar in nerve and muscle, these agents have prominent actions on all types of excitable tissue. Local anesthetics have been used clinically for nearly 100 years. The therapeutic usefulness of these compounds lies in their ability to quantitatively block nerve conduction for a required period of time after which recovery occurs with no apparent neural damage. For a chemical compound to be useful as a local anesthetic, there are several desirable attributes it should possess. The compound should not cause irritation or damage to the tissue. Its systemic toxicity should be low because ultimately it will be absorbed from its site of application. The ideal local anesthetic must be effective irrespective of how it is applied. The onset of its action should be rapid and its duration of action sufficient for performing contemplated surgery, yet allow for rapid recovery following surgery. Desirable physical properties of the local anesthetic are solubility in water, stability in solution, and resistance to inactivation during sterilization.

Local anesthetics possess many different chemical groups (see Figure 1) with no specific structural characteristics. The chemical structures of some of the clinically useful anesthetics and others used in the elucidation of mechanism-of-block of membrane sodium conductance, are shown in Figure 2. It can be seen that most of the compounds which act as local anesthetics consist of three parts: (1) a hydrophilic group connected to (2) a lipophilic aromatic residue by (3) an intermediate chain. In view of this, local anesthetic compounds have the ability to orient at an oil-water interface with their hydrophilic part in water and the lipophilic residue in oil. The accumulation of local anesthetic molecules at the interface will lower the surface tension of water and this in turn will allow the molecules to penetrate the oil phase, the extent of penetration being a function of the lipid solubility. How some of these molecules distribute themselves as free bases between oil (or alcohol) and water (buffer solution) is shown in Table 1. Clinically useful local anesthetics are generally tertiary amines, so they can exist as charged protonated species dependent on their pK_as and the pH of the medium. How the partition or distribution coefficients of these compounds are likely to change with pH is also shown in Table 1. Since the cell can be thought of as a three-phase system: (1) extracellular water phase (pH = 7.4), (2) liphophilic membrane, and (3) intracellular water phase (pH = 7.0), the distribution coefficient, $K_{ph = 7}$, becomes important for comparing cellular uptake of local anesthetics. The greater the partition coefficient at pH 7, the greater will be the accumulation of the local anesthetic in the liphophilic or membrane phase; the relatively acidic intracellular water phase will allow for the accumulation of the protonated local anesthetic. Structural changes of the molecules, their relationship to local anesthetic activity, and physicochemical properties have been discussed by Buchi and Perlia.[2]

There are several books and review articles related to the actions of local anesthetics. Two books of interest are *Local Anesthetics*, Volume 1, edited by Lehcat,[3] and *Progress in Anesthesiology*, Volume 1, edited by Fink.[4] The reviews vary in length and importance, each emphasizing one or several aspects of the subject. Different aspects of local anesthetic action have been covered in the recent reviews by Seeman,[5] Narahashi,[6] Ritchie,[7] and Strichartz.[8] A short account by Lakshminarayanaiah and Bianchi recapitulates some of those aspects of local anesthetics that have received only minor emphasis in the literature.[9]

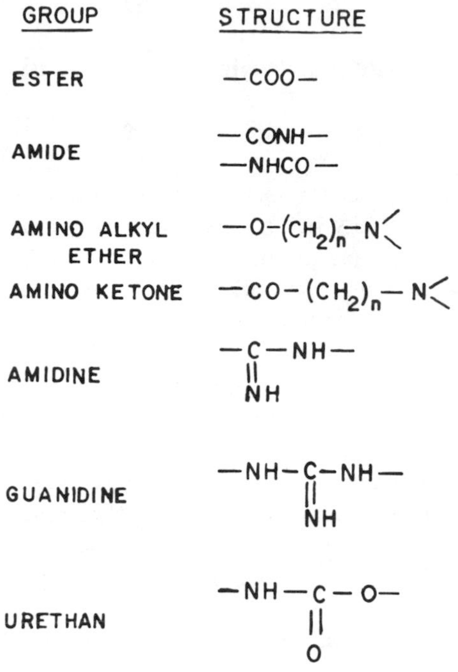

GROUP	STRUCTURE
ESTER	$-COO-$
AMIDE	$-CONH-$ $-NHCO-$
AMINO ALKYL ETHER	$-O-(CH_2)_n-N\!\!<$
AMINO KETONE	$-CO-(CH_2)_n-N\!\!<$
AMIDINE	$-\underset{\underset{NH}{\|\|}}{C}-NH-$
GUANIDINE	$-NH-\underset{\underset{NH}{\|\|}}{C}-NH-$
URETHAN	$-NH-\underset{\underset{O}{\|\|}}{C}-O-$

FIGURE 1.   Several chemical groups present in local anesthetic compounds.

AGING AND LOCAL ANESTHETIC BLOCK

The effect of local anesthetics on excitable cells as a function of age will depend, in large measure, on the susceptibility to block of sodium and calcium channels, the major regulators of inward current. Goldberg et al.[10] and Goldberg and Roberts[11] found that the sodium channels of rat atrial muscle (Fischer 344 rats) become more susceptible to blockade by lidocaine with age. Lidocaine ($1.85 \times 10^{-5}M$) depressed the overshoot of the atrial action potential to a greater extent in rats 28 months of age than in rats 12 months of age. Verapamil ($1 \times 10^{-5}M$), a calcium channel blocker, reduced the atrial action potential plateau duration 50% in rats 24 to 28 months of age compared to a 10% increase in plateau duration for rats 12 months of age.

Our studies (unpublished) on the electrolyte contents of hearts from the same strain of rats indicated that sodium content increased markedly in atria and ventricles as a function of age. The sodium content of left ventricles was found to be 26.9 ± 1.0 μmol/g wet weight for rats 3 to 5 months of age (n = 6), and increased to 41.9 ± 1.5 μmol/g wet weight for rats 24 to 28 months of age (n = 5). Thus the driving force for the generation of inward current due to flow of sodium ions decreased with age as the sodium electrochemical gradient decreased; this may account for the greater susceptibility of the aged excitable cells to local anesthetic blockade of inward sodium currents. Similarly, such a loss of sodium electrochemical gradient in neuronal axons could account for the age-associated decline in conduction velocity observed by Shock.[12] Calcium content was found to increase in rat ventricles from age 3 to 5 months to 24 to 28 months. The younger ventricle contained 0.84 μmol/g wet weight (n = 6) of calcium and the older rat ventricles contained 1.10 μmol/g wet weight (n = 5) of calcium. What effect the increased calcium content would have on local anesthetic action in aged hearts remains to be determined. If the increased calcium content were to reflect an increase in calcium binding to negative charges on the surface of the membrane, then the ventricular cells would become more susceptible to blockade by local anesthetics, since the threshold for excitation would be markedly increased in aged ventricular cells.

129

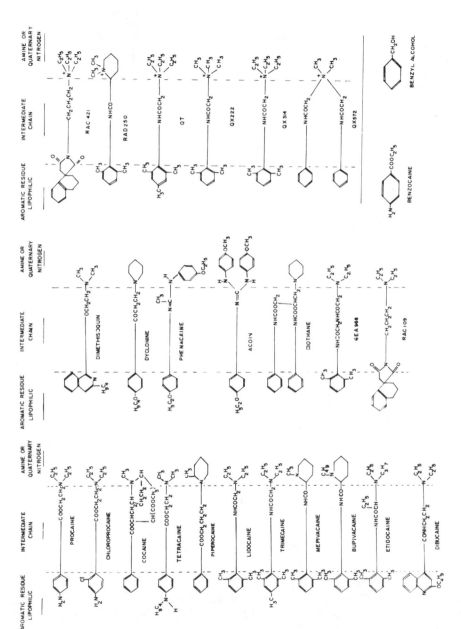

FIGURE 2. Structural formulas of local anesthetics having an amine or a quaternary nitrogen and an alcohol.

Table 1
pK$_a$ AND PARTITION COEFFICIENT (K) OF LOCAL ANESTHETICS

Drug	pK$_a$	K$_{base}$	K$^a_{pH=6}$	K$^a_{pH=7}$	K$^a_{pH=9}$	Medium
Benzocaine	2.6	41	41	41	41	Oleyl alcohol
Lidocaine	7.9	225	2.8	25.2	208	Oleyl alcohol
Tetracaine	8.5	273	0.86	8.4	207	Cod liver oil
Mepivacaine	7.8	46	0.72	6.3	43	Oleyl alcohol
RAC 109	9.4	260	0.10	1.03	74	Cod liver oil
Procaine	8.9	45	0.057	0.56	25	Oleyl alcohol
GEA 968	7.7	1.3	0.025	0.22	1.24	Cod liver oil

[a] K$_{pH}$ values are calculated from the values of K$_{base}$, pK$_a$, and pH.

$$K_{base} = \frac{[B]_{oil}}{[B]_{buffer}}$$

and

$$K_{pH} = \frac{[B]_{oil}}{[B]_{buffer} + [BH^+]_{buffer}}$$

From the reaction, $B + H^+ \rightleftharpoons BH^+$, in the steady-state one gets the relationship,

$$[BH^+] = \frac{[B]\,[H^+]}{K_a}$$

But

$$\frac{[H^+]}{K_a} = \frac{10^{-pH}}{10^{-pK_a}} = 10^{pK_a - pH}$$

Thus,

$$K_{pH} = \frac{[B]_{oil}}{[B]_{buffer}\,(1 + 10^{pK_a - pH})} = \frac{K_{base}}{1 + 10^{pK_a - pH}}$$

Adapted from Hille, B., *J. Gen. Physiol.*, 69, 475, 1977 (Reference 1).

The effect of increased calcium content of aged cells on the threshold for the generation of action potential, and possible synergism with local anesthetics, remains to be determined.

Other factors, e.g., lipophilic properties of plasma membranes, intracellular pH, extracellular pH, have not been studied in relation to aging. The manner in which these factors influence membrane excitability is the subject of the following sections. As will be seen, membrane excitability greatly depends on these and other factors that will be discussed. However, there is virtually no information on how the properties of excitable membranes change with age. Therefore, this area needs much more work.

The primary action of local anesthetics is blockade of impulse initiation and conduction. A brief account of the ionic basis of nervous conduction and of the structural characteristics of nerve membranes is appropriate at this juncture.

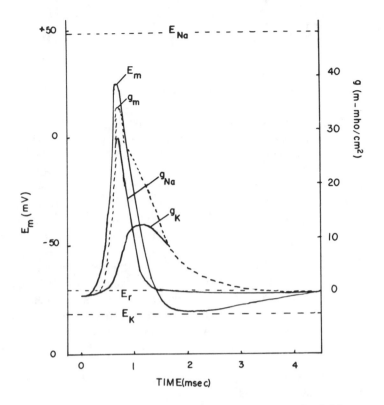

FIGURE 3.   Time course of the propagated action potential and underlying conductances. E_m, E_r, E_{Na}, and E_k are membrane potential, resting potential, sodium
equilibrium potential, and potassium equilibrium potential, respectively; g_m, g_{Na},
and g_K are conductances of the membrane, sodium, and potassium ions, respectively. E_m begins to rise before g_{Na} because of (1) electronic spread from the
arriving spike and (2) time required for g_{Na} to increase. g_{Na} rises, and starts to
fall because of inactivation, at about the time g_K begins to increase appreciably.
The initial part of membrane conductance g_m is predominantly due to Na ions
while the late part is due to K ions. (After Shanes, A. M., *Pharmacol. Rev.*, 10,
165, 1958.)

EXCITABILITY AND IONIC PERMEABILITY OF MEMBRANES

Nerve fibers are excited by an electrical stimulus, which acts to discharge the cell surface
membrane and thus reduce the existing resting membrane potential to a lower (depolarization)
and unstable level at which excitation occurs. If the stimulus is strong enough, the local
electrical effect is propagated without attenuation and with constant velocity as an action
potential along the fiber (Figure 3). The action potential is the result of a transient change
in cell membrane potential which, at rest, is negative relative to the outside. The transient
change in potential reaches zero and becomes positive, reaching an amplitude of about 100
mV and lasting about 1 msec. The propagated action potential or impulse is an all-or-none
event.

Several hypotheses have been advanced to explain the reversal of membrane potential
during excitation. Of these, the ionic hypothesis, proposed by Hodgkin, Huxley, and Katz,[13-20] has been most widely used in the studies of excitable cells. According to this hypothesis,
the plasma membrane on excitation becomes highly permeable to sodium ions, which are
at a higher concentration outside than inside the nerve cell. The membrane potential tem-
porarily approaches the equilibrium potential for sodium ions (Figure 3). The equilibrium
potential for sodium, E_{Na}, is obtained from

$$E_{Na} = \frac{RT}{F} \ln \frac{[Na]_o}{[Na]_i} \qquad (1)$$

where $[Na]_o$ and $[Na]_i$ are the sodium concentrations outside and inside the cell, respectively, and R, T, and F are the gas constant, absolute temperature, and Faraday constant, respectively.

Hodgkin and Katz demonstrated,[13] according to Equation 1, that the amplitude of the action potential decreased with a decrease in $[Na]_o$. The increase in permeability to sodium ions, responsible for the action potential, is also reflected in a transient increase in electrical conductance of the membrane during an impulse. Cole and Curtis showed that during an impulse[21] the membrane resistance fell from its resting value of 10^3 ohmcm^2 to about 25 ohmcm^2 (see Figure 3) without appreciable changes either in the electrical capacitance of the membrane or the resistance of the axoplasm. Further, isotope studies showed that entry of sodium into the cell and exit of potassium from the cell during an impulse were equal, about 4 pmol/cm^2/impulse.[20,22]

The electrical events during an action potential that result in the all-or-none reaction have been examined by Hodgkin and Huxley,[15-18] employing the voltage clamp technique described by Cole.[23,24] The membrane ionic currents are made up of two components — an early transient component due to the inward flow of sodium ions and a late component that levels off to a steady-state due to the outward flow of potassium ions. The maximum values of the early transient current and the steady-state current are dependent on voltage across the membrane.

Several experiments show that early and late currents go through pathways (channels or pores) that are separate entities.[25] Evidence favoring the existence of independent pathways comes from experiments with pharmacological agents that selectively block one component of the membrane current without affecting the other.[6,26] The substance, tetrodotoxin (TTX), blocks the early current without affecting the late component of the membrane current.[27,28] It blocks the channel itself, irrespective of the nature of the ion going through the channel, since it is observed that both the early outward current due to potassium ions[29] and the early inward current due to flow of ions other than sodium[26,30,31] are blocked by TTX. Tetraethylammonium ion (TEA) affects the channel through which the late current is carried, without any effect on the channel for the early current.[32,33] A similar effect is exerted by cesium and rubidium ions when they are applied internally.[34,35] A demonstration of the existence of two distinct channels, one for the early current and one for the late current is obtained by use of the ammonium ion. This ion passes through both channels.[36] The early component of the membrane current due to ammonium is blocked by TTX and the late component, again due to the same ion, is blocked by TEA.

A set of empirical equations have been used by Hodgkin and Huxley to describe the kinetics of conductance change following changes in membrane potential.[18] The early current, I_{Na}, is described by

$$I_{Na} = g_{Na} \, m^3 \, h \, (E - E_{Na}) \qquad (2)$$

where g_{Na} is the maximum early conductance, m and h are the activation and inactivation parameters that describe the kinetics of conductance change, and E is the membrane potential. These parameters follow the equations

$$\frac{dm}{dt} = \frac{m_\infty(E) - m}{\tau_m(E)} \qquad (3)$$

$$\frac{dh}{dt} = \frac{h_\infty(E) - h}{\tau_h(E)} \tag{4}$$

Similarly, the late current, I_K, is described by

$$I_K = g_K n^4 (E - E_K) \tag{5}$$

$$\frac{dn}{dt} = \frac{n_\infty(E) - n}{\tau_n(E)} \tag{6}$$

From voltage clamp data, the functions $m_\infty(E)$, $h_\infty(E)$ $n_\infty(E)$, $\tau_m(E)$, $\tau_h(E)$, and $\tau_n(E)$ have been derived and are shown in Figure 4.

The quantities m, h, and n represent definite physical entities (they may be equated to particles in the membrane). The physical entities m and govern the activation of channels for early and late currents. Channel opening brought about by movement of a particle or dipole in the membrane (i.e., activation or opening of gates) allows sodium and potassium ions to move down their electrochemical gradients. The n gate does not close (i.e., inactivation), whereas the gate controlling the h parameter does open and close. Destruction of inactivation by pronase,[38-39] shows that inactivation is controlled by the physical entity, h (a dipolar protein involving probably arginine or lysine),[40] similar to the way activation is governed by the physical entity, m. The gates open or close in response to changes in membrane potential.[41-43] This means that the chemical structures of the gates must be charged, thus are able to move in the membrane when changes in potential occur, as pointed out very early by Hodgkin and Huxley.[18] This movement of charge is the gating current which has been measured in recent years.[41-52] Total gating charge for squid giant axon at saturation, reported by several investigators, is as follows (in $-e/\mu m^2$): 1882,[44] 1600,[46] 2114,[53] and 1200.[54] On the assumption that 6 electron (e) charges per channel are involved,[18] an average value of 283 (i.e., 1699/6) channels per square micrometer of membrane area can be calculated (also see Armstrong).[41] The number of channels will be doubled (566/μm^2) if the presence of 3 charges in each sodium channel is assumed.[45,46] The latter value is close to the value of 553/μm^2, estimated from measurements of binding of tritiated TTX to squid giant axons.[55] Similarly, measurements of charge displacement in the frog nodal membrane have given a value of 521 sodium channels per square micrometer of the nodal membrane area.[50,51] Measurements of maximum potassium conductance of the squid axon membrane have been used to estimate the potassium channel density. Estimates by Armstrong indicate a value of 100 potassium channels per square micrometer of axon membrane area.[41]

The physical sizes of sodium and potassium channels have been estimated from studies of membrane permeability to inorganic and organic ions of different shapes and different sizes. Hille has given an explicit picture for the sodium channel.[56,57] It is considered to conform to an oxygen lined pore, 3 Å × 5 Å in cross-section. Similarly, the potassium channel diameter has been estimated to be 3.0 to 3.3 Å.[58] Armstrong considered the potassium channel to correspond to a narrow pore (range of diameter 2.6 to 3 Å) with a mouth of 8 Å diameter to just admit the TEA ion.[41] In any case, sodium and potassium channels are now considered to be pores and the open pores provide aqueous pathways for the ions to move across the membrane. A schematic diagram by Hille shows an ionic channel to be a protein macromolecule forming a pore through the lipid bilayer membrane.[59] The pore has on the outside a narrow selectivity filter (to explain the selectivity of the channel to ions) and on the inside a gate whose opening is controlled by a voltage sensor responding to the intramembrane field.

There are no studies available, to our knowledge, describing how the different membrane properties, the gating mechanisms, and the ionic current channels are changing with age.

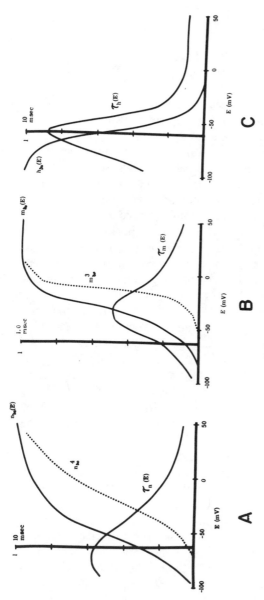

FIGURE 4.   Several parameters of the Hodgkin-Huxley equations. The conductance parameters, n_∞, m_∞, and the inactivation parameter, h_∞, are normalized. The time constants (τ_∞, τ_m, and τ_h) and the conductance parameters (n_∞, m_∞, and h_∞) are shown as functions of voltage for the squid axon membrane whose representative conductances are $g_K = 36$ mho/cm^2 and $g_{Na} = 120$ mho/cm^2. (After Ehrenstein, G. and Lecar, H., *Annu. Rev. Biophys. Bioeng.*, 1, 347, 1972. Reference 37.)

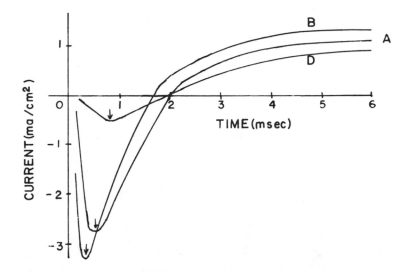

FIGURE 5.   Effect of 3.7 m*M* procaine at pH 7.9 on the membrane currents following a depolarization step. Initially, the membrane was held at a hyperpolarized level and a depolarizing step pulse to — 10 mV was applied. The current curves marked (B), (D), and (A) refer respectively to before, during, and after application of procaine. The arrows indicate the time taken to reach the peak of the inward current. (After Taylor, R. E., *Am. J. Physiol.*, 196(5) 1071, 1959.)

GENERAL ACTIONS OF LOCAL ANESTHETICS

Local anesthetics, in general, increase the threshold for excitation, slow down the propagation of an impulse, reduce the rate of rise of an action potential, and finally block conduction. The process responsible for the generation of an action potential, i.e., large transient increase in membrane permeability to sodium ions, is interfered with by the local anesthetic molecule. Voltage clamp methods were used by Shanes et al.,[60] Taylor,[61] and Blaustein and Goldman[62,63] to investigate the effects of cocaine and procaine on the electrical properties of the membrane of squid and lobster axons. These studies showed that local anesthetics interfered with the sodium-carrying system and prevented the influx of sodium ions (Figure 5). These drugs also reduce the potassium current. But this effect on potassium current is not involved in impulse block since complete block of potassium channels by TEA does not lead to block of the action potential in myelinated fibers.[33] In addition, the procaine effect on the potassium current is smaller than that on the inward sodium current (see Figure 5). All of the drugs depicted in Figure 2 block conduction by interference with the sodium-carrying system.

In addition to the foregoing actions, local anesthetics reduce the permeability of the resting membrane to sodium and potassium ions, without altering the ionic gradients or the resting membrane potential. Voltage clamp techniques have been applied to studies of permeability changes for sodium following application of several local anesthetics to myelinated nerve fibers from Xenopus[64] and to frog node of Ranvier.[65] These studies showed that local anesthetic molecules reacted with a receptor (R), on a one-to-one basis, following first-order kinetics. The dose-response curve followed the equation

$$\frac{P_x}{P_{Na}} = \frac{K}{K + [X]} \tag{7}$$

where P is permeability measured in the presence (P_x) and absence (P_{Na}) of the drug X. K is the equilibrium constant of the reaction

$$R + X \rightleftharpoons RX \tag{8}$$

Thus,

$$K = \frac{[R][X]}{[RX]} \tag{9}$$

In Equation 7, P_x is proportional to "unbound" sites. If P_x is instead redefined as proportional to bound sites, then Equation 7 becomes

$$\frac{P_x}{P_{Na}} = \frac{[X]}{K + [X]} \tag{10}$$

Neither Equation 7 nor Equation 10 is applicable if the amplitude of the action potential is used as a measure of response, since it is known that the spike height is not linearly related to P_{Na}.[66] These equations have been used by Arhem and Frankenhaeuser[64] and Khodorov et al.[65] to derive K values for several local anesthetics. K values found were as follows (in millimolar): procaine, 0.21; lidocaine, 1.18; benzocaine, 0.49; and trimecaine, 0.3. Wagner and Ulbricht,[67] using a Hill plot, found a value of 0.23 mM as the K value in the case of procaine reacting with frog node.

USE OR FREQUENCY-DEPENDENT BLOCK OF TRANSIENT SODIUM CURRENT BY LOCAL ANESTHETICS

Some local anesthetics having a quaternary nitrogen in their structures (QX and QT) are shown in Figure 2. When these compounds were applied to the external membranes of frog node, there was little effect on the membrane currents. However, when QX was allowed to diffuse into the axoplasm by cutting the internode of the nerve fiber, the sodium current diminished by about 90% (QX314, 0.5 mM, in isotonic KCl). Since the reversal (or equilibrium) potential for sodium remained unchanged, it is concluded that QX inhibited the sodium current by lowering the conductance of sodium channels in the node. This large inhibition has been called the "tonic phase" of inhibition by Strichartz.[68] The other component of reversible depression of sodium current, variably termed voltage-sensitive inhibition,[68,69] use-dependent inhibition,[70] frequency-dependent block,[70] or inhibition by slow-sodium inactivation,[65] is brought about by repetitive depolarization of membranes. This is illustrated in Figure 6. The peak current following a test pulse (E_t), that depolarizes the membrane to -45 mV from -75 mV, is the largest current (indicated by 0). The peak current is diminished to different levels when the test pulse, (E_t), was preceded by several conditioning depolarizations (5 or 20) to $+75$ mV, (E_c), lasting 5 msec each and spaced 1 sec apart. The general pattern of voltages applied to bring about voltage-dependent inhibition of sodium current is shown in Figure 7. The value of E_c determined the degree of inhibition: the more positive the value of E_c and the larger the value of n (number of conditioning pulses), the greater was the inhibition. This voltage-dependent phenomenon is completely reversible; but it occurs slowly when the membrane is held at -75 mV. The recovery process can be hastened by using small depolarizing pulses of about 5 msec duration. Rate of reversal is also governed by the voltage of the prepulse preceding the test pulse. In general, hyperpolarizing prepulses accelerate the reversal and depolarizing prepulses slow down the reversal process.[68,69] These phenomena of voltage-dependent block and reversal have been explained by Strichartz,[68] using the Hodgkin-Huxley parameters, m and h, which are functions of both time and voltage. Both parameters have a value of unity when the sodium channels are open, and zero when the sodium channels are closed. In the latter case, sodium channels

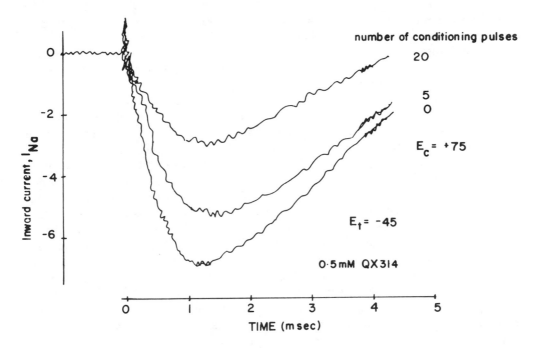

FIGURE 6. The time course of sodium currents with QX314 present inside the nerve. The drug was applied by cutting the internode in 0.12 M KCl containing 0.5 mM QX314. The inhibition of inward Na current increased with an increase in the number of depolarizations. The currents were measured during a depolarizing test pulse, E_t, to -45 mV. Highest peak current was observed when the membrane potential was held at -75 mV and the test pulse to -45 mV was applied (trace 0). Peak currents during the test pulse were reduced when their measurements were preceded by 5 (trace 5) and 20 (trace 20) conditioning depolarizing pulses, E_c to $+75$ mV. The duration of each E_c was 5 msec and spaced 1 sec apart during application of a sequence of E_cs.[68,69]

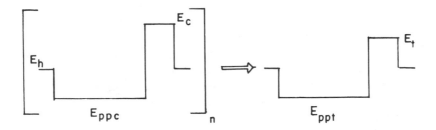

FIGURE 7. The pattern of voltage pulses applied to produce use or frequency-dependent inhibition of inward membrane current. E_h, E_{ppc}, and E_c are respectively the holding potential, conditioning hyperpolarizing prepulse of duration 50 msec, and conditioning depolarizing pulse of short duration (5 msec); n is the number of conditioning pulse sequences, each sequence spaced 1 sec apart. E_{ppt} and E_t are hyperpolarizing (50 msec duration) and depolarizing (5 msec duration) test pulses. (After Strichartz, G. R., *J. Gen. Physiol.*, 62, 37, 1973.)

do not conduct ions. According to Strichartz,[68] the tonic phase of inhibition occurs rapidly when the m gates of the sodium channels are open; but it will be slow if the m gates are closed, even when the h gates are open. Once the tonic phase of inhibition reaches a maximum (90% of the current), it becomes difficult to reverse it. The dependence of voltage-sensitive inhibition on m is difficult to demonstrate in view of the fact that depolarizing pulses necessary to open m gates increase inhibition. Hyperpolarizing prepulses which normally remove inactivation in the sodium-carrying system increase the rate at which voltage-dependent inhibition occurs whereas more positive prepulses bring about inhibition more slowly. This means that h gates must be open for use-dependent inhibition to develop. A train of short depolarizing pulses acting for a certain period of time are more effective than one long depolarizing pulse of equal duration. Strichartz found 5 pulses of 5 msec duration decreased sodium currents by 33% in the presence of internally applied QX compound, compared to only an 11% decrease observed in the case of a 25 msec pulse.[68,69] In the course of one long depolarizing pulse, the sodium channel opens once and eventually closes because of inactivation (h decreases); whereas with short pulses, transient opening of channels occurs with each pulse. This eventually results in greater inhibition. All of the foregoing indicate a direct interaction between the drug molecule and the sodium channels.

Similar phenomena have been noted by Courtney[70] in the case of a tertiary amine local anesthetic, GEA 968, and by Ulbricht et al.[67,71] in the case of procaine and benzocaine applied externally to a frog node. In the study by Courtney,[70] a clear dependence of "use-dependent block" of sodium current on the inactivation parameter, h, has been demonstrated. The drug molecules binding to open sodium channels blocked the channels and shifted the curve relating h to membrane potential by 20 to 40 mV in the hyperpolarizing direction. Similar demonstrations for lidocaine and benzocaine are given by Hille.[72] The intimate relationship of use-dependent inhibition of sodium current to opening and closing of the h gate is clearly shown by the fact that when sodium inactivation is destroyed by pronase[73] or batrachotoxin,[74] use or frequency-dependent drug inhibition is eliminated. In the pronase treated squid giant axon,[73] use-dependent block by QX222 and QX314 was abolished completely; whereas partial elimination occurred in the case of tetracaine and etidocaine.

pH AND LOCAL ANESTHETIC BLOCK

Several studies in the absence of any drug indicate that reduction of pH has basically two effects: (1) reversible depression of sodium and potassium conductances and (2) shifts of sodium and/or potassium conductance-voltage curves in the depolarized direction.[75-84] Århem and Frankenhaeuser found that, in the case of procaine, the sodium permeability-concentration curve was shifted along the concentration axis without any change in shape when the pH was changed.[64] An increase in pH shifted the curve towards lower concentrations, thereby showing that tertiary amine local anesthetics, such as procaine or lidocaine, were more potent in blocking sodium permeability at alkaline pH. Khodorov et al.[65] found that procaine and trimecaine had little effect on sodium permeability when the pH was changed from 7.3 to 6; but the permeability-voltage curve was shifted on the voltage axis in the direction of depolarization. Interestingly the change of pH from 7.3 to 8.5 depressed the sodium permeability and the shift of the permability-voltage curve on the voltage axis was in the direction of hyperpolarization. But the profound effects were on the slow sodium inactivation; the time constant was made larger at low pH.

Changes of pH in the approximate range of 6 to 10 had little effect on the electrical threshold and size of the action potential.[85,86] Consequently, it is presumed that the pH changes brought about in the presence of tertiary amine local anesthetics affected only the amine drugs to different extents, depending on their pK_as according to the relation:

$$pH = pK_a + \log \frac{[B]}{[BH^+]} \tag{11}$$

[B] is the concentration of the basic form of the drug, which on protonation goes into the cationic form, whose concentration is $[BH^+]$.

In the study of the actions of local anesthetics as a function of pH, several biological preparations, such as nerve bundles, desheathed nerve trunk, single nerve, and muscle fibers have been used. The hydrodynamic conditions maintained in the chamber wherein the biological preparation is mounted play a significant role in controlling the biologic response to local anesthetic action. This is due to the presence of unstirred (Nernst stagnant layers) layers close to the membrane surface. Connective tissue, Schwann cells, strands of single fibers in a multifiber preparation, etc., which can trap aqueous layers complicate the problem and make interpretation of experimental results difficult, particularly in the case of local anesthetics which can exist in the two forms, B and BH^+. It is well recognized that B is highly lipid soluble compared to its solubility in aqueous buffer solutions. The reverse is true of BH^+. Consequently, when a pH change is attempted in the bulk phase, the ratio $[B]/[BH^+]$ changes. What this change is at the membrane, site of action is difficult to assess, due to the presence of depots of BH^+ in the unstirred aqueous phase (concentration different from the bulk phase) and of B in the membrane phase and extramembrane phase. In view of these difficulties, conflicting views regarding the active form of local anesthetic and the site of action have been frequently expressed. Hille has summarized some of these views and given his own interpretation.[1]

Generally at high pH, in which the free base, B, predominates, the local anesthetic acts rapidly (within seconds). At low pH, where BH^+ predominates, the rate of local anesthetic action is much slower, taking hundreds of seconds. This has been observed on the frog node[1,87] and in various nerve trunks with intact connective tissue sheaths.[88-92] The opposite has been observed in experiments on nerve trunks from which epineurium has been removed. The block of desheathed rabbit vagus nerves was faster at low pH with dibucaine or with lidocaine (but not with procaine) treatment.[93,94] Similarly, with shorter-acting agents, such as lidocaine or procaine, there was a small enhancement, but it was transient in the case of desheathed sciatic nerves.[95-97] Thus, it was considered that the active form of the drug as the cation, BH^+. For amplification of this, see the several papers by Narahashi et al.[86,98-101] Hille,[1] on the basis of a diffusion model, has refuted that BH^+ is the active form. He has argued that the cation, BH^+, reaches the center of a bundle of nerves quicker by taking a straight hydrophilic route in which it is soluble, than the base, B, which takes a longer time to reach the same point by taking a lipophilic route in which it is soluble. Therefore, the effectiveness of the active form of the drug depends upon its uptake and diffusion. Both forms must be effective, although to different extents, depending on their local concentrations. This conclusion was reached early by Bianchi and Strobel.[95,97] who studied the uptake and washout of labeled procaine and lidocaine as a function of pH. Thus, in the case of tertiary amine anesthetics, both forms, B and BH^+, must be active; otherwise, it becomes difficult to reconcile the action of benzocaine (a drug existing as a base independent of pH) which is equipotent with procaine.[64,65,94] Similarly, Schauf and Agin[102] showed that procaine, at half its minimum blocking concentration (MBC = 8 mM), did not block action potentials, but when mixed with benzyl alcohol at half its MBC (35 mM), did block action potentials.

Narahashi[6] and Narahashi and Frazier[101,103] found that the charged form of local anesthetics acted more effectively from the inside of the squid axon than from the outside. This type of differential action, also noted in the case of pH effects in other preparations, such as barnacle muscle fiber,[82] seems to be due not so much to the drug as to the existence of physically and/or chemically different diffusion barriers at the inside and the outside surfaces of the cell membrane. Further, amine anesthetics perfused internally were found to block less strongly at a high pH than at a low pH.[86,100] The straight inference is that the cationic form blocked better than the basic form. This may be misleading since the stronger block, as Hille has pointed out,[1] is again a problem related to solubility and diffusion rates of BH^+ and B through the stagnant aqueous layers at the membrane surface. As the pH is raised, the percentage of B is increased. But B is less soluble than BH^+ in the stagnant aqueous layer near the membrane surface and thus there is not enough B at the surface to bring about a block. This type of uncertainty can be eliminated by equilibrating the preparation with millimolar quantities of long-lasting drugs such as dibucaine. In such a state, the action potential can be blocked or recovered by switching the outside pH to the neutral or alkaline side.[7,84,90,93,104] Again, uncertainty sets in when short-acting drugs are used. Bianchi and Strobel found that, in the case of procaine or lidocaine applied to desheathed sciatic nerve, a transient increase in block followed by recovery on lowering the pH was obtained.[95-97] On the other hand, Rimmel et al.,[71] in similar experiments with procaine applied to the frog node, observed a monotonic recovery from block. This discrepancy may be an artifact of the stagnant layers since these layers in the experiments of Rimmel et al.[71] would be expected to be very thin compared to those existing in a multifiber preparation used in the experiments by Bianchi and Strobel.[95-97] Even then, Rimmel et al. did find a nonmonotonic time course of block when the alkaline Ringer's solution (pH 8.9, high concentration of buffer) was switched to a solution at pH 7.2 containing 1 mM procaine.

When external pH is lowered, it is possible that internal pH may also be lowered,[86] thus increasing the intracellular concentration of drug in the cationic form, the form in which the drug is considered to be more effective. The effects of both internal and external pH on use-dependent block in muscle have been described by Schwarz et al.[105] Muscles exposed to pH 6 Ringer's solution for 15, 33, and 240 min, on homogenization in distilled water, gave pH values of 7.2, 7.1, and 6.8 for the homogenate. Similarly, muscles exposed to pH 8.8 Ringer's for 20, 50, and 253 min had pH values of 7.04, 7.02, and 7.09. Also, the DMO (5,5-dimethyl-2, 4-oxazoladine dione) technique to evaluate intracellular pH, used by Bianchi and Bolton,[106] showed that when the frog sartorius muscle was in Ringer's solution at pH 7.2 or 8.2, the intracellular pH was 7.09 or 7.49, respectively. Studies related to changes of internal pH in the frog node indicate minor effects on the sodium currents either in the presence or absence of local anesthetics;[105] whereas changes of external pH have profound effects on use-dependent block. Both lidocaine and procaine at pH 6 produced dramatic use-dependent blockade, which vanished when the pH was raised to 8 or 8.8.[105] In contrast, use-dependence with permanently neutral benzocaine or permanently charged QX314 was not sensitive to changes in external pH.

The simple conclusion to be drawn from the foregoing discussion is that both forms of local anesthetics, the charged and uncharged, block the sodium channels. This hypothesis was proposed nearly a decade ago by Bianchi and Strobel.[95-97]

CALCIUM AND LOCAL ANESTHETIC BLOCK

Weidmann showed that in cardiac Purkinje fibers, with elevated calcium, a larger depolarization was needed to initiate a spike.[107] But the rate of rise of the spike was increased, thereby showing that entry of sodium was facilitated. In other words, inactivation was removed. Also it was shown that increased calcium had little effect on the maximum limit for rate of sodium entry into the cell. Similar results were found for squid axon, using voltage clamp, by Frankenhaeuser and Hodgkin.[108] Increases in [Ca]$\rightleftharpoons$ affected both sodium and potassium conductance-versus-voltage curves, shifting them on the voltage axis so that a larger depolarization step was required to attain a given level of conductance. The maximum conductance, however, was unchanged. Decreasing [Ca]$\rightleftharpoons$ shifted the curves in the opposite direction. These shifts have been explained on the basis of a change in surface potential which arises from the screening and/or binding of divalent cations to the negative charges on the outer boundary of the membrane. Even when the transmembrane potential is held constant, the potential profile within the membrane would change, due to binding of calcium ions, making the surface potential more positive. As a result, the electric field within the membrane would change in the same direction. This would be equivalent to hyperpolarizing the membrane. Hydrogen ions too, as their concentration is increased, would bring about the same effect.

Blaustein and Goldman studied the actions of calcium and procaine on lobster axon.[62,63]

They found the magnitude of the response to procaine influenced by $[Ca]\rightleftharpoons$. Increased $[Ca]\rightleftharpoons$ reduced the procaine effect on sodium conductance. Conversely, procaine became more effective when $[Ca]\rightleftharpoons$ was reduced. The in vitro studies of calcium binding to phospholipids in the presence or absence of anionic and cationic anesthetic agents, such as barbiturates and procaine-like drugs, showed that anionic drugs increased the binding of calcium to phospholipids, and cationic drugs decreased calcium binding.[109,110] Based on these findings, the idea emerged that there was a direct competition between calcium and the cationic form of a local anesthetic, such as procaine. In contrast to the findings of Blaustein and Goldman on lobster axon,[62,63] Århem and Frankenhaeuser[64] and Khodorov et al.[65] found no such competition between the local anesthetic (procaine, trimecaine) and calcium on the toad and frog nodes. Similarly, Narahashi et al.[111] found little competition between calcium and local anesthetics on the squid axon membrane. This discrepancy between the results of Blaustein and Goldman[62,63] and the other investigators[64,65,111] was attributed by Khodorov et al.[65] to the maintenance of a less negative holding potential in the experiments of Blaustein and Goldman (i.e., due to existence of slow inactivation). In any case, absence of a direct competitive interaction between calcium and local anesthetics may not completely rule out the possibility that an indirect route might exist by which this apparent competition is mediated.

Hille has shown that the sodium conductance vs. prepulse potential curve is shifted on the voltage axis to more negative potentials in the case of both benzocaine and lidocaine.[72] The effect of increasing $[Ca]\rightleftharpoons$ is to shift the same curve in the opposite direction to more positive potentials. Depending on the conditions maintained before the test pulse which poises the h gate (i.e., slow inactivation or its absence), local anesthetics and calcium can show competition by this mechanism. A direct competition, as revealed by studies on phospholipid model systems, is very unlikely since uncharged benzocaine cannot compete with double charged calcium for the binding sites of phospholipids or lipoproteins.

Again, some experimental results that are apparently contradictory are shown in Figure 8. Rimmel et al.[71] found recovery from benzocaine block in frog node when calcium was increased from 2 to 12 mM (Figure 8A, top panel), whereas Suarez-Kurtz et al.[112] found the opposite in the case of desheathed frog nerve (Figure 8B, bottom panel). The only difference in the two experiments is the rate of stimulation and pH. Assuming that differences in stimulation rate contribute little to this contradiction in experimental findings, the discrepancy probably arises from the difference in pH. It is agreed that raising $[Ca]\rightleftharpoons$ is equivalent to hyperpolarizing the membrane. This occurs primarily by calcium screening and/or binding to surface charges on the membrane. The net effect of this is that the drug effect is lessened (Figure 8A, top panel). In addition, increased $[Ca]\rightleftharpoons$ seems to be a secondary effect, particularly at high pH, through enhancement of the blocking action of the local anesthetic by preventing the drugs escape from the membrane (Figure 8B, bottom panel). There are two lines of evidence for this — one is our preliminary results (unpublished) related to ^{45}Ca uptake in Ringer's solution pH 7.2 and pH 9.0. ^{45}Ca uptake in desheathed frog nerves has been found to be higher at pH 9.0 than at pH 7.2. This means that at pH 9, Ca accumulates and stabilizes the membrane and thus prevents or slows down the escape of the drug from the membrane phase. The second line of evidence, shown in Figure 9, illustrates the actions of 50 μM dibucaine, calcium, and pH on the squid axon held in a single sucrose gap and immersed in artificial sea water (ASW in millimolar: NaCl 455, KCl 15, CaCl$_2$ 44, and tris buffer 30).[104] The results in Figure 9A show that the height of the action potential was decreased when the axon was immersed in 0 Ca ASW, pH 9. Repetitive firing by the axonal membrane, a typical behavior in 0 Ca ASW, was also noted. On application of 50 μM dibucaine in 0 Ca ASW, pH 9, the height of the action potential decreased, repetitive firing was suppressed, and this was followed by block. However, on increasing the threshold stimulus, the spike was restored to 40% of its original amplitude.

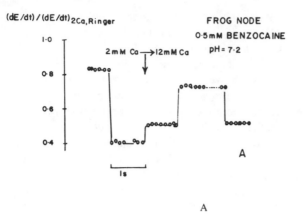

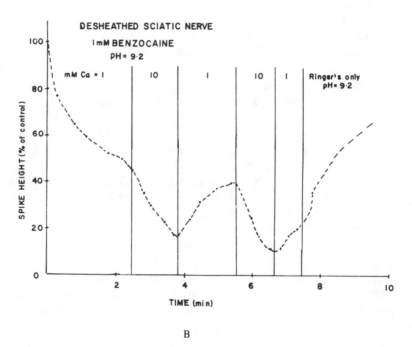

FIGURE 8.   Calcium and benzocaine block at pH 7.2 and 9.2. (A) Top panel: maximum
rate of rise of periodic (10 Hz) action potentials, normalized to the value in Ringer solution
containing 2 mM Ca. Application of 0.5 mM benzocaine gave a reduction (<19%) in
the presence of hyperpolarizing prepulses (18 msec, 20 mV). Removal of these hyperpolarizing prepulses brought about complete block which was relieved partially by raising
calcium from 2 to 12 mM. Now application of hyperpolarizing prepulses further relieved
the block which increased following turning off of the hyperpolarizing prepulses. (After
Rimmel, C., Walle, A., Kebler, H., and Ulbricht, W., *Pflugers Arch.*, 376, 105, 978.)
(B) Bottom panel: spike height normalized to that in absence of benzocaine. Supramaximal
stimulus (0.5 msec, 5 to 10 V) applied every 2.5 min. Increase of calcium from 1 to 10
mM depressed the spike height which recovered on replacement of 1 mM Ca Ringer.
(After Suarez-Kurtz, G., Bianchi, C. P., and Krupp, P., *Eur. J. Pharmacol.*, 10, 91,
1970.)

Application of 44 mM Ca ASW, but at pH 7.2, restored 80% of the spike height, and the
spike stayed at that level irrespective of the pH (7.2 or 9) of the ASW solution. The inference
is that the drug had escaped from the membrane. On the other hand, results of Figure 9B
show that when 44 mM Ca ASW was added at pH 9 instead of pH 7.2, recovery of the

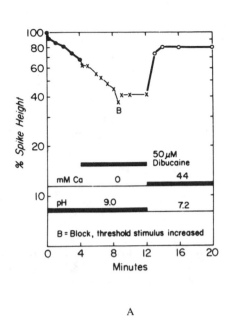

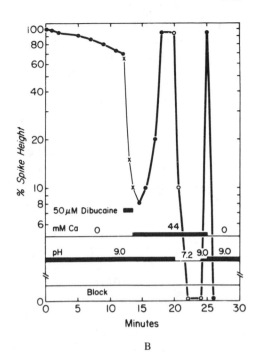

A

B

FIGURE 9. Dibucaine block at pH 7.2 and 9.0 on the squid nerve action potential. Effects of calcium and pH when the nerve is in ASW solutions containing 0 and 44 mM calcium. (A) Application of 44 mM Ca ASW at pH 7.2; (B) application of 44 mM Ca ASW at pH 9.0 (see text for details). (After Lakshminarayanaiah, N. and Bianchi, C. P., *J. Pharm. Pharmacol.*, 27, 787, 1975.)

spike occurred but was eliminated when the solution pH was changed to 7.2. Replacement of the solution by ASW at pH 9 restored the spike. In this case (Figure 9B), when 44 mM Ca was restored at pH 9, drug escape from the membrane was prevented. Obviously, the secondary effect of calcium at high pH (less hydrogen ions to compete for membrane sites) is that calcium probably binds to biopolymeric chains of the membrane and brings them closer, thus trapping the drug. When the biopolymeric chains approach, reducing their distance of separation, drug fixation is probably enhanced by short range forces of the Heitler-London type.

MECHANISMS OF ANESTHETIC BLOCK

It is evident from the foregoing that for the anesthetic molecules to reversibly eliminate the action potential, they should block the channels in the membrane that control the flow of currents carried by sodium and potassium ions. This can be brought about either by physically blocking the channel or by entering the membrane and bringing about a structural change whereby the channel size is so constricted as to prevent ions from moving through the membrane channels. For these actions to occur, the sodium gate must be open and the local anesthetic molecules must possess enough surface activity and lipid solubility so that interfacial tension is reduced to facilitate entry into the membrane phase. In addition, electrical properties of the anesthetic molecules should facilitate their fixation in the membrane. Investigators have discussed this in a general way and consider it to be a hydrophobic interaction which involves entropic changes leading to clustering of apolar groups in the membrane.[113] The question whether the hydrophobic interactions control narcosis in general has been raised without an answer, emphasizing the need to tackle the problem of hydrophobic bonding as it relates to anesthesia in particular.[114] The hydrate formation theory of Pauling[115] and the ordering of water molecules theory put forth by Miller[116] to explain anesthesia have been discarded for lack of evidence.[117] The other important hypotheses to explain the mechanism of local anesthetic action can be put into three groups: (1) those related to electrical properties of the interacting components — membrane and anesthetic molecules, (2) expansion of the plasma membrane, and (3) specific receptor-local anesthetic interaction.

Electrical Theories

Agin et al.[118] considered the short-range interactions between anesthetics and lipoproteins of the biomembrane, which involve only London energies. If the interaction is between two molecules (drug 1 in uncharged form and water molecules, w), then the energy of interaction, E, is given by:

$$E_1 = \frac{3}{2} \frac{\alpha_1 \alpha_w}{r_1^6} \frac{U_1 U_w}{U_1 + U_w} \tag{12}$$

(see also Koski et al.).[119] In this equation, α is the polarizability, U is the zero-point energy, and r_1 is the distance of separation of molecules of drug 1 and w. Agin et al.[118] replaced U_1 and U_w by ionization potential (ev) I_1 and I_w and considered the biomembrane to be equivalent to a conducting wall. Thus the energy of interaction, E_2, between a drug molecule and the membrane is given by:

$$E_2 = \frac{\alpha_1 I_1}{8 r_2^3} \tag{13}$$

Concentration of drug in the membrane, $\overline{C}$, is related to that in the solution, C, by the Boltzmann relation.
Thus,

$$\overline{C} = C \exp \left(\frac{E_2 - E_1}{RT} \right) \tag{14}$$

Substituting for E_2 and E_1 from Equations 12 and 13 into Equation 14 gives, on rearrangement,

$$\ln C = \ln \overline{C} - \frac{\alpha_1 I_1}{2RT} \left(\frac{1}{4r_2^3} - \frac{3\alpha_w I_w}{r_1^6 (I_1 + I_w)} \right) \tag{15}$$

Substituting minimum blocking concentrations of drug in solution, [MBC], and in membrane, $\overline{C}_s$, for C and $\overline{C}$, respectively, Equation 15 becomes:

$$\log [MBC] = \log \overline{C}_s - Q \alpha_1 I_1 \tag{16}$$

where

$$Q = \frac{1}{4.6 \, RT} \left(\frac{1}{4r_2^3} - \frac{3\alpha_w I_w}{r_1^6 (I_1 + I_w)} \right) \tag{17}$$

Q is practically a constant since variation of I_1 from one drug to another is relatively small and α_w, I_w, r_1 and r_2 are constants. A plot of log [MBC] for a variety of chemical compounds with local anesthetic properties vs. the product ($\alpha_1 I_1$) gave a straight line in accordance with Equation 16.[118]

Equation 16 also held for local anesthetics interacting with a model system (monolayer of L-α-dipalmitoyl lecithin). Skou showed that the increase in surface pressure of a monolayer ($d\pi$) is related to the number of molecules of anesthetic agent present per square centimeter of surface (Γ) of the monolayer,[120] with the help of the Gibbs adsorption equation:

$$\Gamma = \frac{C}{RT}\frac{d\pi}{dc} \tag{18}$$

where C is [MBC] in millimole per liter in the solution. If $\overline{C_s}$ is the concentration at a certain depth, t (in cm) of the monolayer, then Equation 18 can be written as:

$$\overline{C}_s = \frac{\Gamma}{t} = \frac{[MBC]}{t\,RT}\frac{d\pi}{dc} \tag{19}$$

Substituting for $\overline{C_s}$ in Equation 16 gives, on rearrangement:

$$\log\frac{d\pi}{dc} = \log(t\,RT) + Q\alpha_1 I_1 \tag{20}$$

Since [MBC] is small, the approximation:

$$\log\frac{d\pi}{dc} \simeq \log\frac{\Delta\pi}{\Delta c} \simeq \log\frac{\Delta\pi}{[MBC]}$$

gives

$$\log\frac{\Delta\pi}{[MBC]} = \log(t\,RT) + Q\alpha_1 I_1 \tag{21}$$

For a series of anesthetic agents (β-napthol, thymol, ephedrine, procaine, tetracaine, phenyltoloxamine, quinine, and dibucaine), Hersh determined the surface pressure vs. area curves for the monolayer formed from L-α-dipalmitoyl lecithin on a subsolution containing [MBC] of the agent.[121] Surface pressure increases ($\Delta\pi$) at an initial area of 100 A^2 per molecule were considered. A plot of log $\Delta\pi$/[MBC] against $\alpha_1 I_1$ gave a straight line according to Equation 21. Thus the interaction that caused surface tension reduction involved London energies.

Another way of treating this problem of local anesthetic action is to consider that the anesthetic molecules in the charged form, BH^+, interact with the membrane, thereby reducing the membrane surface charge density. This would lead to a change (steeper gradient) in the electrical potential profile within the membrane as shown in Figure 10. As shown, though the resting potential has not changed, the transmembrane potential is increased considerably. If this increase is great, the action currents from adjacent unanesthetized nerve membrane areas may not have sufficient strength to reduce the membrane potential to threshold level, thus allowing conduction block to ensue.

Although many of the physiologically important effects of calcium and pH are explained on the basis of interaction with fixed negative charges on the nerve membrane, the evidence for a similar action of local anesthetic agents is largely indirect. It has come from studies on conductance properties of model systems, such as phospholipid bilayer membranes[122] and liposomes.[123,124] In these systems, reduction in surface negativity of the membrane by drug adsorption leads to a decrease in cation conductance and an increase in anion conductance. Unfortunately, the concept of a change in surface charge mediating local anesthetic block cannot explain the action of an uncharged local anesthetic, such as benzocaine, which has little effect on the membrane surface charge.

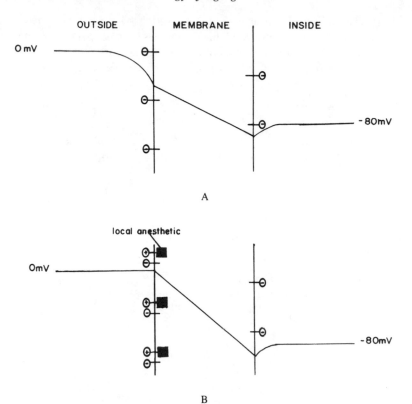

FIGURE 10.   The potential profile in a membrane with fixed negative charges before (A: top) and after (B: bottom) adsorption of local anesthetic molecules to the outside surface of the membrane. In both cases, the membrane potential is the same but the potential profile is steeper in the bottom figure.

Membrane Expansion Theory

The membrane expansion theory, also called the critical volume theory, states that anesthetics adsorb to hydrophobic regions of the membrane, expand some critical region(s) in the membrane, and prevent sodium permeability increase.[125] This is a modification of the Meyer-Overton Theory which states,

"narcosis commences when any chemically indifferent substance has attained a certain molar concentration in the lipoids of the cell. This concentration depends on the nature of the animal or cell but is independent of the narcotic."

Formally, this principle is

$$x_2 P_{50} = \text{Const} = X_{50} \tag{22}$$

where x_2 is the mole fraction solubility per unit pressure of the anesthetic at its site of action, P_{50} is the partial pressure of anesthetic that produces anesthesia in 50% of a group of subjects, and X_{50} is the mole fraction solubility of anesthetic that produces anesthesia in 50% of a group of subjects. Equation 22 follows from Henry's law and can be put in the form of a distribution law:

$$\frac{\text{Concentration of gas in membrane phase}}{\text{Concentration of gas in aqueous phase}} = \text{Constant}$$

that is

$$\frac{X_{50}}{P_{50}} = x_2 \qquad\qquad (23)$$

Ferguson pointed out that the above relationships can be derived in principle from thermodynamic concepts of activity.[127] Recently, a thermodynamic, or rather absolute reaction rate theory, describing the effect of anesthetics on protein conformation, has been advanced to explain general anesthesia.[128,129] Similarly, Hill has advanced a thermodynamic explanation of general anesthetic action based on the Gibbs free energy of the anesthetic site.[130] Mullins has proposed that anesthesia begins when a certain critical volume fraction of an inert substance is attained in membranes.[131,132] Possible interaction of general anesthetic agents and membranes has again been emphasized by Mullins.[133] Other aspects of general anesthetic action have been reviewed by Kaufman.[117]

Absorption of local anesthetics leads to an increase in the volume of nerve membranes[134] and the fluidity of the membrane interior.[135] When local anesthetics in conduction blocking concentrations are absorbed, the volume change in nerve membrane may be at least 4 to 6%.[136] But in phospholipid-cholesterol membranes these changes are considerably less.[137] Presence of protein is apparently necessary to show large volume changes. There is evidence to indicate that local anesthetics modify the dynamic behavior of membrane lipids. During anesthesia, lipid hydrocarbon tails in the membrane have freedom to bend and rotate and thus induce disorder.[135,138-140] In one form of the membrane expansion theory,[141] this disordering effect on lipids is considered to induce a conformational change in proteins closely associated with the lipid. The change in conformation leads to a decrease in membrane permeability to cations, and thus block occurs. Shane's view of the theory is that membrane expansion causes an increase in lateral pressure in the membrane, leading to a constriction of the sodium channel.[142,143] Sodium ions are no longer able to move across the membrane, no action potential can be generated, and conduction block occurs. Antagonism between pressure and anesthesia provides direct evidence for the membrane expansion theory of anesthesia. In 1950, Johnson and Flagler showed that the spontaneous swimming motion of tadpoles, abolished by local anesthetics, was restored by hydrostatic pressures of 150 to 350 atmospheres.[144] This observation has been confirmed in newts.[141] In addition, the ion permeability of liposomes in the presence of anesthetic agents has been counteracted by increasing the pressure.[141] Recently, Kendig and Cohen showed that high atmospheric pressure reversed the depression of the compound action potential produced by halothane, methoxy-flurane, lidocaine, or benzocaine.[145] This is the first demonstration of reversal by pressure of the effect of nitrogeneous local anesthetic agents. Seeman has given a tentative pictorial representation of how pressure would relieve block brought on by anesthetic agents.[146] Pressure reversal of block does not remove the anesthetic from the membrane phase; block reversal is considered to occur by a pressure-induced reconformation of the excitable protein (sodium conductance channel protein). Some role is attributed to the change in the state of water, "melting of the hydrophobic ice-caps and restoration of electrostricted water." However, these changes remain to be demonstrated. One very interesting feature of the membrane expansion theory is that it would, by one mechanism, explain the actions of both general and local anesthetic agents.

Specific Receptor Theory

This hypothesis is based on the fact that the nerve has membrane receptor sites with which local anesthetics may react reversibly, to produce conduction block. Although the membrane expansion theory as envisioned by Shanes[142,143] can explain block of action potentials by the uncharged form of a local anesthetic, it cannot explain the block produced by the charged form. Quaternary analogues of local anesthetics exist only as cations and act from the inside.

They are as active as their tertiary analogues.[68,69,87,99] The mechanism by which they are considered to act is that they form a complex with the sodium channel in the membrane. Sodium ions cannot cross the membrane when the drug-receptor is in the sodium channel. The frequency or use-dependent block cannot be explained without the concept of a specific receptor site or sites. The work of Strichartz showed both the m and h gates of the sodium channel must be open for the sodium current inhibition to occur.[68] Also, reversal of this inhibition when m and h gates are open (membrane depolarization) indicates that drug molecules bind and dissociate from open and not closed sodium channels. Courtney[70] and Hille et al.[87] showed that tertiary amine local anesthetics act in a similar manner. To explain the actions of all forms of local anesthetics (tertiary amine, quaternary compounds, neutral amine), Hille has presented a modulated receptor model.[72] This model uses only one receptor in the sodium channel, accessible to hydrophobic molecules through the membrane phase, and to hydrophilic molecules through the aqueous pore from the axoplasmic side. Hydrophobic molecules can reach the receptor at any time, whereas the hydrophilic molecules can enter only by way of open sodium channels. Both produce sodium inactivation by binding to the receptor on the inside. Similarly, Wagner and Ulbricht,[67] while studying the binding of procaine to a receptor in the presence of saxitoxin (STX), came to the conclusion that procaine had easy access to its receptor located inside the axon. Study of the use or frequency-dependent phenomenon related to procaine-benzocaine interactions at the node of Ranvier also showed that voltage-dependent binding of benzocaine and procaine was to a common receptor.[71]

As opposed to this one receptor model, Khodorov et al.[65] postulate existence of multiple receptors, both outside and inside the axon, to explain their results; particularly the results related to producing or reversing slow sodium inactivation by three types of drugs, neutral, tertiary amine, and quaternary compounds. Colquhoun questions Hille's common receptor site model for not providing experimental evidence of the interactions between ionized and neutral molecules.[147] However, Hille found that benzocaine (neutral) produced the same kind of large negative voltage shift of sodium conductance curve as did lidocaine.[72] But this evidence is considered inadequate, in view of the findings that volatile general anesthetic (trichloroethylene) also produced a similar shift.[148] In keeping with the principle that if two compounds compete for a common site of action, then a mixture of equipotent solutions of the two compounds should have the same effect at equilibrium as either solution by itself, Mrose and Ritchie have demonstrated that lidocaine and mercaine, both partially ionized, act on the same receptor.[149] Nonionized local anesthetics, benzocaine and benzyl alcohol, also followed the principle. But combinations of lidocaine and benzocaine or of lidocaine and benzyl alcohol gave larger responses than those due to solutions of the separate drugs. This suggests that the latter drug combinations do not compete for the same receptor. If benzocaine competes for the lidocaine receptor site, then in order for the combination to produce a larger response it must be acting at another closely related site or it must be producing anesthetic effects through additional mechanisms. In summary, the idea of a common receptor, although useful for explaining several voltage-dependent actions of local anesthetics, cannot explain the experimental results of Khodorov et al.[65] and of Mrose and Ritchie.[149]

CONCLUDING REMARKS

As has been stated earlier, effects of age on excitable membranes have not been studied extensively. It is not known conclusively which ionic channels undergo change during aging, nor what the nature of the changes is. Sensitivity changes to local anesthetic agents with respect to age, outside those mentioned earlier for the action of lidocaine on the heart, have also not been studied extensively. This area is therefore ripe for investigation, both in laboratory animal models and in the clinical setting.

REFERENCES

1. **Hille, B.,** The pH-dependent rate of action of local anesthetics on the node of Ranvier, *J. Gen. Physiol.,* 69, 475, 1977.
2. **Buchi, J. and Perlia, X.,** Structure-activity relations and physio-chemical properties of local anesthetics, in *Local Anesthetics,* Vol. 1, Section 8, International Encyclopedia of Pharmacology and Therapeutics, Lechat, P., Ed., Pergamon Press, Oxford, 1971, 39.
3. *Local Anesthetics,* Vol. 1, Section 8, International Encyclopedia of Pharmacology and Therapeutics, Lechat, P., Ed., Pergamon Press, Oxford, 1971.
4. *Progress in Anesthesiology,* Vol. 1, Molecular Mechanisms of Anesthesia, Fink, B. R., Ed., Raven Press, New York, 1975.
5. **Seeman, P.,** Membrane actions of anesthetics and tranquilizers, *Pharmacol. Rev.,* 24, 583, 1972.
6. **Narahashi, T.,** Drugs affecting axonal membranes, in *Fundamentals of Cell Pharmacology,* Dikstein, S., Ed., Charles C Thomas, Springfield, Ill., 1973, 395.
7. **Ritchie, J. M.,** Mechanisms of action of local anesthetic agents and biotoxins, *Br J. Anaesth.,* 47, 191, 1975.
8. **Strichartz, G.,** Molecular mechanisms of nerve block by local anesthetics, *Anesthesiology,* 45, 421, 1976.
9. **Lakshminarayanaiah, N. and Bianchi, C P.,** Membranes, ions and drugs, in *Advances in General and Cellular Pharmacology,* Vol. II, Narahashi, T. and Bianchi, C. P., Eds., Plenum Press, New York, 1977, 1.
10. **Goldberg, P. B., Stoner, S. A., and Roberts, J.,** Influence of age on activity of antiarrhythmic drugs in rat heart, *Adv. Exp. Med. Biol.,* 97, 309, 1977.
11. **Goldberg, P. B. and Roberts, J.,** Age-related changes in rat atrial sensitivity to lidocaine, *J. Gerontol.,* 36, 520, 1981.
12. **Shock, N. W.,** The science of gerontology, in *Proc. Seminars 1959-61, Durham, N.C.: Council on Gerontology,* E. C. Jeffers, Ed., Duke University Press, Durham, N.C., 1962, 123.
13. **Hodgkin, A. L. and Katz, B.,** The effect of sodium ions on the electrical activity of the giant axon of the squid, *J. Physiol.,* 108, 37, 1949.
14. **Hodgkin, A. L., Huxley, A. F., and Katz, B.,** Measurement of current voltage relations in the membrane of the giant axon of *Loligo, J. Physiol.,* 116, 424, 1952.
15. **Hodgkin, A. L. and Huxley, A. F.,** Currents carried by sodium and potassium ions through the membrane of the giant axon of *Loligo, J Physiol.,* 116, 449, 1952.
16. **Hodgkin, A. L. and Huxley, A. F.,** The components of membrane conductance in the giant axon of *Loligo, J. Physiol.,* 116, 474, 1952.
17. **Hodgkin, A. L. and Huxley, A. F.,** The dual effect of membrane potential on sodium conductance in the giant axon of *Loligo, J. Physiol.,* 116, 497, 1952.
18. **Hodgkin, A. L. and Huxley, A. F.,** A quantitative description of membrane current and its application to conduction and excitation in nerve, *J. Physiol.,* 117, 500, 1952.
19. **Hodgkin, A. L.,** Ionic movements and electrical activity in giant nerve fibers, *Proc. R. Soc. (London),* B148, 1, 1958.
20. **Hodgkin, A. L.,** *The Conduction of the Nervous Impulse,* Charles C Thomas, Springfield, Ill., 1964.
21. **Cole, K. S. and Curtis, H. J.,** Electric impedance of the squid giant axon during activity, *J. Gen. Physiol.,* 22, 649, 1939.
22. **Keynes, R. D. and Lewis, P. R.,** The sodium and potassium content of cephalopod nerve fibres, *J. Physiol.,* 114, 151, 1951.
23. **Cole, K. S.,** Dynamic electrical characteristics of the squid axon membrane, *Arch. Sci. Physiol.,* 3, 253, 1949.
24. **Cole, K. S.,** *Membranes, Ions and Impulses,* University of California Press, Berkeley, 1968.
25. **Keynes, R. D.,** Ion channels in nerve-cell membrane, *Sci. Am.,* 240, 126, 1979.
26. **Hille, B.,** Ionic channels in nerve membranes, *Progr. Biophys. Mol. Biol.,* 21, 1, 1970.
27. **Narahashi, T., Moore, J. W., and Scott, W. R.,** Tetrodotoxin blockage of sodium conductance in lobster giant axons, *J. Gen. Physiol.,* 47, 965, 1964.
28. **Kao, C. Y.,** Tetrodotoxin, Saxitoxin and their significance in the study of excitation phenomena, *Pharmacol. Rev.,* 18, 997, 1966.
29. **Rojas, E. and Atwater, I.,** Effect of tetrodotoxin on the early outward currents in perfused giant axons, *Proc. Natl. Acad. Sci. U.S.A.,* 57, 1350, 1967.
30. **Moore, J. W., Blaustein, M. P., Anderson, N. C., and Narahashi, T.,** Basis of tetrodotoxin's selectivity in blockage of squid axons, *J. Gen. Physiol.,* 50, 1401, 1967.
31. **Hille, B.,** Pharmacological modifications of the sodium channels of frog nerve, *J. Gen. Physiol.,* 51, 199, 1968.
32. **Armstrong, C. M. and Binstock, L.,** Anomalous rectification in the squid giant axon injected with tetraethylammonium chloride, *J. Gen. Physiol.,* 48, 859, 1965.

33. **Hille, B.,** The selective inhibition of delayed potassium currents in nerve by tetraethylammonium ion, *J. Gen. Physiol.*, 50, 1287, 1967.
34. **Chandler, W. K. and Meves, H.,** Voltage clamp experiments on internally perfused giant axons, *J. Physiol.*, 180, 788, 1965.
35. **Adelman, W. J., Jr. and Senft, J. P.,** Voltage clamp studies on the effect of internal cesium ions on sodium and potassium currents in the squid giant axon, *J. Gen. Physiol.*, 50, 279, 1966.
36. **Binstock, L. and Lecar, H.,** Ammonium ion currents in the squid giant axon, *J. Gen. Physiol.*, 53, 342, 1969.
37. **Ehrenstein, G. and Lecar, H.,** The mechanism of signal transmission in nerve axons, *Annu. Rev. Biophys. Bioeng.*, 1, 347, 1972.
38. **Rojas, E. and Armstrong, C. M.,** Sodium conductance activation without inactivation in pronase perfused axons, *Nature (London)*, 229, 177, 1971.
39. **Armstrong, C. M., Rojas, E., and Bezanilla, F.,** Destruction of sodium conductance inactivation in squid axons perfused with pronase, *J. Gen. Physiol.*, 62, 375, 1973.
40. **Rojas, E. and Rudy, B.,** Destruction of sodium conductance inactivation by a specific protease in perfused nerve fibre from *Loligo, J. Physiol,* 262, 501, 1976.
41. **Armstrong, C. M.,** Ionic pores, gates and gating currents, *Q. Rev. Biophys.*, 7, 179, 1974.
42. **Ulbricht, W.,** Ionic channels and gating currents in excitable membranes, *Annu. Rev. Biophys. Bioeng.*, 6, 7, 1977.
43. **Almers, W.,** Gating currents and charge movement in excitable membranes, *Rev. Physiol. Biochem. Pharmacol.*, 82, 96, 1978.
44. **Armstrong, C. M. and Bezanilla, F.,** Charge movement associated with opening and closing of the activation gates of the Na channels, *J. Gen. Physiol.*, 63, 533, 1974.
45. **Keynes, R. D. and Rojas, E.,** Kinetics and steady state properties of the charged system controlling sodium conductance in the squid giant axon, *J. Physiol.*, 239, 393, 1974.
46. **Meves, H.,** The effect of holding potential on the asymmetry currents in squid giant axons, *J. Physiol.*, 243, 847, 1974.
47. **Meves, H.,** Asymmetry currents in intracellularly perfused squid giant axons, *Phil. Trans. R. Soc.*, B270, 493, 1975.
48. **Rojas, E. and Keynes, R. D.,** On the relation between displacement currents and activation of the sodium conductance in the squid giant axon, *Phil. Trans. R. Soc.*, B270, 459, 1975.
49. **Bezanilla, F. and Armstrong, C. M.,** Kinetic properties and inactivation of gating currents of sodium channels in squid axon, *Phil. Trans. R. Soc.*, B270, 449, 1975.
50. **Nonner, W., Rojas, E., and Stämpfli, R.,** Gating currents in the node of Ranvier: voltage and time dependence, *Phil. Trans. R. Soc.*, B270, 483, 1975.
51. **Nonner, W., Rojas, E., and Stämpfli, R.,** Displacement currents in the node of Ranvier: voltage and time dependence, *Pflugers Arch.*, 354, 1, 1975.
52. **Hille, B.,** Gating in sodium channels of nerve, *Annu. Rev. Physiol.*, 38, 139, 1976.
53. **Keynes, R. D. and Rojas, E.,** The temporal and steady state relationships between activation of sodium conductance and movement of the gating particles in the squid giant axon, *J. Physiol.*, 255, 157, 1976.
54. **Armstrong, C. M. and Bezanilla, F.,** Currents associated with the ionic gating structures in nerve membrane, *Ann. N.Y. Acad. Sci.*, 264, 265, 1975.
55. **Levinson, S. R. and Meves, H.,** The binding of tritiated tetrodotoxin to squid giant axons, *Phil. Trans. R. Soc.*, B270, 349, 1975.
56. **Hille, B.,** The permeability of sodium channels to organic cations in myelinated nerves, *J. Gen. Physiol.*, 58, 599, 1971.
57. **Hille, B.,** The permeability of sodium channels to metal cations in myelinated nerves, *J. Gen. Physiol.*, 59, 637, 1972.
58. **Hille, B.,** Potassium channels in myelinated nerves, *J. Gen. Physiol.*, 61, 669, 1973.
59. **Hille, B.,** Ionic channels in excitable membranes: current problems and biophysical approaches, *Biophys. J.*, 22, 283, 1978.
60. **Shanes, A. M., Freygang, W. H., Grundfest, H., and Amatniek, E.,** Anesthetic calcium action in voltage clamped squid giant axon, *J. Gen. Physiol.*, 42, 793, 1959.
61. **Taylor, R. E.,** Effect of procaine on electrical properties of squid axon membrane, *Am. J. Physiol.*, 196, 1071, 1959.
62. **Blaustein, M. P. and Goldman, D. E.,** Competitive action of calcium and procaine on lobster axon, *J. Gen. Physiol.*, 49, 1043, 1966.
63. **Goldman, D. E. and Blaustein, M. P.,** Ions, drugs and the axon membrane, *Ann. N.Y. Acad. Sci.*, 137, 967, 1966.
64. **Århem, P. and Frankenhaeuser, B.,** Local anesthetics: effects on permeability properties of nodal membrane in myelinated nerve fibers from *xenopus, Acta Physiol. Scand.*, 91, 11, 1974.

65. **Khodorov, B., Shishkova, L., Pegnov, E., and Revenko, S.,** Inhibition of sodium currents in frog Ranvier node treated with local anesthetics: role of slow sodium inactivation, *Biochim. Biophys. Acta,* 433, 409, 1976.
66. **Frankenhaeuser, B. and Huxley, A. F.,** The action potential in the myelinated nerve fibre of xenopus laevis as computed on the basis of voltage clamp data, *J. Physiol.,* 171, 302, 1964.
67. **Wagner, H.-H. and Ulbricht, W.,** Saxitoxin and procaine act independently on separate sites of the sodium channel, *Pflugers Arch.,* 364, 65, 1976.
68. **Strichartz, G. R.,** The inhibition of sodium currents in myelinated nerve by quaternary derivatives of lidocaine, *J. Gen. Physiol.,* 62, 37, 1973.
69. **Strichartz, G. R.,** Inhibition of ionic currents in myelinated nerves by quaternary derivatives of lidocaine, in *Progress in Anesthesiology,* Vol. 1, Molecular Mechanisms of Anesthesia, Fink, B. R., Ed., Raven Press, New York, 1975, 1.
70. **Courtney, K. R.,** Mechanism of frequency dependent inhibition of sodium currents in frog myelinated nerve by lidocaine derivative GEA 968, *J. Pharmacol. Exp. Ther.,* 195, 225, 1975.
71. **Rimmel, C., Walle, A., Kebler, H., and Ulbricht, W.,** Rates of block by procaine and benzocaine and the procaine-benzocaine interaction at the node of Ranvier, *Pflugers Arch.,* 376, 105, 1978.
72. **Hille, B.,** Local anesthetics: hydrophilic and hydrophobic pathways for drug-receptor reaction, *J. Gen. Physiol.,* 69, 497, 1977.
73. **Cahalan, M. D.,** Local anesthetic block of sodium channels in normal and pronase treated squid giant axons, *Biophys. J.,* 23, 285, 1978.
74. **Khodorov, B. I.,** Chemicals as tools to study nerve fiber sodium channels: effects of batrachotoxin and some local anesthetics, in *Membrane Transport Processes,* Vol. 2, Tosteson, D. C., Ovachinnikov, Yu. A., and Latorre, R., Eds., Raven Press, New York, 1978, 153.
75. **Hille, B.,** Charges and potentials at the nerve surface. Divalent ions and pH, *J. Gen. Physiol.,* 51, 221, 1968.
76. **Drouin, H. and The, R.,** The effects of reducing extracellular pH on the membrane currents of the Ranvier node, *Pflugers Arch.,* 313, 80, 1968.
77. **Mozhayeva, G. N. and Naumov, A. P.,** Effect of surface charge on the steady state potassium conductance of nodal membrane, *Nature (London),* 228, 164, 1970.
78. **Mozhayeva, G. N. and Naumov, A. P.,** Effect of surface charge on the steady state potassium conductivity of a node of Ranvier. I. Change in pH of external solution, *Biophysics,* 17, 644, 1972.
79. **Stillman, I. M., Gilbert, D. L., and Lipicky, R. J.,** Effect of external pH upon voltage dependent currents of the squid giant axon, *Biophys. J.,* 11, 55a, 1971.
80. **Woodhull, A. M.,** Ionic blockage of sodium channels in nerve, *J. Gen. Physiol.,* 61, 687, 1973.
81. **Shrager, P.,** Ionic conductance changes in voltage clamped crayfish axons at low pH, *J. Gen. Physiol.,* 64, 666, 1974.
82. **Lakshminarayanaiah, N. and Rojas, E.,** Effects of pH and ionic strength on the potassium system in the internally perfused giant barnacle muscle fiber, *Pflugers Arch.,* 358, 349, 1975.
83. **Schauf, C. L. and Davis, F. A.,** Sensitivity of sodium and potassium channels of *Myxicola* giant axons to changes in external pH, *J. Gen. Physiol.,* 67, 185, 1976.
84. **Carbone, E., Fioravanti, R., Prestipino, G., and Wanke, E.,** Action of extracellular pH on Na^+ and K^+ membrane currents in the giant axon of *Loligo Vulgaris, J. Membrane Biol.,* 43, 295, 1978.
85. **Ritchie, J. M. and Greengard, P.,** On the active structure of local anesthetics, *J. Pharmacol. Exp. Ther.,* 133, 241, 1961.
86. **Narahashi, T., Frazier, D. T., and Yamada, M.,** The site of action and active form of local anesthetic. I. Theory and pH experiments with tertiary compounds, *J. Pharmacol. Exp. Ther.,* 171, 32, 1970.
87. **Hille, B., Courtney, K., and Dum, R.,** Rate and site of local anesthetics in myelinated nerve fibers, in *Progress in Anesthesia,* Vol. 1, Molecular Mechanisms of Anesthesia, Fink, B. R., Ed., Raven Press, New York, 1975, 13.
88. **Skou, J. C.,** Local anesthetics, I. The blocking potencies of some local anesthetics and of butyl alcohol determined on peripheral nerves, *Acta Pharmacol. Toxicol.,* 10, 281, 1954.
89. **Rud, J.,** Local anesthetics, *Acta Physiol. Scand.,* 51(Suppl. 1978), 1, 1961.
90. **Ritchie, J. M., Ritchie, B. R., and Greengard, P.,** The effect of nerve sheath on the action of local anesthetics, *J. Pharmacol. Exp. Ther.,* 150, 160, 1965.
91. **Ritchie, J. M. and Greengard, P.,** On the mode of action of local anesthetics, *Annu. Rev. Pharmacol.,* 6, 405, 1966.
92. **Ritchie, J. M.,** The mechanism of action of local anesthetic agents, in *Local Anesthetics,* Vol. 1, Section 8, International Encyclopedia of Pharmacology and Therapeutics, Lechat, P., Ed., Pergamon Press, Oxford, 1971, 131.
93. **Ritchie, J. M., Ritchie, B. R., and Greengard, P.,** The active structure of local anesthetics, *J. Pharmacol. Exp. Ther.,* 150, 152, 1965 .

94. **Ritchie, J. M. and Ritchie, B. R.,** Local anesthetics: effect of pH on activity, *Science,* 162, 1394, 1968.
95. **Bianchi, C. P. and Strobel, G. E.,** Modes of action of local anesthetics in nerve and muscle in relation to their uptake and distribution, *Trans. N.Y. Acad. Sci.,* 30, 1082, 1968.
96. **Strobel, G. E. and Bianchi, C. P.,** The effects of pH gradients on the action of procaine and lidocaine in intact and desheathed sciatic nerves, *J. Pharmacol. Exp. Ther.,* 172, 1, 1970.
97. **Strobel, G. E. and Bianchi, C. P.,** The effects of pH gradients in the uptake and distribution of C^{14}-procaine and lidocaine in intact and desheathed sciatic nerve trunks, *J. Pharmacol. Exp. Ther.,* 172, 18, 1970.
98. **Narahashi, T., Moore, J. W., and Poston, R. N.,** Anesthetic blocking of nerve membrane conductances by internal and external applications, *J. Neurobiol.,* 1, 3, 1969.
99. **Frazier, D. T., Narahashi, T., and Yamada, M.,** The site of action and active form of local anesthetics. II. Experiments with quaternary compounds, *J. Pharmacol. Exp. Ther.,* 171, 45, 1970.
100. **Narahashi, T., Frazier, D. T., Moore, J. W.,** Comparison of tertiary and quaternary amine local anesthetics in their ability to depress membrane ionic conductances, *J. Neurobiol.,* 3, 267, 1972.
101. **Narahashi, T. and Frazier, D. T.,** Site of action and active form of procaine in squid giant axons, *J. Pharmacol. Exp. Ther.,* 194, 506, 1975.
102. **Schauf, C. and Agin, D.,** Cooperative effect of certain anesthetics on the lobster giant axon, *Nature (London),* 221, 768, 1969.
103. **Narahashi, T. and Frazier, D. T.,** Site of action and active form of local anesthetics, in *Neuroscience Research,* Vol. 4, Ehrenpreis, S. and Solnitsky, O. C., Eds., Academic Press, New York, 1971, 65.
104. **Lakshminarayanaiah, N. and Bianchi, C. P.,** Ca^{2+} concentration and interaction of long-lasting local anesthetics with the squid axon membrane, *J. Pharm. Pharmacol.,* 27, 787, 1975.
105. **Schwarz, W., Palade, P. T., and Hille, B.,** Local anesthetics: effect of pH on use-dependent block of sodium channels in frog muscle, *Biophys. J.,* 20, 343, 1977.
106. **Bianchi, C. P. and Bolton, T. C.,** Action of local anesthetics on coupling systems in muscle, *J. Pharmacol. Exp. Ther.,* 157, 388, 1967.
107. **Weidmann, S.,** The effects of calcium ions and local anesthetics on electrical properties of Purkinje fibers, *J. Physiol.,* 129, 568, 1955.
108. **Frankenhaeuser, B. and Hodgkin, A. L.,** The action of calcium on the electrical properties of squid axons, *J. Physiol.,* 137, 218, 1957.
109. **Blaustein, M. P. and Goldman, D. E.,** Action of anionic and cationic nerve blocking agents. Experiment and interpretation, *Science,* 153, 429, 1966.
110. **Blaustein, M. P.,** Phospholipids as ion-exhangers: implications for a possible role in biological membrane excitability and anesthesia, *Biochim. Biophys. Acta,* 135, 653, 1967.
111. **Narahashi, T., Frazier, D. T., and Takeno, K.,** Effects of calcium on the local anesthetic suppression of ionic conductances in squid axon membranes, *J. Pharmacol. Exp. Ther.,* 197, 426, 1976.
112. **Suarez-Kurtz, G., Bianchi, C. P., and Krupp, P.,** Effect of local anesthetics on radiocalcium binding in nerve, *Eur. J. Pharmacol.,* 10, 91, 1970.
113. **Nemathy, G.,** Hydrophobic interactions, *Angew. Chem. Int. Ed.,* 6, 195, 1967.
114. **Hersh, L-S.,** Cellular narcosis and hydrophobic bonding, in *Biosurfaces,* Vol. 1, Hair, M. L., Ed., Marcel Dekker, New York, 1971, 349.
115. **Pauling, L.,** A molecular theory of anesthesia, *Science,* 134, 15, 1961.
116. **Miller, S. L.,** A theory of gaseous anesthesia, *Proc. Natl. Acad. Sci. U.S.A.,* 47, 1515, 1961.
117. **Kaufman, R. D.,** Biophysical mechanisms of anesthetic action: historical perspective and review of current concepts, *Anesthesiology,* 46, 49, 1977.
118. **Agin, D., Hersh, L., and Holtzman, D.,** The action of anesthetics on excitable membranes: a quantum-chemical analysis, *Proc. Natl. Acad. Sci. U.S.A.,* 53, 952, 1965.
119. **Koski, W. S., Wilson, K. M., and Kaufman, J. J.,** Correlation between anesthetic potency and the van der Waals a constant, in *Progress in Anesthesiology,* Vol. 1, Molecular Mechanisms of Anesthesia, Fink, B. R., Ed., Raven Press, New York, 1974, 277.
120. **Skou, J. C.,** Local anesthetics. VI. Relation between blocking potency and penetration of a monomolecular layer of lipoids from nerve, *Acta Pharmacol. Toxicol.,* 10, 325, 1954.
121. **Hersh, L.,** The interaction of local anesthetics with lecithin monolayers, *Mol. Pharmacol.,* 3, 581, 1967.
122. **McLaughlin, S.,** Local anesthetics and the electrical properties of phospholipid bilayer membranes, in *Progress in Anesthesiology,* Vol. 1, Molecular Mechanisms of Anesthesia, Fink, B. R., Ed., Raven Press, New York, 1975, 193.
123. **Bangham, A. D., Standish, M. M., and Miller, N.,** Cation permeability of phospholipid model membranes: effect of narcotics, *Nature (London),* 208, 1295, 1965.
124. **Singer, M.,** Effects of local anesthetics on phospholipid bilayer membranes, in *Progress in Anesthesiology,* Vol. 1, Molecular Mechanisms of Anesthesia, Fink, B. R., Ed., Raven Press, New York, 1975, 223.
125. **Seeman, P.,** The membrane actions of anesthetics and tranquilizers, *Pharmacol. Rev.,* 24, 583, 1972.
126. **Meyer, K. H.,** Contribution to the theory of narcosis, *Trans. Faraday Soc.,* 33, 1062, 1937.

127. **Ferguson, J.,** The use of chemical potentials as indices of toxicity, *Proc. R. Soc.,* B127, 387, 1939.

128. **Eyring, H., Woodbury, J. W., and D'Arrigo, J. S.,** A molecular mechanism of general anesthesia, *Anesthesiology,* 38, 415, 1973.

129. **Woodbury, J. W., D'Arrigo, J. S., and Eyring, H.,** Molecular mechanism of general anesthesia: lipoprotein conformation change theory, in *Progress in Anesthesiology,* Vol. 1, Molecular Mechanisms of Anesthesia, Fink, B. R., Ed., Raven Press, New York, 1975, 253.

130. **Hill, M. W.,** The Gibbs free energy hypothesis of general anesthesia, in *Molecular Mechanisms of General Anesthesia,* Halsey, M. J., Miller, R. A., and Sutton, J. A., Eds., Churchill Livingstone, Edinburgh, 1974, 132.

131. **Mullins, L. J.,** Some physical mechanisms in narcosis, *Chem. Rev.,* 54, 289, 1954.

132. **Mullins, L. J.,** Anesthetics, in *Handbook of Neurochemistry,* Vol. 6, Lajtha, A., Ed., Plenum Press, New York, 1971, 395.

133. **Mullins, L. J.,** Anesthesia: an overview, in *Progress in Anesthesiology,* Vol. 1, Molecular Mechanisms of Anesthesia, Fink, B. R., Ed., Raven Press, New York, 1975, 237.

134. **Roth, S. H. and Seeman, P.,** All lipid soluble anesthetics protect red cells, *Nature (London), New Biol.,* 231, 284, 1971.

135. **Trudell, J. R. and Cohen, E. N.,** Anesthetic induced nerve membrane fluidity as a mechanism of anesthesia, in *Progress in Anesthesiology,* Vol. 1, Molecular Mechanisms of Anesthesia, Fink, B. R., Ed., Raven Press, New York, 1975, 315.

136. **Roth, S. H., Jay, A. W. L., and Beck, J. S.,** Expansion of intact red blood cell membrane by butanol, *Fed. Proc., Fed. Am. Soc. Exp. Biol.,* 33, 2079, 1974.

137. **Seeman, P.,** The membrane expansion theory of anesthesia, in *Progress in Anesthesiology,* Vol. 1, Molecular Mechanisms of Anesthesia, Fink, B. R. Ed., Raven Press, New York, 1975, 243.

138. **Hubbell, W. L. and McConnell, H. M.,** Spin label studies of the excitable membrane of nerve and muscle, *Proc. Natl. Acad. Sci. U.S.A.,* 61, 12, 1968.

139. **Metcalf, J. C., Seeman, P., and Burgen, A. S. V.,** The proton relaxation of benzyl alcohol in erythrocyte membranes, *Mol. Pharmacol.,* 4, 87, 1968.

140. **Metcalf, J. C. and Burgen, A. S. V.,** Relaxation of anesthetics in the presence of cytomembranes, *Nature (London),* 220, 587, 1968.

141. **Johnson, S. M. and Miller, K.,** Antagonism of pressure and anesthesia, *Nature (Lonon),* 228, 75, 1970.

142. **Shanes, A. M.,** Electrochemical aspects of physiological and pharmacological action in excitable cells. I. The resting cell and its alteration by extrinsic factors, *Pharmacol. Rev.,* 10, 59, 1958.

143. **Shanes, A. M.,** Electrochemical aspects of physiological and pharmacological action in excitable cells. II. The action potential and excitation, *Pharmacol. Rev.,* 10, 165, 1958.

144. **Johnson, F. H. and Flagler, E. A.,** Hydrostatic pressure reversal of narcosis in tadpoles, *Science,* 112, 91, 1950.

145. **Kendig, J. J. and Cohen, E. N.,** Pressure antagonism to nerve conduction block by anesthetic agents, *Anesthesiology,* 47, 6, 1977.

146. **Seeman, P.,** Anesthetics and pressure reversal of anesthesia: expansion and recompression of membrane proteins, lipids and water, *Anesthesiology,* 47, 1, 1977.

147. **Colquhoun, D.,** Noise: a tool for drug receptor investigation, in *Cell Membrane Receptors for Drugs and Hormones: a Multi-Disciplinary Approach,* Straub, R. W. and Bolis, L., Eds., Raven Press, New York, 1978, 31.

148. **Shrivastav, B. B., Narahashi, T., Kutz, R. J., and Roberts, J. D.,** Mode of action of trichlorethylene on squid axon membranes, *J. Pharmacol. Exp. Ther.,* 199, 179, 1976.

149. **Mrose, H. E. and Ritchie, J. M.,** Local anesthetics: do benzocaine and lidocaine act at the same single site?, *J. Gen. Physiol.,* 71, 223, 1978.

AUTONOMIC DRUGS

Jay Roberts

INTRODUCTION

Autonomic drugs include adrenergic and cholinergic agonists and antagonists. These drugs can interact directly with specific cellular receptors within the organ system, or indirectly at sites within the autonomic nervous system, i.e., at presynaptic and postsynaptic areas such as ganglia, nerve terminals, or postganglionic fibers. Autonomic activity may be influenced by hormones or modulators of neurotransmisson[1] through positive and negative feedback mechanisms operating locally at the neuroeffector junction (Figure 1). Also, response to autonomic receptor activation may be altered by agents acting on the sequence of events which follow receptor stimulation.

Some drugs which influence autonomic function do so by modifying the afferent input of visceral reflexes, for example, at the chemo- and baroreceptors in the carotid body and sinus. Others influence autonomic function through the centers of the brain such as the hypothalamus and vasomotor centers. Thus, drug effects on the autonomic nervous system can vary, depending on the setting. Effects may differ both quantitatively and qualitatively.

In what follows, an attempt will be made to assess whether drug effects are due to direct or indirect changes. With the exception of the section on neurotransmitters which refers to autonomic function in general, the discussion is organized to examine drug effects on autonomic function, system by system. The systems analyzed had to be restricted to those for which sufficient data have been compiled with respect to age: (1) heart, (2) vasculature, (3) exocrine glands, (4) smooth muscle of the pupil and bronchi, and (5) thermogenesis.

The term "aging" is reserved for that part of the age spectrum which is not developmental, that is, it excludes from the neonatal state into adulthood. For information about drugs that influence transmitters in the central nervous system, the reader is referred to Dr. Horita's chapter in this handbook.

Since the autonomic nervous system regulates visceral function involved in the maintenance of homeostasis, and since breakdown in homeostasis has been suggested as the cause for the demise of the organism with age,[2] it is extremely important to consider how autonomic functions may be influenced by pharmacologic means. This approach should not only aid in defining the role of alterations in autonomic function in the aging process but should provide insight into how the aging process could be manipulated through the autonomic nervous system.

Presentation of data in this review will primarily relate to the three species: man, rat, and mouse, most commonly used for aging investigations. However, the sparser data available for monkeys, rabbits, and chickens will also be mentioned. With respect to definition, Finch[3,4] has attempted to define and measure chronological age in terms of physiological landmarks. In mice and rats, whose normal life span is limited to 3 years (compared to 80 years in man), the first quarter (9 months) of life can be designated as "youth" during which chemical maturity and puberty occur. During months 10 to 12, maximum stable values of skeletal size and body and brain weight (maturity) are achieved; this corresponds to the first 20 to 30 years of human life. The last quarter of life in man as well as in rodents, when many body functions are deteriorated and organs show pathological changes, may be designated as senescence.[5]

NEUROTRANSMITTERS

There is considerable evidence that synthesis of the transmitters and their biotransformation as well as degradation of autonomic agents are influenced by increasing age. Enzymes

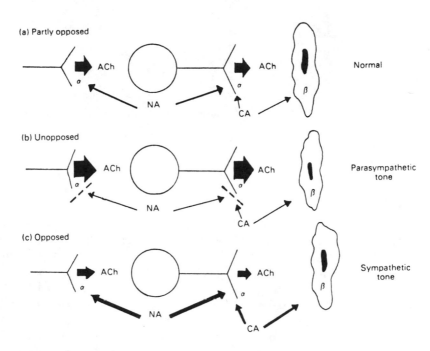

FIGURE 1.   Interneuronal modulation of cholinergic transmission in the gastrointestinal tract. 'Brake' system operates: (a) noradrenaline released from the sympathetic nerves continuously inhibits the release of acetylcholine from Auerbach's plexus which is, in fact, responsible for the motility (normal); (b) when the noradrenergic control is partly or completely removed acetylcholine release becomes higher resulting in a parasympathetic tone; however, when the noradrenergic outflow is increased (shock, stress, etc.) the cholinergic outflow is partly, or completely inhibited producing the symptoms of sympathetic dominance (e.g., obstipation, paralytic ileus). The sympathetic tone can be counteracted by β-receptor blocking drugs. (Taken from Vizi, E. S., *Trends in Pharmacol. Sci.*, (1), 173, 1979-1980. With permission.)

involved in synthesis of transmitters have been studied by Reis et al.[6] They investigated regionally, in the brain, in the adrenal medulla, and in the sympathetic ganglia of young (4 months) and aged (24 to 26 months) rats and mice the effects of aging on the activities of the catecholamine synthesizing enzymes (1) tyrosine hydroxylase (TH), (2) aromatic L-amino acid decarboxylase (DDC), (3) dopamine-β-hydroxylase (DBH), and (4) phenylethanolamine-*N*-methyltransferase (PNMT). They also studied the activity of choline acetyltransferase (CAT), the enzyme synthesizing acetylcholine. Results of this study are shown in Figures 2 to 4. In brain, significant changes in enzyme activity were variable; they were also regional and present only in rats. The changes were small, usually less than 20%. In both species, however, the activities of CAT, TH, and DDC, but not DBH, were increased 1.5 to 2.5-fold in the adrenals of the aged animals compared with the 4-month-old animals. The increase in adrenal TH and DDC activities with aging occurred without a change in the Michaelis rate constant (Km) for substrate or cofactor and could be demonstrated, by immunotitration with specific antibodies, to be due to accumulation of enzyme protein. A comparable pattern of changes in enzyme activities occurred in the superior cervical ganglion of rats. It was concluded that significant elevations in the activities and amounts of several enzyme-synthesizing catecholamines, and acetylcholine, occur in the adrenals of aging rats and mice. These findings were not observed in the enzymes in brain. The pattern of change in adrenal enzymes appear unique for aging since, in most cases, decreased activity occurs.

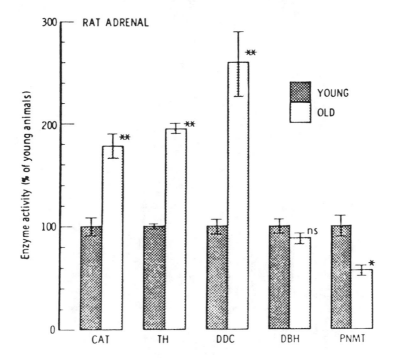

FIGURE 2. Difference in activity of CAT, TH, DDC, DBH, and PNMT in adrenal glands of young and old rats. Each bar represents the mean ± S.E.M. of 6 to 8 rats. Enzyme activity is expressed as percentage of mean ± S.E.M. of activity in adrenal gland of 7 younger rats. Enzyme activity (mean ± S.E.M.) in adrenal glands of young rats is: CAT, 0.53 ± 0.04 nmol ACh formed/adrenal/ h; TH, 42.6 ± 1.0 nmol DOPA formed/adrenal/h; DDC, 26.3 ± 1.7 nmol CO_2 formed/adrenal/h; DBH, 66.5 ± 5.1 nmol phenylethanolamine formed/adrenal/ h; PNMT, 3.7 ± 0.4 nmol N methylphenylethanolamine formed/adrenal/h. **P <0.001, *P <0.01. (Taken from Reis, D. J. et al., *Brain Research*, 1977, 469. With permission.)

The results suggest an increased capacity for biosynthesis of circulating catecholamines. This pattern of change in the adrenal catecholamines was also noted by Kvetnansky et al.[7] These observations may be attributable to decreased influences of sympathetic innervation of heart with age, which results in increased synthesis of adrenal catecholamines according to Gauthier et al.[8]

The absence of changes in brain TH and DBH activity found by Reis et al.,[6] contradicting observations made by others in man and another strain of rat,[9,10] suggests that some changes in brain catecholamine enzymes in aging may be a species and even strain-specific event, and not a universal concomitant of aging. Indeed, Simkins et al.[11] found in the brains of older Wistar rats that catecholamine metabolism decreases, whereas that of serotonin increases. They related these changes to decreased release of gonadotropins and increased release of prolactin with increasing age.

With regard to monoamine oxidase (MAO) activity, the effect of age has been variously reported. Feldman, and Roche[12] studied the effect of aging on MAO activity in tissues of mice and rabbits. There were no alterations in the MAO activity of liver, kidney, pancreas, and brain (adult mice and rabbits) or testis and heart (adult mice) with aging. There were no alterations in the norepinephrine content of the brain, kidney, and heart of older mice. The Feldman study indicates that increased MAO activity is not inevitably associated with aging in all species.[12]

In human beings, Robinson et al.[13,14] reported that MAO activity has a significant positive

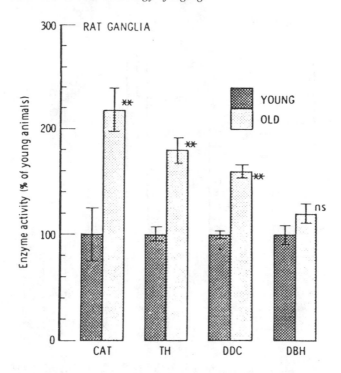

FIGURE 3.   Differences in CAT, TH, DDC, and DBH activity in
superior cervical ganglia of young and old rats. Each bar represents
mean ± S.E.M. of 6 to 8 animals and enzyme activity is expressed
as percentage of mean ± S.E.M. of enzyme activity in young rats.
Enzyme activity (mean ± S.E.M.) in superior cervical ganglia of
young rats is: CAT, 4.27 ± 1.07 nmol ACh formed/ganglia/h; TH,
2.8 ± 0.2 nmol DOPA formed/ganglia/h; DDC, 1.7 ± 0.06 μmol
CO_2 formed/ganglia/h; DBH, 135.4 ± 12.1 nmol octopamine formed/
ganglia/h. (Taken from Reis, D. J. et al., *Brain Research*, 1977, 469.
With permission.)

correlation with age in plasma and blood platelets of normal subjects, and patients suffering
from depressive disorders. According to Robinson, in humans, MAO and increasing age
correlated positively in hindbrain and in eight separate areas of human brains, from patients
who died from a variety of causes. Hindbrain norepinephrine concentration progressively
decreased with advancing age (r = −0.44 p<0.01) while no changes were noted for
serotonin (5-HT) and 5-hydroxyindoleacetic acid (5-HIAA). Hindbrain norepinephrine concentration has a significant negative correlation with MAO (r = −0.41 p<0.025) and
hindbrain 5-HIAA had a significant positive correlation with MAO (r = +0.66 p = <0.05).
These studies suggest that the aging process may affect significantly monoamine mechanisms
and may be a predisposing factor to the development in man of clinical diseases, such as
depression, Parkinsonism and other disorders of central nervous system homeostasis.

In Wistar rats, Inagaki and Tanaka reported changes in the activities of L-aromatic amino
acid decarboxylase (AADC) and MAO (Table 1).[15] The enzyme activity was measured in
kidney, liver, brain, and heart of the rat from neonatal to senescent stages. Rapid neonatal
increase to adult level was observed in the specific activity of AADC in the kidney, liver,
and brain. The total activity of AADC continued to increase in the brain for 3 weeks after
birth and for 20 weeks in the kidney and liver. In the heart, the specific activity of AADC
increased up to the 10th day after birth, then decreased to the mature level during the next
10 days. Senescent decreases both in specific and total activities of AADC were observed
in all organs examined. Similarly, neonatal increment to the adult level was observed in the
specific and total activities of MAO in kidney, liver, and brain. Senescent decrement in

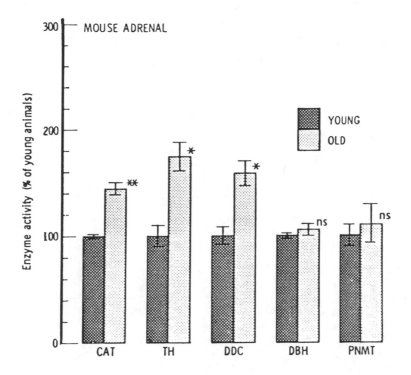

FIGURE 4.   Differences in CAT, TH, DDC, DBH, and PNMT activity in adrenal glands of young and old mice. Each bar represents mean ± S.E.M. of 6 mice and enzyme activity is expressed as a percentage of mean ± S.E.M. of enzyme activity in young mice. Enzyme activity (mean ± S.E.M.) in adrenal glands of young mice is: CAT, 4.0 ± 0.1 nmol ACh/adrenal/h; TH, 12.4 ± 1.3 nmol DOPA/adrenal/h; DDC, 5.17 ± 0.42 μmol CO_2/adrenal/h, DBH, 5.44 ± 0.12 nmol phenylethanolamine/adrenal/h; PNMT, 11.6 ± 1.2 nmol N-methylphenylethanolamine/adrenal/h.** P <0.001, * P < 0.01, ns, not significant. (Taken from Reis, D. J. et al., *Brain Research,* 1977, 469. With permission.)

specific and total MAO activities was demonstrated in the kidney, but changes in liver and brain were not observed. The MAO activity in heart continued to increase in linear fashion for 70 weeks after birth. The concentration of 5HT in kidney, liver, and brain of the 10-day old rats was much less than that in the adult. Senescent decrease of 5HT content was not evident in any organ examined. These findings suggest an age-related change of amine metabolism may occur in some organ systems, but not in others.

In addition to MAO and AADC, catecholamine-o-methyltransferase (COMT) shows changes with aging. Prange et al.[16] found that in the liver of Sprague Dawley rats of 2 to 9 weeks (Group I), 9 to 35 weeks (Group II), and 35 to 100 weeks (Group III) of age COMT and MAO activity increased in Group II compared to Group I but the activity in Group III was similar to that of Group I. In the heart,[16] only MAO increased with aging; COMT activity in the kidney decreased. The activity of both enzymes in brain was constant across all age groups.

Evidence that not only the metabolism of transmitters is affected by age but also by drugs which affect transmitter function is provided by the observation that, in human beings,[17] propranolol metabolism in smokers who are older is decreased, compared to its metabolism by young smokers. This was attributed to the possibility that there is decreased induction of drug metabolizing enzymes with aging.[17,18] Mueller and Shideman,[19] studying infant male Sprague Dawley rats (20 to 24 g) and adult male rats (350 to 379 g), found that in infant brain, reserpine is readily metabolized. In the case of nicotine, older female mice (18 months) were able to produce cotinine (oxidative metabolite of nicotine) at the same rate as younger mice (2 to 12 months).[18]

Table 1
5HT LEVELS AND ENZYME ACTIVITIES PER GRAM OF RAT TISSUES AT VARIOUS AGES

		10 Days[a]	6 Weeks	20 Weeks	Over 70 weeks
Kidney	5HT	0.083 ± 0.000[b]	0.204 ± 0.045	0.200 ± 0.024	0.319 ± 0.114
	AADC	3.53 ± 0.67[b]	11.07 ± 1.35	8.74 ± 0.65	4.66 ± 1.35[b]
	MAO	0.073 ± 0.002[b]	0.334 ± 0.081	0.258 ± 0.026	0.105 ± 0.025[b]
Liver	5HT	0.185 ± 0.032[b]	0.417 ± 0.041	0.883 ± 0.123	0.882 ± 0.259
	AADC	2.40 ± 0.49[b]	6.50 ± 0.68	7.47 ± 0.64	3.77 ± 0.08[b]
	MAO	0.600 ± 0.179[b]	2.589 ± 0.618	1.001 ± 0.190	1.050 ± 0.132
Brain	5HT	0.249 ± 0.010[b]	0.563 ± 0.030	0.576 ± 0.022	0.537 ± 0.017
	AADC	0.281 ± 0.028[b]	0.527 ± 0.075	0.548 ± 0.076	0.253 ± 0.083[b]
	MAO	0.130 ± 0.019[c]	0.352 ± 0.054	0.329 ± 0.060	0.294 ± 0.025

Note: 5HT: μg 5HT/g of tissue.
AADC (L-aromatic amino acid decarboxylase): μmol 5HT/g of tissue/hr.
MAO (monoamine oxidase) activity: μmol 5HIAA/g of tissue/hr.
Means ± S.E. of values from 6 to 8 rats.

[a] Means ± SE of 3-4 determination from 9 to 12 rats.
[b] p <0.01.
[c] p <0.05 as compared to the corresponding value at 20 weeks of age.

Taken from Tanaka, C. and Inagaki, C., *Jpn. J. Pharmacol.*, 24, 439, 1074. With permission.

ACTIONS ON THE HEART

Certain autonomic substances affecting the heart have been studied with regard to age differences. These can be divided into the following groups: (1) the sympathomimetic amines, e.g., epinephrine and norepinephrine; (2) sympathetic antagonists, e.g., propranolol; (3) parasympathomimetic agonists, e.g., acetylcholine; and (4) parasympathetic antagonists, e.g., atropine (Table 2).[20] Other substances within the groups just mentioned (e.g., tyramine, which acts through release of norepinephrine from prejunctional sympathetic nerve terminals) have been studied primarily as pharmacological tools for investigating drug action in tissue, but not with respect to age.

Sympathetic Agonists and Antagonists

In the whole animal, sensitivity to sympathomimetics has been found to increase with increasing age[21,22] although there are many opposite findings and there is confusion between maturational and senescent changes. For example, the LD$_{50}$ for epinephrine was found to decrease significantly with increasing age in mice.[23] In contrast, the LD$_{50}$ for ephedrine was found to decrease significantly during maturation between young (4 months old) and adult (12 months old) rats, then to increase somewhat in old (24 months) rats.[24] If it is assumed that cardiac toxicity of the substance contributes to its lethality, then it is expected that cardiac sensitivity to the substance has changed as a function of age. Other evidence of increased sensitivity is obtained from measurements of blood pressure and heart rate changes. Thus, it has been shown that old rabbits require lower intravenous doses of epinephrine and norepinephrine than do adult rabbits to evoke equivalent changes in arterial blood pressure.[25] Similarly, in rats, it was found that for a given dose of epinephrine and norepinephrine, greater blood pressure changes were evoked in adult (14 months) than in young adult (3

Table 2
EFFECT OF INCREASING AGE ON CARDIOVASCULAR SENSITIVITY TO AUTONOMIC DRUGS

Drug	Species	Effect studied	Effect of increasing age
Sympathetic			
Epinephrine	Mouse	LD_{50}	Decrease
	Rat	Increase blood pressure	Increase
	Rabbit	Increase blood pressure	Increase
	Man	Increase heart rate	Increase
Norepinephrine	Rat	Increase blood pressure	Increase
		Increase ventricular active tension	Decrease
		Increase ventricular maximum rate of tension development	Decrease
		Decrease ventricular contraction duration	Decrease
		Relax aortic smooth muscle	Decrease
	Rabbit	Increase blood pressure	Increase
Isoproterenol	Rat	Increase ventricular active tension	Decrease
		Increase ventricular maximum rate of tension development	Decrease
		Decrease ventricular contraction duration	Decrease
		Relax aortic smooth muscle	Decrease
	Rabbit	Relax aortic smooth muscle	Decrease
	Dog	Increase heart rate	Decrease
	Man	Increase heart rate	Decrease
Phenylephrine	Rat	Reflex decrease heart rate	Decrease
	Man	Reflex decrease heart rate	Decrease
Ephedrine	Rat	LD_{50}	Decrease, young to adult, increase adult to old
Reserpine	Cat	Deplete cardiac catecholamines	Decrease, young to adult
Tyramine	Rabbit	Increase heart rate (in vitro) due to release of cardiac neuronal catecholamines	Decrease, young to adult
Propranolol	Man	Decrease systolic and diastolic blood pressure	Increase
		Decrease cardiac index	Increase
Parasympathetic			
Acetylcholine	Rabbit	Decrease blood pressure	Increase
		Decrease cardiac output	Increase
		Decrease atrial rate (in vitro)	Decrease, neonatal to adult
Methacholine	Man	Decrease blood pressure	Increase
Atropine	Man	Increase heart rate	Decrease

Based on Goldberg, P. B. and Roberts, J., Pharmacology, in *The Aging Heart, Aging,* Vol. 12, Weisfeldt, M. L., Ed., Raven Press, New York, 1980, 238. With permission.

months) rats.[26] Corresponding results have been obtained in humans, where it was found that infusion of a standard dose of catecholamines increased heart rate in older individuals (67.5 years mean age) to a greater extent than in young individuals (25.5 years mean age).[27] However, opposite results with respect to catecholamines have been found in aging dogs.[28] Conway found that propranolol,[29] a beta-adrenergic receptor antagonist, used in younger and older human subjects in comparable doses, produced significant decreases in systolic and diastolic blood pressure, as well as in cardiac index — in persons 50 to 65 years of age; but it did not produce these changes in humans 18 to 35 years of age.

The above observations indicate that alterations of the pharmacological effects of sympathetic agonists and antagonists occur as aging progresses. However, because of the complexity of the in vivo situation, it cannot be ascertained whether the changes occur in the heart per se, in the vasculature, in the cardiovascular reflex mechanisms, or some combination of these. Indeed, it has been shown that the baroreceptor reflex is more reactive in young animals and man than in old individuals,[30,31] indicating that reflex influences and autonomic regulation of cardiac function diminishes with increasing age. In these studies, phenylephrine was used as the pressor agent; and, since it has negligible direct effects on the heart, the observed changes in heart rate can reasonably be assumed to result from reflex pathway activation. Rothbaum et al.[30] further pursued the question of whether the diminished baroreceptor reflex in the old animals was attributable to a differential aging effect on sympathetic or parasympathetic control of the heart. This was accomplished by the use of a beta-adrenergic receptor antagonist (propranolol), and a parasympathetic antagonist (atropine). They found that with increasing age, both sympathetic and parasympathetic influences on the heart decreased, but that the latter decreased to a greater extent. However, this conclusion was based on the assumption that the antagonists have similar blocking potentials in young and old hearts (i.e., the affinity and the number of cardiac receptors for these antagonists do not change with increasing age). The validity of this assumption is open to question, based on the observations of Conway et al.[29] discussed above. Rothbaum et al.[30] also concluded that the decline in cardiac output and stroke volume with increasing age was not related to differences in sympathetic nervous system tone. However, since dose-response relationships were not performed with propranolol, their conclusion requires further validation.

Age also influences the response of hypertensive persons to beta-adrenergic blocking agent. In 83% of patients aged under 40 years, oxyprenolol caused a reduction in diastolic pressure to < 95 mmHg, while it produced this effect in only 50% of those in the 40- to 56-year-old group.[32] This work has been extended to show that the beta blocking agents, propranolol and oxyprenolol, normalized blood pressure (< 96 mmHg diastolic) in 75% of those younger than 40 years; in about half of those aged 40 to 60 years, but in only 20% of those over 60 years of age.[33,34] This seems to indicate that older patients, who often have low renin, exhibit a relatively hypoadrenergic state. Those with a normal or high renin for a given age, concomitant with elevated blood pressure, have a relatively increased adrenergic nervous activity.[33] However, Buhler found that in persons with low renin,[34] hypertension progressively increased with increasing age, there being no difference between the sexes. It should be noted that in the elderly (64 to 84 years), treatment of hypertension may not always be appropriate; reducing pressure with methyldopa, oxyprenolol, and cyclopenthiazide in six of six patients caused episodes of unconsciousness requiring hospitalization.[35] This study is supported by another which pointed to the need to use extreme care in treating the elderly with antihypertensive agents.[36] The effect of the beta blocking agent, metoprolol, given to 12 geriatric patients, age greater than 60 years, seems to be more variable than in those who are younger. This may be due to differences in body weight, absorption, and/or degradation of the drug by the liver.[37]

Along with increased blood pressure levels, there seems to be an increase in plasma norepinephrine with age (Figures 5 and 6).[38-41] Although the incidence of hypertension

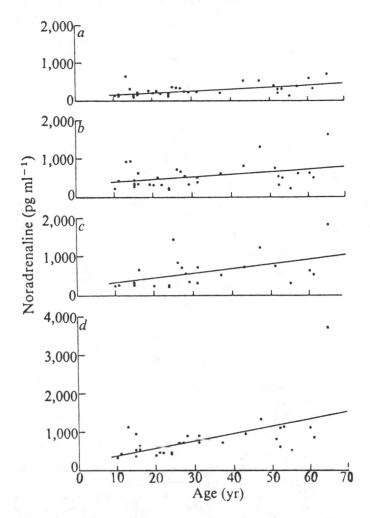

FIGURE 5.   Plasma noradrenaline in pg mℓ⁻¹ of subjects aged 10 to 65 years
while supine and resting (a), standing for 5 (b) or 10 (c) min or performing
isometric exercise (d). (Taken from Ziegler, M. G., Lake, C. R., and Kopin,
I. J., *Nature (London)*, 261, 334, 1976. With permission.)

increased with increasing age, in most reports of elevated plasma levels of norepinephrine
in hypertension, the control subjects have not been age-matched.[41] However, in the study
of Young et al.,[42] it is apparent that there is an increase in plasma norepinephrine in older
people. It has been suggested that in studies of plasma levels of norepinephrine or of the
responsiveness of the sympathetic nervous system to stress or drugs, age should be considered
in choosing appropriate controls.

There are alterations in cardiac responsiveness to sympathetic drugs in human beings
during aging, as indicated in the studies of Harris and Bluestone.[43] Harris treated 39 patients
over 75 years of age, suffering from symptoms of chronic atrioventricular block, over a 5-
year period, using artificial pacemakers and isoproterenol. Long-acting isoproterenol, i.e.,
preparation providing action of the drug for several hours, was used to maintain 17 patients;
of these, 7 remained well and active for an average time of 8 months (range 2 months to 2
years). After an average time of 9 months (range 2 days to 3 years), 10 patients died, 7 of
them from Stokes-Adams attacks. Of 22 patients treated with long-term artificial pacing,
15 were still surviving when the report was made (16 months into the study); most of them
were fully active and well. After an average time of 9 months (range 2 days to 2.5 years),

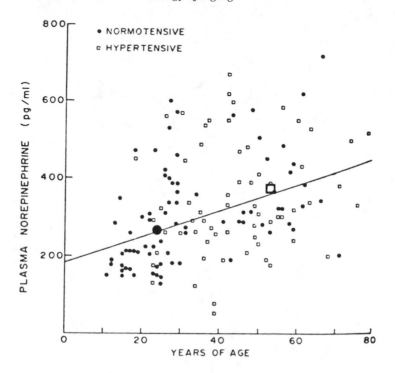

FIGURE 6.   Distribution of plasma norepinephrine levels with age in normotensive and hypertensive subjects. The regression line for level of norepinephrine vs. age (norepinephrine = 195 + 3.09 × age: r = 0.28, P <0.001) is indicated. The mean values (± S.E.M.) for catecholamine levels in hypertensive subjects over the age of 40 (large open square) and normotensive subjects between the ages of 16 and 30 years (large closed circle) are indicated at the mean age of each of the groups. When the norepinephrine levels of these two groups were corrected with a one-way analysis of covariance to account for the age disparity, there was no statistically significant difference between levels in the normotensive (16 to 30 years of age) and those in the hypertensive group (ages over 40) with use of the Student t-test. (Three hypertensive subjects are obscured by mean symbols.) (Taken from Lake, C. R., Ziegler, M. G., Coleman, M. D., and Kopin, I. J., *N. Engl. J. Med.*, 296, 208, 1977. With permission.)

7 of the paced patients died; 5 from failure or complications of their pacing system. It was Harris' conclusion that all elderly patients with symptoms from heart block should be treated initially with large doses of long-acting isoproterenol, and if this fails to control symptoms, long-term artificial pacing is recommended. Harris' results suggest a decreased effectiveness of isoproterenol in older people, supporting the contention that there is a decreased effect of catecholamines on the heart with increasing age.

It has been reported that aging results in a decrease in the maximum heart rate during exercise and in the response to isoproterenol.[28] To determine if the age-associated decline in maximal heart rate might be due to a decreased chronotropic response to catecholamines, the maximum heart rate induced by systemic injections of isoproterenol was compared in unanesthetized mature (1 to 4 years) and senescent (8 to 12 years) beagle dogs. Maximum rate was also assessed under pentobarbital anesthesia before and after cholinergic blockade with atropine. The unanesthetized baseline heart rates in the mature and senescent groups did not differ [148 ± 6 vs. 147 ± 7 beats per minute (bpm)] but the maximum isoproterenol induced heart rate was lower in the senescent compared to the mature group (249 ± 7 vs. 286 ± 13 bpm, p < 0.03). After pentobarbital anesthesia, the baseline heart rates did not differ and the age difference in maximum heart rate persisted (senescent: 220 ± 8 bpm;

mature: 260 ± 10 bpm; p < 0.02). The maximum heart rates were not affected by atropine. In contrast to the age difference in maximum rate after isoproterenol, both mature and senescent dogs could be paced electrically to a rate greater tha two times the maximum drug-induced heart rate. In anesthetized dogs, dose-response curves of isoproterenol, as in the unanesthetized animal, demonstrated a diminished response to this catecholamine in the aged group. These studies indicate an age-associated decline in chronotropic response to catecholamines and suggest that the mechanism responsible is located in the beta-adrenergic system and is not due to an age decrement in response of the pacemaker cells to direct electrical stimulation.

The effect of age on sensitivity to both isoproterenol and propranolol has been investigated in 27 male volunteers aged 21 to 73 years.[17] The dose of isoproterenol (given as a rapid intravenous injection) required to increase the resting heart rate by 25 bpm (I_{25}) increased with increasing age. The I_{25} was repeated during an intravenous infusion of propranolol and the dose ratio (I_{25} after propranolol divided by the control I_{25}) determined. This was related to the concentration of free propranolol in plasma. It was found that the effectiveness of any given free concentration diminished progressively with age. These data are consistent with a diminished responsiveness of the beta-adrenoreceptor to both agonist and antagonist drugs with advancing years.

The changes in response to adrenergic agonists and antagonists may be associated with the age decrease in ventricular response to hemodynamic stress during beta-adrenergic blockade.[44] The left ventricular response to hemodynamic stress was compared in 17 normal young (mean 29 years) and 11 normal old (mean 68 years) men. Echocardiographic measurements of left ventricular end-diastolic dimension, left ventricular endsystolic dimension, and velocity of circumferential fiber shortening were made at rest and during 30 mmHg increases in systolic blood pressure, induced by handgrip exercise or phenylephrine infusion. At rest, there was no age difference in heart rate, left ventricular end-diastolic dimension, lcft ventricular end-systolic dimension, or circumferential fiber shortening. Both handgrip and phenylephrine induced significant changes in these indices in both age groups, but no age difference in thc responses could be elicited. To eliminate the influence of beta-adrenergic receptor activation, the measurements were repeated during propranolol block. While there was no age difference in ventricular response during beta blockade at rest, phenylephrine infusion during beta-blockade induced greater increase in left ventricular end-diastolic dimension in the elderly group compared with the young group (Table 3). This increase in the elderly group occurred despite a significantly smaller decrease in heart rate than in the young group. It was concluded that aged human heart performs as well as a young heart at rest and during beta-blockade, but it has a greater reliance on beta-adrenergic activity during hemodynamic stress.

The importance of considering "stress" in the response to adrenergic neurotransmitters is further illustrated by the work of Palmer et al.[45] They found that while at rest, young human subjects had lower mean arterial blood pressure than old subjects and lower circulating levels of the neurotransmitter of the sympathetic nervous system, norepinephrine (NE). After standing and performing in isometric exercise, young persons increased their circulating levels of NE less than old persons. Palmer et al.[45] found that young subjects had a much smaller pressor response than old subjects to commonly used stimuli of the sympathetic nervous system. Also, in response to uniform stresses, young subjects secreted less NE and had a smaller blood pressure response than old subjects.

Although studies performed in vivo have been extremely valuable, many of the questions concerned with whether there are changes in responsiveness of the heart to drugs are better resolved through studies of the heart in vitro.

The effect of increasing age on myocardial contractile responsiveness to catecholamines was studied in rat hearts.[46] In the absence of exogenously added drugs, it was found that

Table 3
EFFECT OF PHENYLEPHRINE INFUSION ON LEFT VENTRICULAR PERFORMANCE AND DIMENSIONS

Group	ΔHeart rate/min	ΔSystolic blood pressure (mmHg)	ΔLVDD (mm)	ΔLVSD (mm)	ΔVCF (circ/s)	ΔVPW (cm/s)
Before beta-blockade[a]						
Old	−16 ± 4.0[b]	34 ± 3.0[b]	0.3 ± 0.5	2.0 ± 0.6[b]	−0.33 ± 0.05[b,d]	−1.10 ± 0.31[b,d]
Young	−19 ± 1.6[b]	28 ± 1.4[b]	0.2 ± 0.5	1.6 ± 0.5[b]	−0.26 ± 0.05[b,d]	−1.23 ± 0.24[b,d]
P (O vs. Y)	NS	NS	NS	NS	NS	NS
During beta-blockade[a]						
Old	−8 ± 1.6[b]	33 ± 1.2[b]	2.3 ± 0.6[b]	2.4 ± 0.7[b]	−0.13 ± 0.03[b]	−0.42 ± 0.15[c]
Young	−19 ± 1.6[b]	31 ± 1.8[b]	0.1 ± 0.5	1.0 ± 0.3[c]	−0.15 ± 0.03[b]	−0.52 ± 0.09[e]
P (O vs. Y)	<0.01	NS	<0.01	NS	NS	NS

a Numbers are differences between the intervention and its control value. A positive difference indicates an increase.
b $P < 0.01$.
c $P < 0.05$, compared with the corresponding resting value.
d $P < 0.05$.
e $P < 0.01$, compared with the corresponding change during handgrip listed in Table 2.

Taken from Yin, F., Raizes, G., Guarnieri, T., Spurgeon, H., Lakatta, E., Fortuin, N., and Weisfeldt, M., *Br. Heart J.*, 40, 1349, 1978. With permission.

contraction duration (for electrically elicited twitches) of rat cardiac ventricular muscle increased with increasiing age between 12 and 25 months. Norepinephrine, in this study, increased active tension and the maximum rate of tension development, but decreased contraction duraton; the magnitude of these effects were directly related to the concentration. The increase in active tension and the rate of tension rise with norepinephrine were significantly reduced in muscles from old rat hearts (25 months) compared to muscles from younger rat hearts (6 and 12 months). Contraction duration shortened proportionately in both age groups. Similar age-dependent effects were observed with isoproterenol as with norepinephrine; however, when calcium effects were studied also, no differences were observed in contractile responsiveness to calcium. It may be concluded from these observations that the ability of the cell to respond to calcium as an inotropic agent is unimpaired by aging, while increasing age seems to impair the positive inotropic response to catecholamines. The latter does not appear to result from tachyphylaxis or differences in tissue uptake of catecholamines, or the ability of the contractile proteins to respond to increasing concentrations of calcium; instead, it may result from a decreased ability of catecholamines to increase the intracellular calcium available for contraction. Since the catecholamines bring about their cellular effects (e.g., membrane depolarization, increased levels of cyclic AMP, increased calcium concentrations, increased contractility, etc.) by interacting with beta-adrenergic receptors on the plasma membrane surface, it may be that aging contributes to a decreased affinity of these receptors for catecholamines, or that the total number of receptors is decreased. Indeed, where beta-adrenergic receptors have been studied in other tissues, i.e., vascular smooth muscle,[47-49] cerebellum, corpus striatum, and pineal gland,[50] it has been found that the number of functional receptors decreases with increasing age. If this is the case for the heart as well, then it would be expected that responsiveness to beta-adrenergic agonists would decrease as a function of increasing age and conversely, that responsiveness to beta-adrenergic antagonists would increase with increasing age. The study of Conway,[29] described above, indeed showed an increased effectiveness of beta-adrenergic antagonists in older human beings. Study of cardiac muscle by means of drug-receptor interaction techniques[51-54] might prove fruitful in elucidating the underlying mechanisms for altered sensitivity to catecholamines and their antagonists brought on by increasing age. So far, the experiments using radioligand study methods which measure binding to the receptors suggest that decreases in response to catecholamines are not at the receptor level.[55,56] The density of receptors and their affinity for the transmitter do not seem to change with age. Thus, other sites along the pathway of beta-receptor agonists will have to be explored to determine the nature of the decreased response. The need for this type of approach has recently been reviewed by Lakatta.[57]

There are a number of papers which describe the effects of autonomic drugs on the hearts of young and adult animals, but they are not particularly relevant to the senescent stage. Some of these are described in what follows. The negative inotropic effect of different concentrations of secobarbital was studied on isolated hearts of reserpinized newborn and adult guinea pigs (Effendi et al).[58] This effect was expressed as the percentage of reduction of contraction height, from which the sensitivity of the heart was obtained, as the reciprocal of the secobarbital concentration needed to yield a 50% reduction. It was found that in adults depletion of catecholamines increased this sensitivity, but not in newborns. It was concluded that the age effects are not due to an effect of reserpine on contractility. The responsiveness of isolated perfused newborn (7 to 10 days old) and adult rabbit hearts to norepinephrine (NE), tyramine, and acetylcholine has been studied by Brus and Jacobowitz.[59] Heart rates of adult and immature animals are similarly responsive to NE. The fact that the effect of tyramine on the chronotropic responses is greater in young hearts and that many fewer adrenergic nerves are present in newborn hearts, suggests that proportionally greater amounts of catecholamines are released.

The chronotropic response to noradrenaline, tyramine, acetylcholine, and transmural electrical stimulation was compared in atria isolated from rabbits at different stages of development after birth (day 2 to day 210) (Toda et al.).[60] Pacemaker rates under steady-state conditions were related inversely to days after birth; the contraction rate in atria from rabbits at day 2 was significantly greater than that at days 10 to 210. The rate of neonatal rabbit atria was not significantly reduced by propranolol and the positive chronotropic response to noradrenaline was not siginficantly different in atria from different ages of rabbits, as far as threshold concentrations for inducing tachycardia and ED_{50s} were concerned. The maximum rate induced by noradrenaline was higher in neonatal rabbit atria than in adult rabbit atria. The effect of tyramine was approximately the same regardless of age. Increase in the pacemaker rate induced by transmural neural stimulation varied directly with age.

The effect of acebutolol (beta-blocking agent) on active isometric force generation has been studied in isolated papillary muscle preparations from adult cats and kittens less than 24-hours old.[61] Statistically significant reduction in active force occurred at a concentration of 0.27 nmol/ℓ in the adult preparations and at 1.34 nmol/ℓ in the infant ones. At 2.87 nmol/ℓ active force had fallen to 43.4% $\pm$ 2.2 (SEM) of the control value in the adults and to 52.4% $\pm$ 3.3 (SEM) in the infants. It was concluded that the infant myocardium is no more sensitive to the negative inotropic effect of acebutolol than is the adult myocardium.

A number of reports have described the effects of increasing age on cardiac catecholamine content and metabolism.[62,63] Although a review of this literature might be appropriate to a discussion of transmitters and age (see previous section), the data are presented here to gain a better understanding of the effects of sympathetic agonists and antagonists on the heart, and to speculate about possible development of postsynaptic receptor sensitivity changes.

Cardiac catecholamine content has been shown to undergo age-related changes. From birth through early development, catecholamines in the heart appear to increase with increasing age.[64] The increase in catecholamines during development is associated with the elaboration of sympathetic innervation to the heart. During development, Davidson and Innes found that reserpine,[65] a catecholamine-depleting agent, is more effective in reducing catecholamine content in hearts from young cats than in hearts from older cats. Brus and Jacobowitz found that the indirectly acting sympathomimetic, tyramine,[59] appeared to be more effective in releasing neuronal catecholamines in young rabbits than in adult rabbits, as indicated by the concentration of this agent necessary to produce half-maximal and maximal increases of heart rate in vitro. However, the absolute maximal response to tyramine in these studies was greater in the adult rabbits. It appears, therefore, that although the intraneuronal pools of catecholamines are more labile in the young animals (i.e., more completely depleted by reserpine and more readily released by tyramine), the responsiveness of the heart to catecholamines is greater in the adults (the adults being capable of attaining a greater increase in heart rate response than the young). Increased cardiac responsiveness during this phase of life may be due to the development of cardiac receptors in parallel with innervation, or to a general development of physiological and biochemical function.

Differences in transmitter content have been revealed in studies using injected nicotine (Table 4).[66] As reported by Goldberg and Roberts,[62] cardiac norepinephrine decreased with age although the effect of nicotine on the transmitter was not influenced by age. During later phases of aging, that is, with increasing age from maturity through old age, catecholamine content in the heart decreases.[63,66] For the late phase of the life span, neurotransmitter regulating enzymes, such as DOPA decarboxylase in the synthetic pathway and monoamine oxidase in the degradation pathway, decrease in activity.[63]

Uptake of catecholamines has been reported to be delayed in the old heart by Gey et al.,[67] but Hody et al.[68] have reported otherwise. Age-related delays in the uptake of norepinephrine (NE) by the rat myocardium were observed after subcutaneous injection of NE by Gey et al.[67] Hody et al.[68] reported that in vitro, uptake of ³H-NE by myocardia slices from healthy

Table 4

UPTAKE OF [³H] SEROTONIN AND [³H] NOREPINEPHRINE INTO VARIOUS RAT TISSUES AFTER NICOTINE[a]

Tissue	Injections for 2 months			Injections for 22 months		
	Control (6)[b]	Nicotine (6)	P	Control (4)	Nicotine (14)[c]	P
Serotonin						
Heart	5.4 ± 0.58	5.2 ± 0.45	NS[d]	4.1 ± 0.38	4.0 ± 0.25[e]	NS
Oxyntic gland area mucosa	1.9 ± 0.12	2.3 ± 0.28	NS	2.2 ± 0.47	1.8 ± 0.21	NS
Pyloric gland area mucosa	2.4 ± 0.24	2.6 ± 0.15	NS	2.2 ± 0.16	2.4 ± 0.14	NS
Small bowel mucosa	1.9 ± 0.41	2.1 ± 0.35	NS	2.8 ± 1.07	2.8 ± 0.67	NS
Descending colon mucosa	1.4 ± 0.14	1.4 ± 0.07	NS	1.8 ± 0.25	1.8 ± 0.16	NS
Norepinephrine						
Heart	15.0 ± 1.51	13.9 ± 1.10	NS	7.1 ± 0.73[f]	6.9 ± 0.37[g]	NS
Thoracic aorta	3.7 ± 0.21	3.6 ± 0.13	NS	4.1 ± 1.02	28 ± 0.11[f]	NS

a   Data reported as mean ± SE, in mℓ of bath fluid cleared/g wet tissue/hr.

b   Number of animals sampled is indicated in parentheses.

c   18 rats used for [³H] norepinephrine uptake.

d   NS, not significant.

e   Difference significant at $p < 0.02$ between 2- and 22-month control, or between 2- and 22-month nicotine-treated groups.

f   Difference significant at $p < 0.005$ between 2- and 22-month control, or between 2- and 22-month nicotine-treated groups.

g   Difference significant at $p < 0.001$ between 2- and 22-month control, or between 2- and 22-month nicotine-treated groups.

Taken from Thompson, J. H., Su, C., Shih, J. C. et al., *Toxicol. Appl. Pharmacol.*, 27, 41, 1974. With permission.

C57BL/6J male mice is not impaired by aging (8 to 28 months). The uptake of 0.1 ng/mℓ, 2.0 ng/mℓ or 1000 ng/mℓ of NE was explored. Additionally, no age-related changes of inulin space in myocardial slices were observed. Hence, the delayed uptake observed in vivo by Gey et al.[67] may be attributed to age-related changes in absorption from the subcutaneous site. Taken collectively, the evidence indicates that the net effect of all the catecholamine metabolic changes is a decreased neurotransmitter content. A summary of neurotransmitter substances changes with aging is given by Samorajski.[69]

It appears that with increasing age cardiac sympathetic nerve terminals become increasingly less efficient in storing catecholamines in the granular compartment, and eventually begin to lose catecholamines from the nongranular compartment.[70] The overall pattern of decreasing catecholamine availability in sympathetic nerve terminals of the heart explains, at least in part, the decreasing sympathetic control of the heart as aging progresses, observed in the studies on the baroreceptor reflex[30,71] discussed above. Changes in the sensitivity of tissues to adrenergic nervous effects during aging may be explained in the same manner. In experiments on 47 cats between 2 to 3 and 10 to 13 years of age, the following were determined: (1) the threshold values for sympathetic nerve stimulation and (2) the dosages of intravenously administered epinephrine and norepinephrine which elicited contraction of the nictitating membrane.[72] It was shown that the contraction of the nictitating membrane in old cats required a 42.1% greater stimulation of the sympathetic nerve than in young animals. In 10- to 13-year-old cats, the contraction of the nictitating membrane occurred with the administration of 2.7 $\pm$ 1.1 μg/kg of norepinephrine; whereas, the 2- to 3-year-old cats required 26.2 $\pm$ 5.3 μg/kg of norepinephrine. Thus, it is possible that in the nictitating membrane supersensitivity still may develop when there is a decrease in nervous input in older animals. Within the framework of decreasing nervous input to the heart, postsynaptic receptor-sensitivity (receptor density and/or affinity for drugs) changes would be expected to take place. We can speculate that the change may be a compensatory supersensitivity initially, whereas later, it is conceivable that homeostatic mechanisms fail and that subsensitivity results. Such receptor sensitivity changes, initiated by a failing innervation, would be consistent with the results of Lakatta et al.[46] However, since beta-receptor density and affinity do not appear to change in cardiac tissue,[55,56] alternatives must be considered to explain the decreased cardiac response to catecholamines as age increases.

Evidence that age-associated loss of beta-receptors occur in humans has been provided by the work of Schocken and Roth.[73] In lymphocytes, these investigators showed a reduced binding of (H^3) dihydroalprenolol (Table 5).[74] Other changes in beta-adrenergic responses are indicated in studies using isoproterenol in large doses on submandibular glands.[75] The age-dependency of isoproterenol (Iso)-induced DNA synthesis was investigated in different organs of Balb/c mice; the results indicated changes in the beta receptor mechanism with age. Although modifications of the physiologic rate of DNA synthesis after Iso injection occurred also in liver and spleen, a quasi-linear decrease of the peak of Iso response with advancing age was observed only in submandibular glands. Such a decrease was observed when animals were injected with 10^{-4} g Iso per gram of body weight, lower doses being unable to discriminate between young and old mice. In spite of some differences between mice and rats, the early appearance and linearity of the age-dependency remain common features of Iso response.

Finally, in the discussion of the effects of adrenergic transmitters on the heart and other organs innervated by the autonomic nervous system, some reference should be made to the control from higher centers.[76,77] Control of transmitter action in the autonomic nervous system originates from the hypothalamus and vasomotor centers. In the hypothalamus of the male rat, both the content of dopamine and norepinephrine were significantly less in the aged than in the young groups. Average dopamine content of the young and aged groups was 32.0 $\pm$ 9.3 μg and 15.6 $\pm$ 2.5 μg per hypothalamus, respectively. Norepinephrine

Table 5

AGE-GROUP ANALYSIS OF SPECIFIC ($-$)
[^{3}H]DIHYDROALPRENOLOL BINDING TO
MONONUCLEAR CELL MEMBRANES

	Age (years)	fmol/mg protein	Molecules × 10³/cell
Young	29.4 ± 1.7 n = 11	572 ± 58	28.3 ± 4.7
Old	63.0 ± 3.4 n = 14	318 ± 42	11.3 ± 1.5
	p <0.001	p <0.002	p <0.001

Note: All figures indicate means ± S.E.M.

Taken from Schocken, D. D. and Roth, G. S., *Adv. Exp. Med. Biol.*, 97, 273, 1978. With permission.

content averaged 47.6 ± 10.7 and 22.8 ± 1.8 μg per hypothalamus in the young and aged groups (Figure 7).[77] In this context, it is interesting that improvement of central function by administration of alpha blockers of the ergotamine group (Hydergine®) in humans has been reported by Jennings[78] and Rosen.[79]

Parasympathetic Agonists and Antagonists

Work on pharmacological effects of parasympathetic agonists and antagonists on the heart, in relation to aging, is less extensive than work on sympathetic agonists and antagonists.

The pharmacological effects of parasympathomimetics in whole animal studies have been shown to increase with increasing age (see Table 2).[22] In old rabbits (4.5 to 5 years), a lower intravenous dose of acetylcholine was required to produce a hypotensive response than in adult rabbits (1 to 1.5 years).[20,22] A dose of acetylcholine (0.05 μg/kg) produced a greater decrease in blood pressure and cardiac output in old rabbits than in adults.[72] Similarly, a study in humans has shown that methacholine elicited greater hypotensive responses in older subjects (over 45 years) than in young subjects (under 45 years).[80] The effect of parasympathomimetics in the whole animal result from a direct negative chronotropic action on the heart and a direct vasodilator effect on vascular smooth muscle. Depending on the dose of acetylcholine, its direct parasympathetic effects on the heart may be attenuated by cardiovascular reflexes and its ability to release catecholamines from the adrenal medulla and sympathetic postganglionic nerve fibers. The role of reflex control of cardiac function has been discussed above, where it was suggested that parasympathetic control of the heart very likely decreased with increasing age.[31] It has also been shown by Dauchot and Gravenstein that in humans,[81] atropine, a parasympathetic antagonist, elicits progressively smaller increases in heart rate with advancing age; this lends further support to the hypothesis that parasympathetic control diminishes as age increases. It is possible that supersensitivity to acetylcholine may develop during aging, which would account for the reduced effect of atropine. However, there is little experimental evidence, as yet, documenting the development of supersensitivity of parasympathetic receptors in older animals. In one report,[82] it was shown that the sensitivity to pilocarpine topically applied to the eyes of monkeys is greater in older monkeys.

Evidence exists which clearly indicates parasympathetic nervous control of the heart decreases with aging. Experiments were conducted by Froklis on rats (ages 1 month, 10 to 12 months, and 28 to 32 months), rabbits (ages 10 to 12 months and 48 to 62 months), and cats (ages 2 to 3 years and 10 to 13 years).[72] in 10- to 12-month-old rats, the excitation

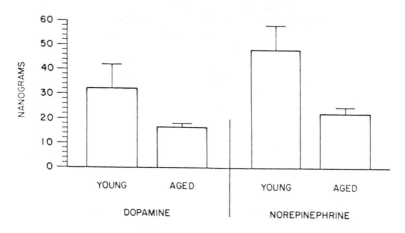

HYPOTHALAMIC CATECHOLAMINES (CONTENT)

FIGURE 7.   Hypothalamic content of dopamine and norepinephrine from young and aged male rats. Dopamine and norepinephrine concentrations are expressed as average concentrations (ng/hypothalamus; n = 8) with the standard error of the mean. (Taken from Miller, A. E. et al., *Exp. Aging Res.*, 2(5), 478, 1976. With permission.)

threshold of the vagus nerve, as indicated by bradycardia was 0.52 ± 0.121 V and in 28- to 32-month-old rats, it was 1.15 ± 2.010 V. In addition, the quantity of the cholinomimetic substances required (acetylcholine and carbochol) was smaller in old than in young animals. Although Kelliher and Conahan concur with the data obtained with vagus nerve,[83] they found in older animals that methacholine is less effective than in younger ones. Other studies showing that cholinergic neurons become less responsive with increased age were made with respect to ganglionic transmission. In ganglia of 25 cats of various ages (upper cervical sympathetic ganglion, sympathetic nerve, and the ganglia of the cardiac vagus nerve), the excitability of the ganglia decreased with age. In old cats excitablity was 0.3 ± 0.045 V, minimal frequency 108.5 ± 11.37 impulses per second and in the adult it was 0.11 ± 0.041 V, while minimal effective frequency was 266.7 ± 47.73 impulses per second. In old cats, excitation of the upper cervical sympathetic ganglia occurred with 1.1 ± 0.19 μg/kg of acetylcholine and in the adult with the administration of 6.3 ± 1.3 μg/kg.[72]

Blockade of the ganglionic transmission occurred with the administration of 86.5 ± 7.81 μg/kg of hexamethonium in old animals, and with 241.7 ± 24.48 μg/kg in adults.

In vitro studies on the effects of increasing age on cardiac responsiveness to parasympathetic drugs are very few. During early growth and development, it appears that acetylcholine activity decreases. For example, Brus and Jacobowitz[59] have shown that in rabbit atria, the ED_{50} (dose producing 50% of the maximum response) of acetylcholine in producing bradycardia increased approximately 100-fold from the neonatal to the adult (3 months) phase. Another study indicates that the ED_{50} for acetylcholine-induced bradycardia in rabbit atria increased approximately 4- to 5-fold during development from neonate to adult (6 months).[60] In the latter study, initial atrial rate decreased during this time period, so that the actual change (beats per minute) in atrial rate was greater in the young animals than in the older ones. The manner of expressing data notwithstanding, the results of these studies are somewhat ambiguous, since cholinesterases were not inhibited in either study.

Effects of acetylcholine on automaticity of isolated cardiac Purkinje fibers from neonatal and adult dogs, and on the idioventricular rhythm of adult dogs with complete atrioventricular block, were explored.[84] Isolated Purkinje fibers were studied with standard microelectrode techniques during superfusion with Tyrode's solution at 37°C. For both age groups, spontaneous rate was decreased by acetylcholine, an effect that was reduced by atropine. The

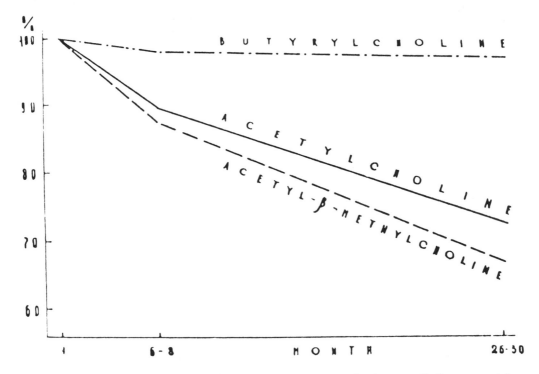

FIGURE 8.   Changes in cholinesterase activity in the auricle in white rats of various ages. Cholinesterase activity in 1-month-old animals is taken as 100%. (Taken from Frolkis, V. V. et al., *J. Gerontol.*, 21, 161, 1966. With permission.)

magnitude of the effect was equal in both neonatal and adult dogs. The negative chronotropic effect of acetylcholine was not prevented by phentolamine, indicating that an α-adrenergic mechanism was not invovled.

Since acetylcholine is highly susceptible to hydrolysis by tissue cholinesterases and the latter may change with old age, it cannot be said with certainty whether the decreased effectiveness of acetylcholine with old age is due to altered cholinesterase activity, to altered sensitivity of cardiac parasympathetic receptors, or to both phenomena unless these various factors are controlled. It has been shown that changes in acetylcholine metabolism accompany the observed age-dependent changes in tissue sensitivity.[72] In experiments on rabbits and rats, it was shown that alterations in total, true, and pseudocholinesterase activities take place in the auricles, ventricles, skeletal muscles, and liver with age; a decrease in cholinesterase activity occurred with increasing age in animals.[72] In auricular tissues, as in those of other organs, the greatest decrease was found in true cholinesterase activity and the least in pseudocholinesterase activity (Figure 8). In old rats there were changes not only in cholinesterase activity but also in its distribution in the cell, which was determined by histochemical methods.[72]

Not only does cholinesterase activity decrease with age, but there is evidence that the synthesis of acetylcholine and its content also decreases.[72] The acetylcholine content of the auricles of 1-month-old, 8- to 12-month-old, and 28- to 32-month -old rats was 5.61 ± 0.83, 4.69 ± 0.53, and 2.65 ± 0.42 μg/g of tissue, respectively.[72] After incubation with choline, the acetylcholine content of the auricles increased to 11.8 ± 1.38, 6.33 ± 0.32, and 2.99 ± 0.52 μg/g, respectively.

ACTIONS ON THE VASCULATURE

As might be expected from the age effects on cardiac muscle function and blood pressure, increasing age has had a profound effect on the response of the vasculature to autonomic

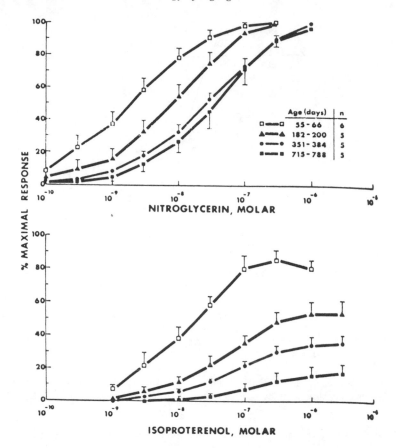

FIGURE 9. Effect of age on the relaxation response of male rabbit thoracic aortas to both isoproterenol and nitroglycerin. There is a decreased response in the aged aortas to isoproterenol, but not to nitroglycerin. (Taken from Fleisch, J. H. and Hooker, C. S., *Circ. Res.*, 38, 243, 1976. With permission.)

agents. When catecholamines are applied directly to the mesentery of anesthetized rats, the old rats showed a much smaller constriction than the young ones (3 months).[26] The response of aortas of rats (47 to 375 days) and rabbits (56 to 1835 days) to relaxation induced by pharmacologic means has also been studied by Fleisch et al.[48] Strips of aortas were initially contracted with histamine or serotonin (5-HT) and given an alpha-adrenergic blocking agent. The relaxation response to the beta-adrenergic agonist, isoproterenol, was then tested. They found regional differences in the relaxation response. The thoracic aortas of rabbits and rats relaxed when isoproterenol was administered. The abdominal aortas did not relax with beta-adrenergic stimulus, but did relax with sodium nitrate. The response of rabbit was greater than that of rat. With increasing age, the response to isoproterenol decreased in both species, but the relaxation response to nitrates was unchanged in the rat (Figure 9). It was concluded that the relaxation deficit with increasing age was somewhere along the beta-adrenergic receptor-response system, but that the relaxation mechanism itself was intact since there was no age difference in response to the nonspecific relaxation caused by nitrates.

Tuttle[49] measured the response of rat aortas to norepinephrine and found an increase in the threshold and decrease maximum response in 2-year-old as compared to 1-year-old rats. Cox[85] also demonstrated a decreased response to norepinephrine in 24-month-old as compared to 2- or 12-month-old rat aortas.

Cohen and Berkowitz studied the effects of various contracting and relaxing agents in old and young rat aortas.[86] They reported different results from Tuttle.[49] They found that the old aortas had a greater contractile response to 5-HT, potassium chloride, and norepinephrine than did the young ones. This age difference was thought not to be due to an adrenergic receptor change since it was present with the nonadrenergic drugs. Relaxation response was tested by administering cyclic AMP to aortic strips previously contracted with 5-HT. They found that the young relaxed 50 to 60%, whereas the old relaxed only 10%. Dibutyryl cyclic AMP, which permeates cell membranes, caused a similar age decline in relaxation, as did administration of a phosphodiesterase inhibitor. However, there was no age difference in relaxation to nitroglycerin. They concluded that the age-associated decrease in relaxation response was due to a specific decrease in the vascular response to cyclic nucleotides rather than to age differences in cell permeability.

As was the case with the smooth muscle of the aorta, Fleisch and Hooker[87] found that the relaxation response to isoproterenol was decreased 50% in old compared to young pulmonary arteries. There was no age difference in relaxation to the nonadrenergically mediated relaxant, nitroglycerin.

Even in a comparison of the effects of aortas taken from immature and mature animals, but not from old animals, there is the suggestion that beta-receptor induced relaxation is impaired with aging.

Taken collectively, the above studies indicate changes in the beta-adrenergic receptor-response system as an explanation for the decreased ability of aged vascular muscle to relax. The exact site or sites of the age defect have not been unequivocally determined. Age differences in the alpha-adrenergic contraction mechanism may also be present.

Aside from these age changes in receptors, there are other sites in the link from central nervous system to muscle which could exhibit age changes, in particular, differences in adrenergic innervation of the vascular smooth muscle in old and young rabbits. Shibata et al.[88] found that the young had specific catecholamine fluorescence in the muscle of the media. The old, however, had specific fluorescence only in the adventitia and adventitia-media junction. The young also had levels of tissue catecholamines twice as high as those of the old rabbits. They attributed their findings to degeneration with age in the adrenergic innervation of the media. Similar findings were reported for the decrease in innervation of cardiac tissue.[89] In these studies, there seems to be increased degeneration of adrenergic nerve terminals in the atrium and this may account for the decrease in neural effect in this organ.

A decreased innervation would explain a decreased in vivo response to adrenergic neural stimulation, but still would not explain the decreased pharmacologic responsiveness described above as increased responsiveness usually accompanies denervation. Perhaps, as Weiss et al.[90] have noted in the pineal gland, denervation does not lead to supersensitivity to adrenergic stimuli in many tissues of older animals.

ACTIONS ON NONCARDIOVASCULAR TISSUES

Pupil of the Eye

There is evidence that sympathetic tone to the pupil of the eye becomes diminished with increasing age (Table 6).[91] It is clear that drugs which act, in part or in whole, through mechanisms affecting the transmitter release, such as cocaine and hydroxyamphetamine, show a dramatic decrease in effect in the elderly. Phenylephrine, however, produced dilatation of the pupils to the same extent in the young and the elderly. This suggests that the receptor mechanisms in the dilator pupillae muscle remain intact in older individuals while the transmitter release processes are diminished.

Trachea

The beta-adrenoceptor activity in the tracheal muscle of rats and guinea pigs diminishes with increasing age, as in the smooth muscle of aorta.[92] In Sprague-Dawley rats (45, 90,

Table 6
PUPILLARY DIAMETERS (MEAN ± SD) BEFORE AND AFTER
VARIOUS DRUGS IN 23 YOUNG (Y) AND 15 ELDERLY (E) SUBJECTS

Treatment	Age group	Pupil diameter (mm)	MR
Control	Y	4.60 ± 0.83	—
	E	3.75 ± 0.67[a]	—
Phenylephrine	Y	8.28 ± 0.75	1.83 ± 0.23
	E	8.21 ± 0.84	2.23 ± 0.33[a]
Hydroxyamphetamine	Y	8.17 ± 0.82	1.80 ± 0.21
	E	6.96 ± 0.66[a]	1.88 ± 0.22
Cocaine	Y	8.36 ± 0.69	1.85 ± 0.24
	E	5.50 ± 0.78[a]	1.48 ± 0.22[a]

Note: MR mydriatic ratio (mean ± SD).

[a]   Statistically significant difference between the two age groups (p. <0.01).

Taken from Korczyn, A. D., Laor, N., and Nemet, P., *Arch. Ophthalmol.*, 94, 1905, 1976. With permission.

and 210 days old) and in guinea pigs (3 weeks, 4 months, and 27 months old), the tracheal muscle response during maturation (ages 45 to 90 days in the rat, and 18 to 120 days in the guinea pig) showed a reduced responsiveness to isoproterenol induced relaxation, but this did not occur during further aging; that is, after maturation, the response to isoproterenol remained the same in the older animals. These results underscore the importance of defining the age parameters involved in a given study and the organ system which is being explored.

Other Smooth Muscle

Other types of smooth muscle, e.g., vas deferens of the rat, ileum, colon and uterine horn of the guinea pig, also appear to exhibit significant changes in sensitivity to a variety of agonists (e.g., norepinephrine, acetylcholine, histamine, and serotonin) on aging.[93] Most frequently, smooth muscle from adult animals displayed a greater contractile activity to norepinephrine and acetylcholine than did tissue from young animals, while the reverse was found for serotonin- and histamine-induced contractions. Botting reported that for histamine-induced contractile responses on rabbit ileum the responses were greatest with the tissues from young animals.[94] More recently, Goldberg and Roberts[95] found that with age there is a decreased response of the rat stomach to carbamylcholine and that this is due to decrease in receptor number. Collectively, such data would seem to suggest that the aging process not only can influence responses of vascular smooth muscle to a variety of agonists but that this may apply to all types of mammalian smooth muscle. It is obvious that much work remains to be done in this area before one will be able to state with conviction: (a) exactly when these changes take place during the aging process, (b) whether regional differences exist with respect to aging and reactivity of smooth muscles, and (c) whether only certain contractile and relaxant agonists are affected by the aging process.

Salivary Glands

It appears that a relationship similar to that in the eye exists with innervation of the salivary glands.[96] In mice (NIH, male) of different ages (1, 6, and 9 months), there is a reduced salivary response to d-amphetamine (an indirect acting amine) in the older animals, but aging does not affect salivation produced by the directly acting adrenergic sialogogue (1-norepinephrine). This suggests that the receptor mechanisms in the salivary gland remains intact but that transmitter release is the mechanism by which amphetamine action is depressed with increasing age. It should be noted that the response to a cholinergic sialogogue, pilcarpine, is also not affected by age (Figure 10).[96]

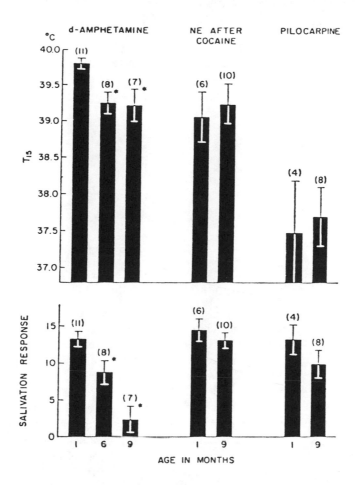

FIGURE 10.   The first three bars on the left represent salivation responses and T_{15} values for d-amphetamine (7.3 mg/kg) in mice 1, 6, and 9 months old. The two middle bars represent salivation responses and T_{15} values for l-norepinephrine (0.5 mg/kg) 5 min after cocaine (18 mg/kg), in 1- and 9-month-old mice. The two bars on the right represent salivation responses and T_{15} values for pilocarpine (15 mg/kg) and 1- and 9-month-old mice. Bars represent mean values $\pm$ SE for the number of mice indicated in parentheses. An asterisk indicates that the value differs significantly from that in 1-month-old mice (p $<$0.05). (Taken from Maling, H. M. and Koppanyi, T., *Proc. Soc. Exp. Biol. Med.*, 140, 794, 1972. With permission.)

ROLE IN THERMOGENESIS

Another function in which drugs affecting the autonomic system are involved is thermogenesis. It is well known that ability to maintain thermal homeostasis is suppressed with age. One of the major sites involved in thermogenesis is the fat cell. Nakano et al.[97] described the effect of age on basal lipolysis in isolated fat cells and on levels of norepinephrine, ACTH, and on theophylline and dibutyryl cyclic AMP-induced lipolysis in the rat. They found that both basal and norepinephrine-induced lipolysis decrease with advance of age (Figure 11). In addition, the lipolytic effect of ACTH, theophylline, and dibutyryl cyclic AMP was significantly greater in younger rats than in older rats. The reduction in the lipolytic action observed in the fat cells isolated from the older rats was reversible since starvation was able to restore the lipolytic action of norepinephrine, ACTH, and theophylline.

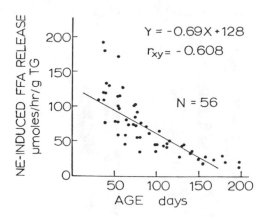

FIGURE 11.   Effect of age of Holtzman male rats on norepinephrine (NE)-induced free fatty acid release in isolated rat fat cells. The concentration of NE was 5.9 × 10⁻¹M. (Taken from Nakano, J. et al., *J. Gerontol.*, 26, 8, 1971. With permission.)

These observations indicate that senescence may decrease the activity of hormone-sensitive lipase in rats although the mechanism is not known. However, Estler seemed to find the opposite. He found that the plasma nonesterified fatty acid rise in old mice was even higher than that in juvenile mice, after methamphetamine.[98] Furthermore, in contrast to juvenile mice, old mice treated with methamphetamine are unable to adequately mobilize their carbohydrate reserves. These observations are difficult to reconcile with reports that the lipolytic response to sympathomimetics decreases during aging. One possible explanation as mentioned by Estler may be obtained by considering a parallel situation in cold-stressed mice, i.e., that plasma levels of free fatty acids are the resultant of the rate of lipolysis and uptake of fatty acids by the various organs, and that the oxidation of fatty acids in the citric acid cycle is dependent on the simultaneous degradation of an adequate amount of carbo-hydrates.[98] Carbohydrates are required to provide the oxaloacetate necessary to enter the citric acid for the two-carbon fragments of fatty acids. Therefore, utilization of fatty acids is necessarily also impeded when carbohydrates are lacking. Thus, in Estler's experiments a similar defect in utilization is indicated.

Gonzalez and DeMartinis[99] seemed to confirm the results of Nakano et al.[97] Isolated fat cells from 3-, 12-, and 28-month-old rats were compared for their lipolytic response to various doses of 1-epinephrine. With increasing age, a progressive decline in response occurred when comparing rats with unmatched mean adipocyte diameters. However, this apparently age-related decrease was no longer evident if the diameters were matched, since the 28-month-old animals had a lipolytic response less than that of the 3-month-old rats, but greater than that of rats 12 months old. Similar results have been reported by Jolly et al.;[100] body weight differences between the given ages may account for these observations. Within each age group, the initial lag in glycerol release decreased and the lipolytic response increased as mean cell size increased. The rate of hormone-stimulated glycerol release varied inversely with incubations of 3,700 to 25,000 cells per milliliter and aging had no effect on this parameter; DNA content per fat cell remained constant with age.

The effect on the adenylate-cyclase-cAMP system is the basis for the lipolytic effect of many agents. Decreases in hormone-sensitive adenylate cyclase activities of the fat cell of the rat have been reported with age. The response to epinephrine declines modestly during senescence.[101-103] The content of cAMP, the release of glycerol and nonesterified fatty acids (NEFA), of adipose tissue with and without the stimulation of ACTH were determined in young and old rats.[103] The lipid-mobilizing hormones resulted in lowered concentration of cAMP and there was an impaired stimulation of lipolytic activity in old rats (Figure 12).[104]

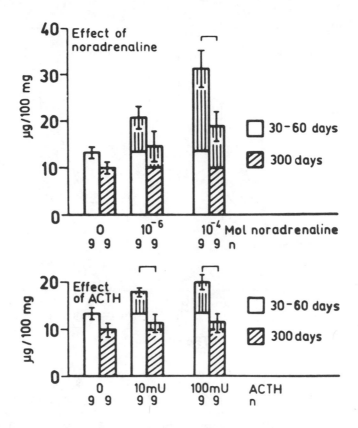

FIGURE 12.   The concentration of cAMP in adipose tissue of rats at different age after the stimulation with ACTH or noradrenaline (M ± S. E.), n = number of animals, age in days, ⌐⌐ = P <0.05. (Taken from Kolena, L. M., *Endocrinol. Exp.*, 9, 93, 1975. With permission.)

Furthermore, less stimulation of glycerol and NEFA release by cAMP was observed in these animals. These results suggested to the investigator that in old animals a lower lipolytic activity per tissue and smaller lipid mass is available in intact and hormone-stimulated fat tissue and, therefore, the accumulation of lipids in fat depots is facilitated.

The liver plays an important role in thermogenesis. Age changes in the liver response to autonomic agents have been noted by Bitensky et al.[103] The referenced study presents data which indicate that the activities of the glucagon and epinephrine responsive components of hepatic adenylate-cyclase vary separately as a function of aging, sex, and steroid hormone levels in the rat. These observations lend support to the hypothesis that the two hormonally sensitive adenylate-cyclase systems in liver are independent. Indeed, the older males responded much less to epinephrine than to glucagon stimulation of hepatic adenylate cyclase. However, Kalish et al.[105] reported different findings. The influence of postmaturational aging on the activity and stability of rat liver epinephrine and glucagon-sensitive adenylate cyclases [ATP pyrophosphate-lyase (cyclizing), EC 4.6.1.1] was studied in liver homogenates from male and female Wistar rats ages 3, 12, and 24 months. Enzyme activity was measured in the unstimulated (basal) state and with fluoride activation as well as with a range of concentrations of glucagon and epinephrine. Basal activity was the same at 3 and 12 months, but at 24 months was 1.4 times higher in both sexes. Fluoride and glucagon (1 nM to 10 µM) activities were slightly but significantly greater (1.2 times) in females at 24 months compared with their levels at 3 and 12 months. This increase did not occur in males. In contrast, epinephrine-stimulated activity doubled from 3 to 24 months in both males and females, with most of the increase occurring between 12 and 24 months.

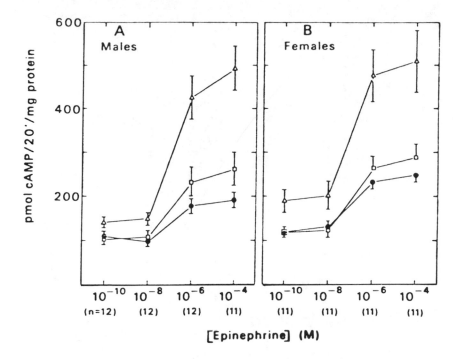

FIGURE 13.   Epinephrine stimulation of liver homogenate adenylate cyclase from 3-, 12-, and 24-month-old rats, males (A) and females (B). Each plotted value represents the mean stimulated activity ± S.E. of n experiments each comparing liver homogenates from three single rats ages 3 (●—●), 12 (□—□), and 24 (△—△) months. For males 12 vs. 24 months. P <0.02, <0.01, <0.005, <0.005 for 10^{-10}, 10^{-8}, 10^{-6}, and $10^{-4}M$, respectively. For females 12 vs. 24 months, P <0.005, <0.005, <0.001, <0.005. Significance of differences between 3 and 24 months is comparable. Basal values are not shown. (Taken from Kalish, M. S. et al., *Biochim, Biophys. Acta,* 483, 452, 1977. With permission.)

Because Bitensky used Sprague-Dawley rats, and the ages were based on weight, (old rats weighed more than 200 g),[103] it seems that the effect that Bitensky was examining was that of maturation rather than aging. It also appears that Bitensky used a particulate preparation, whereas the Kalish group (Katz et al.) used homogenates.[106] Another study by Kalish et al.[105] (Figure 13) showed that adenylate cyclase activity in rat liver is best quantified in homogenates, and he suggests caution in making comparisons of enzyme activity based on particulate or membrane preparations from animals of differing physiological states.

In addition to an effect on adenylate cyclase, cAMP, changes in the glycolytic cycle have been noted.[107] The influence of various adrenergic agonists and antagonists on pyruvate kinase activity and lactate production from endogenous glycogen reserves was investigated in hepatocytes isolated from young and old rats.[108] The results showed that with hepatocytes prepared from juvenile rats (100 to 150 g) 10 μM epinephrine and 10 μM isoproterenol (beta-adrenergic agonist) inhibit pyruvate kinase activity and lactate production; whereas, 10 μM phenylephrine (an alpha-adrenergic agonist) has no influence on either (Table 7). With hepatocytes from fully mature adults (300 g and up), epinephrine, isoproterenol, and phenylephrine were all without influence on lactate production from endogenous glycogen reserves. Epinephrine produced a small but reproducible inhibition of pyruvate kinase activity in hepatocytes from adult rats, but isoproterenol and phenylephrine have no significant influence on the enzyme activity. In the presence of 0.5 mM theophylline, epinephrine and phenylephrine give a significant inhibition of pyruvate kinase activity and lactate production, using hepatocytes from both young and adult rats. Theophylline alone had no significant influence on pyruvate kinase activity, but it did give approximately 20% inhibition of lactate

Table 7
GLUCOSE AND LACTATE PRODUCTION FROM ENDOGENOUS GLYCOGEN RESERVES IN HEPATOCYTES FROM YOUNG AND OLD RATS

Additions	Glucose production		Lactate production	
	100—150 g	300 g and up	100—150 g	300 g and up
	μmol/10⁸ cell			
C	14.7 ± 1.8 (7)	23.1 ± 1.7 (16)	16.8 ± 2.4 (7)	21.2 ± 1.6 (16)
T	15.4 ± 2.3 (5)	19.5 ± 1.3 (9)	12.2 ± 1.5 (5)[a]	19.1 ± 1.3 (9)[a]
E	24.8 ± 3.3 (5)[a]	46.8 ± 4.6 (11)[a]	10.0 ± 1.8 (5)[a]	20.8 ± 1.8 (11)
E + T	29.4 ± 4.0 (6)[a]	57.0 ± 5.6 (11)[a,b]	3.4 ± 0.5 (6)[a,b]	8.7 ± 1.1 (11)[a,b]
G	32.6 ± 4.1 (8)[a]	72.2 ± 5.1 (16)[a,c]	0.1 ± 0.9 (7)[a]	−1.5 ± 0.4 (16)[a,c]

Note: Hepatocytes were prepared from juvenile (100 to 150 g) and mature (300 g and up) rats as indicated. The cells were preincubated for 10 min at 37°C. Individual cell suspensions then received a control vehicle (C), 0.5 m*M* theophylline (T), 10 μ*M* L-epinephrine (E), or 1 μ*M* glucagon, as indicated. The incubation was continued an additional 20 min, then terminated by addition of perchloric acid. Samples were also taken at the end of the 10-min preincubation period. The amount of glucose and lactate produced over the final 20-min period was then determined. The results are presented as micromoles of glucose or lactate produced per 10⁸ cells over the 20-min period. Each value represents the mean ± S.E. of results from the number of cell preparations shown in parentheses.

[a] p <0.01 vs. control, paired *t* analysis.
[b] p <0.01 vs. E alone, paired *t* analysis.
[c] p <0.01 vs. E + T combination.

Taken from Blair, J. B., James, M. E., and Foster, J. L., *J. Biol. Chem.*, 254, 7585, 1979. With permission.

production. The results of this investigator demonstrate that selective changes in the metabolic response of the hepatocyte to various adrenergic agonists occur as the rat matures; however, similar changes were not observed with glucagon. The selective changes in the metabolic response of the hepatocytes appear to be related to changes in the adrenergic receptor system which occur during development and aging.

It appears from the observations reported in this section that, in general, metabolic response to autonomic drugs and transmitters decreases with age. This may in part explain the susceptibility of the aged to the cold stress.

REFERENCES

1. **Vizi, E. S.,** Non-synaptic modulation of transmitter release: pharmacological implications, *Trends Pharmacol. Sci.*, 1, 172, 1979/80.
2. **Shock, N. W.,** System integration, in, *Handbook of the Biology of Aging*, Finch, C. B. and Hayflick, L., Ed., Van Nostrand, Reinhold, New York, 1977, 639.
3. **Finch, C. E.,** The regulation of physiological changes during mammalian aging, *Cl. Rev. Biol.*, 51, 49, 1976.
4. **Finch, C. E.,** The relationship of aging changes in the basal ganglia to manifestations of Huntington's chorea, *Ann. Neurol.*, 7, 406, 1980.
5. **Pradhan, S. N.,** Central neurotransmitters and aging, *Life Sci.*, 26, 1643, 1980.
6. **Reis, D. J., Ross, R. A., and Joh, T. H.,** Changes in the activity and amounts of enzyme synthesizing catecholamines and acetylcholine in brain, adrenal medulla and sympathetic ganglia of aged rat and mouse, *Brain Res.*, 136, 465, 1977.

7. **Kvetnansky, R., Jahnova, E., Torda, T., Strbak, V., Balaz, V., and Macho, L.,** Changes of adrenal catecholamines and their synthesizing enzymes during ontogenesis and aging in rats, *Mech. Ageing Dev.,* 7, 209, 1978.

8. **Gauthier, P., Nadeau, R., and deChamplain J.,** Acute and chronic cardiovascular effects of 6-hydroxy-dopamine in dogs, *Circ. Res.,* 31, 307, 1972.

9. **McGeer, E. G., McGeer, P. L., and Wada, J. A.,** Distribution of tyrosine hydroxylase in human and animal brain, *J. Neurochem.,* 18, 1647, 1971.

10. **McGeer, E. G., Fibiger, H. C., McGeer, P. L., and Wickson, V.,** Aging and brain enzymes, *Exp. Gerontol.,* 6, 391, 1971.

11. **Simpkins, J. W., Mueller, G. P., Huang, H. H., and Meites, J.,** Evidence for depressed catecholamine and enhanced serotonin metabolism in aging male rats: possible relation to gonadotropin secretion, *Endocrinology,* 100, 1672, 1977.

12. **Feldman, J. M. and Roche, J. M.,** Effects of aging on monamine oxidase activity of mouse and rabbit tissues, *Exp. Aging Res.,* 4, 97, 1978.

13. **Robinson, D. S.,** Changes in monoamine oxidase and monoamines with human development and aging, *Fed. Proc., Fed. Am. Soc. Exp. Biol.,* 34, 103, 1975.

14. **Robinson, D. S., Nies, A., Davis, J. N. et al.,** Aging, monoamines and monoamine oxidase levels, *Lancet,* 1, 290, 1972.

15. **Inagaki, C. and Tanaka, C.,** Neonatal and senescent changes in L-aromatic amino acid decarboxylase and monamine oxidase activities in kidney, liver, brain and heart of the rat, *Jpn. J. Pharmacol.,* 24, 439, 1974.

16. **Prange, A. J., Jr., White, J. E., Lipton, M. A., and Kinkead, A. M.,** Influence of age on monamine oxidase and catechol-*o*-methyl transferase in rat tissues, *Life Sci.,* 6, 581, 1967.

17. **Vestal, R. E., Wood, A. J. J., Branch, R. A., Shand, D. G., and Wilkinson, G. R.,** Effects of age and cigarette smoking on propranolol disposition, *Clin. Pharmacol. Ther.,* 26, 8, 1979.

18. **Slanina P. and Stalhandske, T.,** *In vitro* metabolism of nicotine in liver of ageing mice, *Arch. Int. Pharmacodyn.,* 226, 258, 1977.

19. **Mueller, R. A. and Shideman, F. A.,** A comparison of the absorption, distribution and metabolism of reserpine in infant and adult rats, *J. Pharmacol. Exp. Ther.,* 163, 91, 1968.

20. **Goldberg, P. B. and Roberts, J.,** Pharmacology, in, *The Aging Heart, Aging,* Vol. 12, Weisfeldt, M. L., Ed., Raven Press, New York, 1980, 215.

21. **Bender, A. D.,** The influence of age on the activity of catecholamines and related therapeutic agents, *J. Am. Geriatr. Soc.,* 18, 220, 1970.

22. **Goldberg, P. B. and Roberts, J.,** Influence of age on the pharmacology and physiology of the cardio-vascular system, in, *Special Review of Experimental Aging Research, Progress in Biology,* Elias, M. F., Eleftheriou, B. F., and Elias, P. K., Eds., Experimental Aging Research, Bar Harbor, Maine, 1976, 71.

23. **Frolkis, V. V.,** The autonomic nervous system in the aging organism, *Triangle,* 8, 322, 1968.

24. **Chen, K. K. and Robbins, E. B.,** Age of animal and drug action, *J. Am. Pharm. Assoc.,* 33, 80, 1944.

25. **Frolkis, V. V.,** The autonomic nervous system in the aging organism, *Farmakol. Toksikol.,* 28, 612, 1969.

26. **Hrouza, Z. and Zweifach, B. W.,** Effect of age on vascular reactivity to catecholamines in rats, *J. Gerontol.,* 22, 469, 1967.

27. **Hoffman, V. H., Kiesewetter, R., Krohs, G. and Schmitz, C.,** Dependence on age of the effects of catecholamines in man. I. Effect of noradrenaline, adrenaline and isoprenaline on blood pressure and heart rate, *Z. Gesamte Inn. Med.,* 30, 89, 1975.

28. **Yin, F. C. P., Spurgeon, H. A., Greene H. L., Lakatta, E. G., and Weisfeldt, M. L.,** Age-associated decrease in heart rate response to isoproterenol in dogs, *Mech. Ageing Develop.,* 10, 17, 1979.

29. **Conway, J.,** Effect of age on the response to propranolol, *Int. Z. Klin. Pharmakol. Ther. Toxicol.,* 4, 148, 1970.

30. **Rothbaum, D. A., Shaw, D. J., Angell, C. S., and Shock, N. W.,** Age differences in baroreceptor response of rats, *J. Gerontol.,* 29, 488, 1974.

31. **Rothbaum, D. A., Shaw, D. J., Angell, C. S., and Shock, N. W.,** Cardiac performance in the una-nesthetized senescent male rat, *J. Gerontol.,* 28, 287, 1973.

32. **Bühler, F. R., Lutold, B. E., Kung, M., and Koller, F. J.,** Once daily dosage — beta-blockade antihypertensive efficacy of slow release oxprenolol as related to renin and age, *Aust. N.Z. J. Med.,* 6, 37, 1976.

33. **Bühler, F. R. and Lutold, B. E.,** A beta-blocker-based antihypertensive drug program guided by age and renin, *Aust. N.Z. J. Med.,* 6, 29, 1976.

34. **Buhler, F. R., Burkhart, F., Lutold, B. E., Kung, M., Marbet, G., and Pfisterer, M.,** Antihypertensive beta blocking action as related to renin and age: a pharmacologic tool to identify pathogenetic mechanisms in essential hypertension, *Am. J. Cardiol.,* 36, 653, 1975.

35. **Jackson, G., Pierscianowski, T. A., Mahon, W., and Condon, J.,** Inappropriate hypertensive therapy in the elderly, *Lancet,* 2, 1317, 1976.

36. **Chrysant, S. G., Frohlich, E. D., and Papper, S.,** Why hypertension is so prevalent in the elderly and how to treat it, *Geriatrics,* 31, 101, 1976.
37. **Lundborg, P. and Steen, B.,** Plasma levels and effect on heart rate and blood pressure of metoprolol after acute oral administration in 12 geriatric patients, *Acta Med. Scand.,* 200, 397, 1976.
38. **Ziegler, M. G., Lake, C. R., and Kopin, I. J.,** Plasma noradrenaline increases with age, *Nature (London),* 261, 333, 1976.
39. **Jones, D. H., Hamilton C. A., and Reid, J. L.,** Plasma noradrenaline, age and blood pressure: a population study, *Clin. Sci. Mol. Med.,* 55, 73S, 1978.
40. **Brecht, H. M. and Schoeppe, W.,** Relation of plasma noradrenaline to blood pressure, age, sex and sodium balance in patients with stable essential hypertension and in normotensive subjects, *Clin. Sci. Mol. Med.,* 55, 81S, 1978.
41. **Lake, C. R., Ziegler, M. G., Coleman, M. D., and Kopin, I. J.,** Age-adjusted plasma norepinephrine levels are similar in normotensive and hypertensive subjects, *N. Engl. J. Med.,* 296, 208, 1977.
42. **Young, J. B., Rowe, J. W., Pallotta, J. A., Sparrow, D., and Landsberg, L.,** Enhanced plasma norepinephrine response to upright posture and oral glucose administration in elderly human subjects, *Metabolism,* 29, 532, 1980.
43. **Harris, A. and Bluestone, R.,** The treatment of heart block in the elderly, *J. Chronic Dis.,* 19, 689, 1966.
44. **Yin, F. C. P., Raizes, E. S., Guarnieri, T., Spurgeon, H. A., Lakatta, E. G., Fortuin, N. J., and Weisfeldt, M. L.,** Age-associated decrease in ventricular response to haemodynamic stress during beta-adrenergic blockade, *Br. Heart J.,* 40, 1344, 1978.
45. **Palmer, G. J., Ziegler, M. G., and Lake, C. R.,** Response of norepinephrine and blood pressure to stress increases with age, *J. Gerontol.,* 33, 482, 1980.
46. **Lakatta, E. G., Gerstenblith, G., Angell, C. S., Shock, N. W., and Weisfeldt, M. L.,** Diminished inotropic response of aged myocardium to catecholamines, *Circ. Res.,* 36, 262, 1975.
47. **Fleisch, J. H.,** Pharmacology of the aorta. A brief review, *Blood Vessels,* 11, 193, 1974.
48. **Fleisch, J. H., Maling, H. M., and Brodie, B. B.,** Beta-receptor activity in aorta variations with age and species, *Circ. Res.,* 26, 151, 1970.
49. **Tuttle, R. S.,** Age-related changes in the sensitivity of rat aortic strips to norepinephrine and associated chemical structural alterations, *J. Gerontol.,* 21, 510, 1966.
50. **Greenberg, L. H. and Weiss, B.,** Beta-adrenergic receptors in aged rat brain: reduced number and capacity of pineal gland to develop supersensitivity, *Science,* 201, 61, 1978.
51. **Furchgott, R. F.,** Pharmacological characterization of receptors: its relation to radioligand-binding studies, *Fed. Proc., Fed. Am. Soc. Exp. Biol.,* 37, 115, 1978.
52. **Furchgott, R. F. and Bursztyn, P.,** Comparison of dissociation constants and of relative efficacies of selected agonists acting on parasympathetic receptors, *Ann. N.Y. Acad. Sci.,* 144, 882, 1967.
53. **Karlin, A., Damle, V., Valderamma, R., Hamilton, S., Wise, D., and McLaughlin, M.,** Interactions among binding sites on acetylcholine receptors in membrane and in detergent solution, *Fed. Proc., Fed. Am. Soc. Exp. Biol.,* 37, 121, 1978.
54. **Lefkowitz, R. J.,** Identification and regulation of alpha- and beta-adrenergic receptors, *Fed. Proc., Fed. Am. Soc. Exp. Biol.,* 37, 123, 1978.
55. **Guarnieri, T., Filburn, C., Zitnik, G., Roth, G., and Lakatta, E.,** Diminished contractile response to catecholamines in senescent myocardium, but unaltered β-receptors, cyclic AMP, or protein kinase activation, *Clin. Res.,* 27, 172A, 1979.
56. **Scarpace, P. J. and Abrass, I. B.,** Beta-adrenergic receptors in aged rats, *Fed. Proc., Fed. Am. Soc. Exp. Biol.,* 38, 361, 1979.
57. **Lakatta, E. G.,** Age-related alterations in the cardiovascular response to adrenergic mediated stress, *Fed. Proc., Fed. Am. Soc. Exp. Biol.,* 39, 3175, 1980.
58. **Effendi, H., Versprille, A., and Wise, M. E.,** The negative inotropic effect of secobarbital on the heart of reserpinized newborn and adult guinea pigs, *Arch. Int. Pharmacodyn.,* 215, 276, 1975.
59. **Brus, R. and Jacobowitz, D.,** The influence of norepinephrine, tyramine and acetylcholine upon isolated perfused hearts of immature and adult rabbits, *Arch. Int. Pharmacodyn. Ther.,* 200, 266, 1972.
60. **Toda, N., Ju, W. L. H., and Osumi, Y.,** Age-dependence of the chronotropic response to noradrenaline, acetylcholine and transmural stimulation in isolated rabbit atria, *Jpn. J. Pharmacol.,* 26, 356, 1976.
61. **Sheridan, D. and Tynan, M.,** Direct effect of acebutolol on force generation in immature and adult myocardium, *Cardiovas. Res.,* 11, 247, 1977.
62. **Goldberg, P. B. and Roberts, J.,** Changes in the biochemistry of the rat heart with increasing age, *Exp. Aging Res.,* 2, 519, 1976.
63. **Roberts, J. and Goldberg, P. B.,** Changes in basic cardiovascular activities during the lifetime of the rat, *Exp. Aging Res.,* 2, 487, 1976.
64. **Lee, W. C., Lew, J. M., and Yoo, C. S.,** Studies on myocardial catecholamines related to species ages and sex, *Arch. Int. Pharmacodyn. Ther.,* 185, 259, 1970.

65. **Davidson, W. J. and Innes, S. R.,** Increased depletion of catecholamines by reserpine in immature cats, *Can. J. Physiol. Pharmacol.,* 50, 612, 1972.
66. **Thompson, J. H., Su, C., Shih, J. C. et al.,** Effects of chronic nicotine administration and age on various neurotransmitters and associated enzymes in male Fischer 344 rats, *Toxicol. Appl. Pharmacol.,* 27, 41, 1974.
67. **Gey, K. F., Burkard, W. P., and Pletscher, A.,** Variation of the norepinephrine metabolism of the rat heart with age, *Gerontologia,* 11, 1, 1965.
68. **Hody, G., Jonec, V., Morton-Smith, W., and Finch, C. E.,** Norepinephrine uptake by the myocardium of the senescent mouse *in vitro, J. Gerontol.,* 30, 275, 1975.
69. **Samorajski, T.,** Central neurotransmitter substances and aging: a review, *J. Am. Geriatr. Soc.,* 25, 337, 1977.
70. **Limas, C. J.,** Comparison of the handling of norepinephrine in myocardium of adult and old rats, *Circ. Res.,* 9, 644, 1975.
71. **Gribbin, B., Pickering, T. G., Sleight, P., and Peto, R.,** Effect of age and high blood pressure on baroreflex sensitivity in man, *Circ. Res.,* 29, 424, 1971.
72. **Froklis, V. V.,** Neuro-humoral regulations in the aging organism, *J. Gerontol.,* 21, 161, 1966.
73. **Schocken, D. D. and Roth, G. S.,** Reduced β-adrenergic receptor concentrations in ageing man, *Nature (London),* 267, 856, 1977.
74. **Schocken, D. D. and Roth, G. S.,** Age-associated loss of beta-adrenergic receptors from human lymphocytes *in vivo, Adv. Exp. Med. Biol.,* 97, 273, 1978.
75. **Piantanelli, L., Brogli, R., Bevilacqua, P., and Fabris, N.,** Age-dependence of isoproterenol-induced DNA synthesis in submandibular glands of BALB/C mice, *Mech. Ageing Dev.,* 7, 163, 1978.
76. **Frolkis, V. V., Bezrukov, V. V., Duplenko, Y. K., Shchegoleva, I. V., Shevtchuk, V. G., and Verkhrotsky, N. S.,** Acetylcholine metabolism and cholinergic regulation of functions in aging, *Gerontologia,* 19, 45, 1973.
77. **Miller, A. E., Shaar, C. J., and Riegle, G. D.,** Aging effects on hypothalamic dopamine and norepinephrine content in the male rat, *Exp. Aging Res.,* 2, 4/5, 1976.
78. **Jennings, W. G.,** An ergot alkaloid preparation (Hydergine) versus placebo for treatment of symptoms of cerebrovascular insufficiency: double-blind study, *J. Geriatr. Soc.,* 20, 407, 1972.
79. **Rosen, H. J.,** Mental decline in the elderly: pharmacotherapy (ergot alkaloids vs. Papaverine), *J. Am. Geriatr. Soc.,* 23, 169, 1975.
80. **Nelson, R. and Gellhorn, E.,** The action of autonomic drugs on normal persons and neuropsychiatric patients, the role of age, *Psychosom. Med.,* 19, 486, 1957.
81. **Dauchot, P. and Gravenstein, J. S.,** Effects of atropine on the electrocardiogram in different age groups, *Clin. Pharmacol. Ther.,* 12, 274, 1971.
82. **Bito, L. Z. and Baroody, R. A.,** Gradual changes in the sensitivity of rhesus monkey eyes to miotics and the dependence of these changes on the regimen of topical cholinesterase inhibitor treatment, *Invest. Ophthalmol. Vis. Sci.,* 18, 794, 1979.
83. **Kelliher, G. J. and Conahan, S. T.,** Changes in vagal activity and response to muscarinic receptor agonists with age, *J. Gerontol.,* 35, 842, 1980.
84. **Danilo, P., Jr., Rosen, M. R., and Hordof, A. J.,** Effects of acetylcholine on the ventricular specialized conducting system of neonatal and adult dogs, *Circ. Res.,* 43, 77, 1978.
85. **Cox, R. H.,** Arterial wall mechanics and composition and the effect of smooth muscle activation, *Am. J. Physiol.,* 229, 807, 1975.
86. **Cohen, M. L. and Berkowitz, B. A.,** Age-related changes in vascular responsiveness to cyclic nucleotides and contractile agonists, *J. Pharmacol. Exp. Ther.,* 191, 147, 1974.
87. **Fleisch, J. H. and Hooker, C. S.,** The relationship between age and relaxation of vascular smooth muscle in the rabbit and the rat, *Circ. Res.,* 58, 243, 1976.
88. **Shibata, S., Hattori, K., Sakavai, I., Mori, J., and Fujiware, M.,** Adrenergic innervation and cocaine-induced potentiation of adrenergic responses of aortic strips from young and old rabbits, *J. Pharmacol. Exp. Ther.,* 177, 621, 1971.
89. **McLean, M. R., Goldberg, P. B., and Roberts, J.,** Fine structure and reduced adrenergic control in the senescent rat heart: axon terminal-cardiac cell relationships, *Fed. Proc., Fed. Am. Soc. Exp. Biol.,* 38, 361, 1979.
90. **Weiss, B., Greenberg, L., and Cantor, E.,** Age-related alterations in the development of adrenergic denervation supersensitivity, *Fed. Proc., Fed. Am. Soc. Exp. Biol.,* 30, 1915, 1979.
91. **Korczyn, A. D.,** Sympathetic pupillary tone in old age, *Arch. Ophthalmol.,* 94, 1905, 1976.
92. **Aberg, G., Adler, G., and Ericsson, E.,** The effect of age on β-adrenergic activity in tracheal smooth muscle, *Br. J. Pharmacol.,* 47, 181, 1973.
93. **Petkov, V., Todorov, S., and Kotova, E.,** Differences in the effects of transmitters on smooth muscles from adult and young guinea pigs and rats, *Agressologie,* 16, 95, 1975.
94. **Botting, J. H.,** Sensitivity of neonatal rabbit ileum to histamines, *Br. J. Pharmacol.,* 53, 428, 1975.

95. **Goldberg, P. B. and Roberts, J.,** Age-related changes in rat stomach smooth muscle sensitivity to a cholinergic agonist, *Pharmacologist,* 22, 167, 1980.
96. **Maling, H. M. and Koppanyi, T.,** The effect of age on adrenergic and cholinergic salivation, *Proc. Soc. Exp. Biol. Med.,* 140, 794, 1972.
97. **Nakano, J., Gin, A. C., and Ishii, T.,** Effect of age on norepinephrine-, ACTH-, theophylline- and dibutryl cyclic AMP-induced lipolysis in isolated rat fat cells, *J. Gerontol.,* 26, 8, 1971.
98. **Estler, C. J.,** Dependence on age of methamphetamine-produced changes in thermoregulation and metabolism, *Experientia,* 31, 1436, 1975.
99. **Gonzales, J. and DeMartinis, F. D.,** Lipolytic response of rat adipocytes to epinephrine: effect of age and cell size, *Exp. Aging Res.,* 4, 455, 1978.
100. **Jolly, S. R., Lombardo, Y. B., Lech, J. J., and Menahan, L. A.,** Effect of aging and cellularity on lipolysis in isolated mouse fat cells, *J. Lipid Res.,* 21, 44, 1980.
101. **Cooper, B. and Gregerman, R. I.,** Hormone-sensitive fat cell adenylate cyclase in the rat, *J. Clin. Invest.,* 57, 161, 1976.
102. **Cooper, B., Weinblatt, F., and Gregerman, R. I.,** Enhanced activity on hormone-sensitive adenylate cyclase during dietary restriction in the rat: dependence on age and relation to cell size, *J. Clin. Invest.,* 59, 467, 1977.
103. **Bitensky, M. W., Russell, V., and Blanco, M.,** Independent variation of glucagon and epinephrine responsive components of hepatic adenyl cyclase as a function of age, sex and steroid hormones, *Endocrinology,* 86, 154, 1970.
104. **Kolena, L. M.,** Lipolysis and cyclic-3′, 5′-AMP content in rat adipose tissue at different ages, *Endocrinol. Exp.,* 9, 93, 1975.
105. **Kalish, M. D., Katz, M. S., Pineyro, M. A., and Gregerman, R. I.,** Epinephrine- and glucagon-sensitive adenylate cyclases of rat liver during aging. Evidence for membrane instability associated with increased enzymatic activity, *Biochim. Biophys. Acta,* 483, 452, 1977.
106. **Katz, M. S., Kalish, M. D., Pineyro, M. A., and Gregerman, R. I.,** Quantitation of epinephrine- and glucagon-sensitive adenylate cyclases of liver. Implications of alterations of enzymatic activities during preparation of particular fractions and membranes, *Biochim. Biophys. Acta,* 540, 205, 1978.
107. **Blair, J. B., James, M. E., and Foster, J. L.,** Adrenergic control of glycolysis and pyruvate kinase activity in hepatocytes from young and old rats, *J. Biol. Chem.,* 254, 7585, 1979.

NEUROMUSCULAR BLOCKING DRUGS*

Frank G. Standaert and Kitt Booher

INTRODUCTION

Practical experience does not reveal decreased response of the elderly to neuromuscular blocking drugs administered during surgery. It seems that any changes in the neuromuscular system are such that some diminish transmission while others enhance it, and these tend to compensate for each other. Similarly, the clinician's intuitively cautious approach to anesthetizing the elderly seems to compensate for the altered pharmacodynamics.

ANATOMY AND PHYSIOLOGY OF THE AGING NEUROMUSCULAR SYSTEM

Motoneurons degenerate with increasing age and the neuromuscular junctions of old muscles resemble those of denervated or incompletely innervated muscles. Aged peripheral nerves commonly have

1. Accumulation of lipofuscin pigment[1]
2. Myelin degeneration[2,3]
3. Infolding and thickening of the basement membrane[4]
4. Accumulation of glycogen in axonal vacuoles[3] and increased lysomal activity in Schwann cells[5]
5. Decreased internodal length to axon diameter ratio[6-8]
6. Schwann cell bands, some of which are devoid of axons[4]
7. Replacement of the parenchyma with connective tissue[3,9]
8. A reduction in the number and density of axons[4,7,10-12]

Analyses of electromyograms suggest there is a decrease in the number of axons supplying peripheral muscles and a decrease in the number of muscles innervated by each axon, i.e., the motor units are fewer (Figure 1) and smaller (Figure 2).[13-16] The threshold for stimulation of the remaining nerve fibers is increased,[17,18] and some,[12,16,19,20] but not all,[21-23] investigators have found conduction velocity to be decreased.

Other aspects of the aging sequence may be seen at the neuromuscular junction. Presynaptic nerve terminals at aging motor endplates undergo a variety of alterations in structural features.[24-27] Axon terminals contain conspicuous neurotubules and neurofilaments. Synaptic vesicles are increased[26] but are clumped in patterns resembling the "agglutination" characteristic of early denervation.[28,29] Numerous Schwann cells surround the axon terminal but do not insert between the nerve and the end plate;[29] degeneration and eventual loss of the terminal endings appears to be accomplished by a process of shrinkage and condensation without involvement of adjacent Schwann cells in phagocytic activity.[30] The junctional folds of the end plate are more branched, and the basement membrane is thickened. Unfolding of the subneural pallisades results in a notably enlarged synaptic cleft.[28,31,32] Collagen content is increased and irregular patches of cholinesterase are scattered over the deformed endplates.[28,32]

Degeneration with age does not occur equally in all species or in all muscles. Human beings are more severely afflicted than rats[30,33] and distal muscles suffer more than proximal ones.[9,16,32] The diaphragm seems to be affected less than other muscles[33,34-36] and this may be a major explanation of the observation that the respiratory response of the elderly to

* Supported, in part, by USPHS grant NS12566.

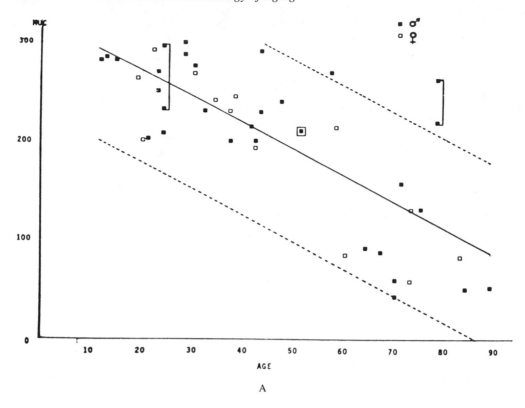

A

FIGURE 1.   (A) Plot of motor unit count against age. Regression line shown ± 2 S.E. Vertical bars connect values in both hands of the same patient. (From **Brown, W. F.**, *J. Neurol. Neurosurg. Psychiatry*, 35, 845, 1972. With permission.) (B) Functioning motor units in thenar, hypothenar, soleus, and extensor digitorum brevis muscles in healthy people. (From **McComas, A. J., Upton, A. R. M., and Sica, R. E. P.**, *Lancet*, 2, 1477, 1973. With permission.)

neuromuscular blocking drugs is not much different from the response of younger patients. Also, it may help to explain why studies of neuromuscular transmission in vitro, where the rat phrenic nerve-diaphragm is the most frequently used preparation, do not show changes with increased age as great as might be expected from observation of human peripheral muscles.

Aging motoneurons seem to have a decreased capacity to synthesize choline acetyltransferase;[18,34] perhaps because there is a reduced availability of substrates such as acetyl coenzyme A and choline,[37] the precursors of acetylcholine, or because amino acids are not transported efficiently into the neuron.[38-41] There is evidence also that the rate of axonal transport of neuroproteins, possibly including a trophic factor, is diminished with aging.[39,41,42]

Although diminished function, degeneration, and death of motor axons is the most likely cause of the changes in neuromuscular junctions that occur with aging, it is not clear that the process is entirely neurogenic. Some of the earliest effects occur in perineural tissues, particularly Schwann cells.[4] Furthermore, the fact that human nerves are affected more than those of rats, and that distal muscles are affected more than proximal ones, suggests that in human beings, circulatory[7,9] or metabolic (e.g., diabetes) derangements[14,32,43] may cause a peripheral neuropathy that does more damage to motoneurons than the primary effects of age. Whatever the cause, the result is a reduction in the efficiency of the coupling of nerve to muscle, then a reduction in the number of muscle cells innervated by an axon, and, eventually, complete denervation and atrophy of the muscle.

Even though aging animals eventually lose the nerve supply to their muscles, there is

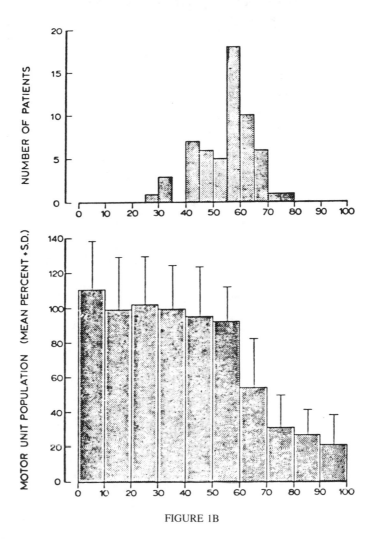

FIGURE 1B

abundant evidence that denervation is not a steadily progressive, inexorable process. Even the oldest nerves seem to have the capacity to regenerate terminals, sprout new branches, and successfully reinnervate muscle cells. A marked increase in the incidence of axonal nodal sprouts, some of which may undergo myelination, is a characteristic feature of the motoneurons of old animals.[4,24,44,45] Many of these new branches contact muscle cells to form fully functional neuromuscular junctions which are distinguishable from those in younger animals only by the increasingly condensed grouping of muscle types which occurs with age.[36,45-49] Other branches are not as successful in establishing functional synaptic contact; the thickened and vesicular swellings at the terminal endings of the reinnervating growth configurations,[28,50] or the thinner diameter of these endings,[4,25] suggests that they failed to establish functional contact with muscle. Other branches form functional but abnormal junctions; a markedly increased incidence of complex and bizarre terminals is one of the most noticeable features of aged muscles.[24,44] Appearance of erratic patterns of cholinesterase distribution (demonstrated with cholinesterase staining techniques) and of endplates in abnormally distal parts of the muscle confirms the random nature of the reinnervation process.[28,45]

Senile muscle has a reduced mass, muscle fiber number,[51,52] often an increased fiber diameter,[51,52] and diminished fiber length reflecting a reduced sacromere number.[51] They undergo peripheral cellular degeneration of myofilaments and proliferation of T and SR

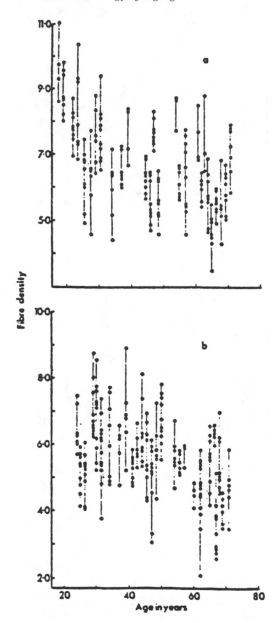

FIGURE 2.   Fiber density [thousand fibers (millimeter squared)] of individual fascicles of the radial nerve (a) and the sural nerve (b) plotted against the subject's age. Values for different fascicles of the same nerve are joined by a line. (From **O'Sullivan, D. J. and Swallow, M.**, *J. Neurol. Neurosurg. Psychiatry*, 31, 464, 1968. With permission.)

cisternae,[29] while numerous deformed and rounded sarcolemnal nucleoli aggregate at endplate areas.[28,32,53] Satellite cells are conspicuous and dense in appearance.[29,32] Aging muscle fiber is further characterized by the appearance of lipopigment, abnormal mitochondria,[53] or tubular aggregates and an increased incidence of rod-like material.[32] These are similar to those found in subjects with neuromuscular disease and are suggestive of impaired innervation.[54] Some cells show considerable disintegration, with disorganization of structure, vacuolization, and signs of pinocytosis and autophagocytosis, while others contain features such as thin filaments, microtubules, and immature sarcoplasmic reticulum, which are more characteristic of embryonal than adult muscle.[29,33] Accelerated protein degradation and reduced protein synthesis,[46,55] delayed recovery of RNA synthesis,[56,57] and shifts in glycolytic and aerobic pathways[33,36,58,59] also occur and further affect the contractile properties of old muscles. Electromyograms from rat,[60,61] from dog,[60] and man[23,62-65] show the muscle action potential to be decreased in amplitude and to have a slow rise and prolonged duration. The direct electrical excitability of the muscle fibers is diminished.[65] Even though there is no consistent change in resting membrane potential,[29,60,66,67] the absolute refractory period is prolonged.[60] A markedly increased incidence of multiple or polyphasic action potentials, which is a common feature of the electromyogram of individuals far advanced in age,[23,60,63,65,68,69] suggests delayed transmission at the endplate and reflects the uncertain synaptic conditions which result from the repeated denervation and innervation occurring in senile muscles.

The sequence of progressive denervation interrupted by repeated episodes of reinnervation also is reflected in the distribution of fiber types. The differences in metabolic and contractile properties which distinguish muscle types become less sharp with age and the muscle fibers become histochemically and functionally more uniform, assuming characteristics that are intermediate between typical fast and slow fibers.[12,33] There is a particularly striking loss of type II (fast) fibers (Figure 3) and a relative increase in slow and undifferentiated types.[32,47,49,70,71] There is also less mixing of fiber types within a muscle, with an increased tendency for fibers of a particular type to be grouped close together.[33] The diminished proportion of fast muscle cells is reflected in the contraction characteristics of old muscles, for example, prolonged latencies, decreased maximum rates of tension development and increased contraction and relaxation times (Table 1).[16,29,35,58,66]

MICROPHYSIOLOGY OF THE AGING NEUROMUSCULAR JUNCTION

The alteration in structure of neuromuscular junctions that accompanies age should cause a corresponding alteration in the efficiency of neuromuscular transmission. Tortuous nerve endings suggest that less transmitter should be released, while enlarged synaptic clefts and flattened postjunctional membranes suggest more transmitter should escape by diffusion from the cleft and that transduction of the chemical signal into an action potential should be less efficient. Only a few detailed analyses of the effects of age on neuromuscular transmission have been reported, and while they indicate that age is accompanied by deteriorated function, they do not document changes as great as those that would be expected from the appearance of the neuromuscular apparatus. This discrepancy is not difficult to reconcile. The deterioration of neuromuscular structure makes it difficult to get an accurate electrophysiologic assessment of the state of neuromuscular transmission; many of the bizarre junctions may be nonfunctional while others may function weakly and these will not be located by the physiologist's probing microelectrode. The electrode is more likely to locate and record from one of the relatively normal junctions and thus produce results biased toward the normal. Furthering this tendency is the frequent use of the rat diaphragm as an experimental model; this muscle seems to be among those least affected by age.

Despite the experimental handicaps, the published results clearly show that age leads to a decreased capacity of motor nerve endings to conduct action potentials and to synthesize, mobilize, and release transmitter. Spontaneous release determined indirectly through measurements of miniature endplate potentials (mepp) is not affected as much or as consistently as evoked release; the diaphragm is not affected as strongly as more peripheral muscles; and high frequency activity is subject to more deterioration than low frequency activity.

Smith reported a twofold increase in mepp frequency in diaphragms from 24- to 26-month-old rats.[72] Vyskocil and Gutmann reported a similarly sized decrease in diaphragms of 30-

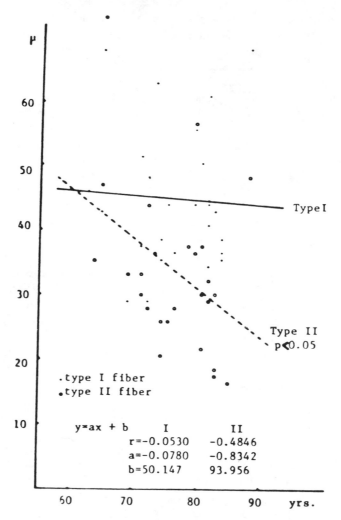

FIGURE 3.   Diameter of type-I and type-II fibers vs. age of the subjects. (From **Tomonaga, M.**, *J. Am. Geriatr. Soc.*, 25, 125, 1977. With permission.)

to 33-month-old rats.[35] The conclusions cited may be misleading, however, since the absolute frequencies were nearly the same in both experiments (2.03 ± 0.40 and 1.73 ± 0.08 mepps/ sec, respectively) but the rats used as controls by Vyskocil and Gutmann were younger than those used by Smith, and had a fourfold greater frequency of mepp activity. In contrast, mepp frequency in levator ani[66] and soleus[35] muscles of old rats clearly were reduced (to 0.30 ± 0.05 and 0.12 ± 0.1 mepps/sec, respectively). Smith noted the frequent occurrence of giant mepps in his preparations and Frolkis et al.[60] remarked on the heterogeneity of mepp activity in old animals; some junctions are almost silent while others have greater than normal activity. Gutmann speculated that the release of a trophic factor may be reduced in proportion to synaptic activity and this may contribute to the loss of integrity which is characteristic of junctional and postjunctional structures in the peripheral muscles of aged animals.[33,48] The resting membrane potential of endplates in old muscles is described as not changed,[29] or else slightly decreased.[67,72] Again, the different conclusions are due to dif- ferences among the animals used as controls. The amplitude of the mepp is increased, apparently because the diameter of the muscle fiber is less and, therefore, membrane imped- ence is greater in old animals, but there is no change in its rate of rise or fall.[29]

Table 1
EFFECTS OF AGE ON PROPERTIES OF MUSCLE CONTRACTION

	Soleus		Diaphragm	
	Young	Old	Young	Old
Frequency of transmitter release per sec	1.52 ± 0.10	0.12 ± 0.01	3.82 ± 0.16	1.73 ± 0.08
%	−92.1		−54.7	
FCT	35.0 ± 1.2	41.6 ± 0.7	16.1 ± 0.4	20.7 ± 0.6
%	+18.9		+28.6	
HCT	12.8 ± 0.43	15.0 ± 0.22	8.2 ± 0.1	9.4 ± 0.4
%	+17.2		+14.6	
TCC	5.2 ± 0.39	11.5 ± 0.39	5.4 ± 0.17	6.4 ± 0.2
%	+32.2		+18.5	
HRT	38.2 ± 0.95	53.9 ± 1.0	14.2 ± 0.6	22.3 ± 1.0
%	+41.1		+57.0	
LP	3.4 ± 0.16	4.2 ± 0.14	3.0 ± 0.1	3.8 ± 0.13
%	+23.5		+26.7	

Note: FCT, full contraction time (time to peak); HCT, half relaxation time; TCC, maximal rate of tension development; HRT, half relaxation time and LP, latency period. Absolute and relative (%) values of these parameters are indicated, the values of the muscles of young animals being 100%. Number of observations on contraction properties was 7 for both the diaphragm and soleus muscles.

From **Vyskocil, F. and Gutmann, E.,** *Experienta,* 28, 280, 1972. With permission.

The release of transmitter in response to repetitive stimulation of the nerve was studied by Smith,[72] who measured endplate potentials (epp) in diaphragms from 12- to 13-month-old and 30- to 33-month-old rats. He found that it took less magnesium or tubocurarine to block transmission in the older muscles. He also found that the fall in amplitude of successive epps evoked by repetitive stimulation was greater in the muscles from the older animals than in those from the younger ones and that tubocurarine induced a greater degree of synaptic depression, as measured by the response to the second of a pair of stimuli, in the older junctions. He documented a decreased capacity for action potentials to propagate into the terminal branches of motor axons from aged rats and showed that junctions from these animals do not transmit high frequency activity (50 Hz or more) as well as do junctions from younger animals. These observations are consistent with earlier ones: that Wedensky inhibition occurs at a lower frequency in older animals,[60,62] and that increased synaptic "jitter" and delay in transmission is evident in electromyograms of old human beings.[67] Smith did not tabulate the results of his calculations, but his report implies that age reduces (1) quantal content of the evoked end plate potentials, (2) readily releasable store of transmitter, and (3) mobilization of stores in response to stimulation. It is unfortunate that the full power of available techniques has not been applied to the study of motor endplates in aged muscles because the continuous cycle of denervation and reinnervation that occurs in muscles of old animals provides an unusually interesting situation.

Most investigators report that muscles of older animals are more sensitive to acetylcholine than those of young adults.[17,18,37] Intra-arterial injections of acetylcholine into the legs of 48- to 62-month-old rabbits showed that the threshold dose for excitation is reduced by a factor of about 2.5, when compared to those of 16- to 20-month-old controls.[17] A contrary result was reported by Gutmann et al. who did not see a change in acetylcholine sensitivity in levators ani of old rats.[29,41]

Supersensitivity to acetylcholine may be due, in part, to the reduction in junctional acetylcholinesterase that occurs with age.[17,18,37,60] It also may be related to a change in cholinergic receptors ionophores. In studies with soleus muscle, Pestronk et al. reported the total junctional acetylcholine (ACh) receptor number to be no different in mature and 28-month-old rats;[25] Courtney and Steinbach calculated a gradual decline in the number of ACh receptors at the endplate of aging sternomastoid muscle.[27] Some increase in the extrajunctional ACh receptor density was found in both muscle types from aged rats.[25,27] Vyskocil measured a spread of receptive area beyond the normal bounds and concluded that extrajunctional receptors,[67] resembling those in denervated muscle, had proliferated in his preparations. Gutmann et al. found no difference in acetylcholine sensitivity or receptive area in levators ani from old and young rats.[29] Vyskocil made the interesting observation that tetrodotoxin blocks the end plate current in diaphragms from 28- to 30-month-old rats.[67] Tetrodotoxin sensitivity is present in embryonic muscle, but disappears from the endplate soon after neuromuscular contact is made in the embryo. Its reappearance in old age may be due to attempted innervation of undifferentiated muscle or satellite cells by the new branches that sprout from motor axons.

This diversity of results is not hard to reconcile. Degeneration of the neuromuscular apparatus occurs over an animal's lifetime. At any instant, most of the remaining junctions will be normal, or nearly normal, and only a small fraction will be in an active state of degeneration or regeneration. Since normal, degenerating, and regenerating junctions are present simultaneously, a variety of responses may be observed. Heterogeneity of function, as of structure, should be characteristic of aging neuromuscular junctions.

Taken together, the observations cited above fit into a dynamic picture. Neuromuscular units fail with age, but their loss is offset by collateral sprouting from motor axons and innervation of denervated or undifferentiated muscle cells. The capacity to synthesize, mobilize, and release transmitter diminishes with age, but there is substantial excess capacity for transmission in young nerve endings and much can be lost before function is impaired. When transmitter release falls significantly, receptor supersensitivity develops in the muscle and increases the response to whatever transmitter is released. The compensatory phenomena are effective in offsetting the effects of degeneration of neuromuscular junctions for a long time and significant functional loss is not apparent until late in life. When it begins to become manifest, it is most noticeable at high rates of neural drive and in the most peripheral muscles.

CHANGES IN EFFECTOR ORGAN SENSITIVITY

Quantitative study of the neuromuscular blocking drugs in old animals has not yet received the attention that the subject deserves. The changes with age in structure and microphysiology of the neuromuscular junction suggest that there is much to be learned from pharmacologic analysis but only a few experiments have been reported. Among the depolarizing compounds only acetylcholine has been used. As reviewed above, the evidence suggests that muscles from aged animals are more sensitive to acetylcholine than muscles from younger animals.

The response of older muscle to acetylcholine is similar to that of denervated or embryonic muscle and seems to be due to the simultaneous development of receptor supersensitivity in some cells and embryonic receptor-ionophore complexes in others. By analogy with other situations wherein neuromuscular junctions are distorted and transmission is inefficient, e.g., myasthenia gravis, it might be expected that muscles from aged animals would be unusually resistant to succinylcholine or decamethonium, but there are no data on the matter.

Nondepolarizing drugs seem to be more effective in blocking neuromuscular transmission in preparations from old animals than in those from young adults. Smith noted that the amount of curare or magnesium required to block contractions of the diaphragm was less for muscles from old rats than for those from young ones.[72] Frolkis et al.[60] showed that only about two thirds as much diplacin (a bis-pyrrolizinium derivative: Chem. Abstr. Service Registry #19918-85-5) was required to prevent neurally stimulated contraction of gastrocnemius muscles from 26- to 28-month-old rats as was required to block contraction of muscles from 8- to 10-month-old animals. He reported, without giving data, that d-tubocurarine also was more effective in old animals. Both Smith and Frolkis et al. noted that high-frequency stimulation was particularly susceptible to curariform drugs given to old animals.

Frolkis et al.[60] are the only ones to mention the use of neostigmine or related compounds in older animals. They noted that the administration of 1.2 to 1.5 µg of neostigmine per 100 g of body weight, to old animals, produced effects equivalent to doses of 2.5 to 3.0 µg/100 g of body weight to younger rats.

These data are not adequate to assess accurately the efficacy of neuromuscular blocking drugs in older animals. While they suggest that nondepolarizing compounds may be more effective, they also suggest that the effective doses are changed by a factor smaller than two, a change that may not be detected easily in clinical research or be meaningful in the ordinary situation of a human being in the operating room.

CHANGES IN PHARMACOKINETICS

All neuromuscular blocking drugs used clinically are quaternary ammonium compounds that are restricted in distribution to the extracellular fluid. They bind only moderately to plasma proteins and to tissues. Consequently, their volumes of distribution are small — about twice that of the extracellular water — and their distribution is accomplished quickly. Since these drugs always are injected intravenously, the time to onset of action is determined by the time to circulate drug to neuromuscular junctions and that consumed in binding to receptors. Succinylcholine is eliminated by intravascular hydrolysis via plasma cholinesterase.[73,74] But since the other compounds are eliminated via the kidney and/or the hepatobiliary system, their durations of action depend upon the function of these organs. The elimination of gallamine,[75] decamethonium,[76] and alcuronium,[77,78] is almost entirely via glomerular filtration in the kidney. Tubocurarine and pancuronium normally are eliminated mostly by the kidney. However, the former also is excreted in bile,[79] and the latter is hydrolyzed slowly in the liver;[80,81] these routes of elimination become more important when renal function is impaired.

Along with aging comes a decrease in (1) intracellular and total body water,[82] (2) plasma albumin,[83,84] (3) cardiac output and circulatory rate,[85] (4) glomerular filtration, (5) creatine clearance,[86] and (6) hepatic blood flow (see Chapter by Dr. Richey).[85] Some older individuals also may produce less plasma cholinesterase than do younger individuals.[87,88] Disease and concurrent use of other drugs may further diminish cardiac, renal, or hepatic function and/or produce changes in fluid and electrolyte balance that may affect the pharmacokinetics of the neuromuscular blocking drugs.

On theoretical grounds, the diminished circulatory and eliminative functions of older individuals should change the time course of action of neuromuscular blocking drugs by increasing the times to onset and offset of action. The dehydration and diminution of plasma protein that accompany age might increase the concentration of drug in plasma water and at the receptor site, but this effect would be relatively small and could be offset by the greater time available for distribution to tissues that follows from the reduced cardiac output and circulatory efficiency. A potentially more intense action of the drugs could also be offset by the anesthetist's choice of a smaller dose or a slower rate of administration when dealing with old people.

Quantitative analysis of the pharmacokinetics of this group of drugs was impeded for a long time by the lack of sensitive methods for measuring the compounds in biological fluids. Appropriate methods have been developed in recent years and reports of studies on animals and normal and diseased young human beings are now appearing. An increasing number of reports include information on the pharmacokinetic features of these drugs in the aged. Agoston et al.[80] measured plasma concentrations and biliary and renal elimination in 7 patients aged 64 to 77 years who were given 6 mg of pancuronium. Despite a wide range of variation among individuals, there was no evidence of prolonged plasma drug concentrations or deviations from normal in the elimination of the drug by either the hepatic or renal pathways. Similar results were found in pharmacokinetic studies in 7 patients between 64 and 76 years of age receiving average doses of 6.5 mg of pancuronium as a combined bolus and constant infusion.[89] Somogyi concluded the decline in the rate of pancuronium clearance from the plasma underwent no reduction with increasing age.[90]

Some studies in aged subjects do find a trend which suggests aging influences the pharmacokinetics of neuromuscular blocking drugs. Duvaldestin et al. measured the effect of pancuronium over a dose range of 70 to 175 µg/kg in a group of 28 patients free of hepatic or circulatory disease whose age exceeded 75 years. Neither dose requirements or plasma concentrations of the relaxant necessary to produce a fixed depression of twitch height was different when aged patients were compared with younger. However, despite a wide range in individual variation the average rate of recovery from neuromuscular blockade was slower in the older age group. The average plasma clearance rate was 1.18 ± 0.39 m$\ell\cdot$min$^{-1}\cdot$kg^{-1} in aged subjects compared to 1.81 ± 0.36 m$\ell\cdot$min$^{-1}\cdot$kg^{-1} in a younger aged group. The amount of pancuronium recovered in the urine was lower in older subjects than in younger within 2 hr after the relaxant but was not changed in the 24 hr cumulative collection. In older subjects the elimination half life of pancuronium was an average 201 ± 69 min in contrast to 107 ± 24 min in younger patients. The prolonged duration of neuromuscular blockade in the aged was attributed to a slower pancuronium elimination kinetics.[91] Similar conclusions were made by McLeod et al. who administered pancuronium (4 mg/kg) to 7 patients between 75 and 86 years of age. The rate of plasma clearance of pancuronium decreased more slowly with increasing age.[92] Matteo et al. described the effect of metocurine in 6 patients 74 to 81 years of age, who received a single dose of 0.3 mg/kg of the relaxant. Neither elemination half life nor plasma clearance rates were different in older patients. A rather notable increase in urinary output of metocurine was found in the older subjects with $70 \pm 7\%$ of the administered dose recovered in a cumulated 24-hr period compared with only $44 \pm 8\%$ in younger subjects. A reduction in the volume of distribution and sustained elevation of plasma metocurine concentration in elderly patients were suggested to influence the urinary output of the muscle relaxant. No attempt was made to correlate neuromuscular blockade and pancuronium elemination kinetics.[93]

Quantitative studies of the efficacy of neuromuscular blocking drugs in human beings are difficult to do under the best of circumstances. Only a few investigators have attempted to do them during surgery on the aged where the situation is complicated by a greater than usual incidence of debilitation, electrolyte imbalance, cardiovascular, renal, and respiratory deficiencies and concurrent use of other drugs. Nevertheless, the published reports are strikingly uniform in concluding that age does not have a major effect on the efficacy of neuromuscular blocking drugs.

The duration of apnea is the most important practical indicator of the effect of a neuromuscular blocking drug. This parameter has been used by several investigators. Dripps,[94] describing his experience with 468 surgical patients between the ages of 60 and 89, who were given a variety of neuromuscular blocking agents, reported only 3 cases of prolonged apnea. He found no obvious correlation between age and unexpected respiratory responses. Miller et al.,[95] using neuromuscular blocking drugs as an adjunct to anesthesia in patients of well-advanced age (over 90 years), remarked on the lack of "dramatic complications". Studies attempting to correlate dose of blocking drugs with age-related variations in body weight and muscle mass[96] or body surface[97] showed these variables to have no greater influence on the response to tubocurarine in the elderly than they did in the young. Walts and Dillon found no significant correlation between age and the duration of neuromuscular block produced by tubocurarine or gallamine.[98]

Measurement of muscle contractile force would be a more sensitive indicator of neuromuscular competency than those discussed above. It was found that age has little influence on the dose of pancuronium needed to abolish the twitch response.[91,99]

However, the time course for abolition of the twitch response was observed to change in old people. The time needed to abolish the twitch response by pancuronium was an average of 11.2 min in 13 patients aged 70 to 86, compared to a range of 3.59 to 8.83 min in 18- to 69-year-old individuals.[99] In the same experiment, there was no significant correlation between the age of the patient and the time to hypoventilation, time to recovery, or the need for incremental doses of pancuronium. Similarly, a delayed onset of muscle relaxation was noticed as assessed by the ease of intubation 3 and 5 min after a bolus injection of pancuronium into 61 patients who ranged between 60 and 86 years of age. Vaughan and Cobb noted that the relaxation at 3 min was poorer in older patients than in younger adults,[99] but that after 5 min the effect was equivalent in both age groups. On the other hand, Lorhan and Lippman studied a population of 75 patients aged 65 to 93 years and reported that sufficient relaxation for intubation was obtained in 90%, 3 min after administration of 2 to 6 mg of pancuronium.[100] This dose produced surgical relaxation for an average of 80 min. Tubocurarine (unspecified dose) produced neuromuscular blockade for a shorter time (45 to 60 min) in a similar group of geriatric patients.

There is less published experience with the use of succinylcholine in aged individuals; however, the data suggest there is no correlation between increasing age and the occurrence of prolonged recovery from neuromuscular blockade. Durrans expressed "surprise" at the tolerance to neuromuscular blocking drugs of aged and very sick patients,[101] including those aged over 70. Furthermore, 65 patients between 70 and 100 years of age undergoing treatment for femoral fractures were found to tolerate well 50 mg of succinylcholine; the duration of apnea was no longer than in younger adults.[102] There have been several individual cases of prolonged apnea,[103] apparently in patients whose diseased livers made less cholinesterase than usual. Fasciculations and post-succinylcholine pain seem to be less severe than in younger patients and there are antedotal suggestions that phase II blockade is more likely to occur in older patients, but little else has been reported.

There is a greater risk of adverse effects upon the cardiovascular system, particularly hypotension and cardiac dysrhythmias, associated with the use of either depolarizing or nondepolarizing compounds in the elderly, apparently because protective reflexes are not as efficient in old age and because more potassium may be released from the partly denervated muscles. Consequently, most authorities recommend that the initial dose of muscle relaxant be smaller than usual and that it be given more slowly.[104,105] Authorities also caution that cardiovascular, renal, hepatic, neural, or other diseases are common among the elderly and can change markedly the response to neuromuscular blocking drugs.[106]

The capacity of neostigmine or pyridostigmine to reverse neuromuscular blockade has been assessed in the elderly. Hunter reported that in six patients who were elderly and "dilapidated", neostigmine failed to reverse the effects of gallamine or d-tubocurarine.[107]

The failure was laid to a "reflection of some major abnormality of the physiology of the myoneural junction." More recently, other investigators have attempted to quantify the reversibility by recording twitch response. Lippman and Rogoff found pyridostigmine produced adequate reversal in 14 patients, age 60 to 74, but not in 2 others, who had received antibiotics and large doses of relaxants.[108] Vaughan and Cobb working with a group of 61 patients who ranged in age from 68 to 86,[99] found neostigmine adequate for reversing the effects of pancuronium. Chmielewski et al.[109] found neostigmine to be equally effective in antagonizing tubocurarine in young and old (68 to 92 years) patients. Conceding that neostigmine is effective in reversing either pancuronium or tubocurarine in the elderly, Owens et al.[110] caution that the elderly are more likely to have adverse cardiovascular effects from this drug than from pyridostigmine. Reporting on 93 patients over the age of 65, all of whom had compromised cardiac function, Owens et al.[110] described an unusually high incidence of cardiac dysrhythmias after the administration of neostigmine.

REFERENCES

1. **Samorajski, T., Ordy, J. M., and Keefe, J. R.,** The fine structure of lipofuscin age pigment in the nervous system of aged mice, *J. Cell. Biol.,* 26, 779, 1965.
2. **Berg, B. N., Wolf, A., and Simms, H. S.,** Degenerative lesion of spinal roots and peripheral nerves in aging rats, *Gerontologia,* 6, 72, 1962.
3. **Grover-Johnson, N. and Spencer, P. S.,** Peripheral nerve abnormalities in aging rats, *J. Neuropathol. Exp. Neurol.,* 40, 155, 1981.
4. **Ochoa, J. and Mair, W. G. P.,** The normal sural nerve in man. II. Changes in the axons and Schwann cells due to aging, *Acta Neuropathol.,* 13, 217, 1969.
5. **Hanzlikova, V. and Gutmann, E.,** Retardation of development and involution of the pudendal nerve in female rat, *J. Ultrastr. Res.,* 38, 302, 1972.
6. **Vizoso, A. D.,** The relationship between internodal length and growth in human nerves, *J. Anat.,* 84, 342, 1950.
7. **Lascelles, R. G. and Thomas, P. K.,** Changes due to age in internodal length in the sural nerve in man, *J. Neurol. Neurosurg. Psychiatry,* 29, 40, 1966.
8. **Arnold, N. and Harriman, D. G. F.,** The incidence of abnormality in control human peripheral nerve studied by single axon dissection, *J. Neurol. Neurosurg. Psychiatry,* 33, 55, 1970.
9. **Cottrell, L.,** Histologic variations with age in apparently normal peripheral nerve trunks, *Arch. Neurol. Psychiatry,* 43, 1138, 1940.
10. **O'Sullivan, D. J. and Swallow, M.,** The fibre size and content of the radial and sural nerves, *J. Neurol. Neurosurg. Psychiatry,* 31, 464, 1968.
11. **Swallow, M.,** Fibre Size and content of anterior tibial nerve of the foot, *J. Neurol. Neurosurg. Psychiatry,* 29, 205, 1966.
12. **Caccia, M. R., Harris, J. B., and Johnson, M. A.,** Morphology and physiology of skeletal muscle in aging rodents, *Muscle Nerve,* 2, 202, 1979.
13. **Brown, W. F.,** A method of estimating the number of motor units in thenar muscles and the changes in motor unit count with ageing, *J. Neurol. Neurosurg. Psychiatry,* 35, 845, 1972.
14. **Brown, W. F.,** Functional compensation of human motor units in health and disease, *J. Neurol. Sci.,* 20, 199, 1973.
15. **McComas, A. J., Upton, A. R. M., and Sica, R. E. P.,** Motoneurone disease and aging, *Lancet,* 2, 1477, 1973.
16. **Campbell, M. J., McComas, A. J., and Petito, F.,** Physiological changes in aging muscles, *J. Neurol. Neurosurg. Psychiatry,* 36, 174, 1973.
17. **Frolkis, V. V.,** Neuro-humoral regulations in the aging organism, *J. Gerontol.,* 21, 161, 1966.
18. **Frolkis, V. V., Bezrukov, V. V., Duplenko, Y. K., Shchegoleva, I. V., Shevtchuk, F. G., and Verkhratsky, N. S.,** Acetylcholine metabolism and cholinergic regulation of functions in aging, *Gerontologia,* 19, 45, 1973.

19. **Norris, A. H., Shock, N. W., and Wagman, I. H.,** Age changes in the maximum conduction velocity of motor fibers of human ulnar nerves, *J. Appl. Physiol.,* 5, 589, 1953.
20. **Wagman I. H. and Lesse, H.,** Maximum conduction velocities of motor fibers of ulnar nerve in human subjects of various ages and sizes, *J. Neurophysiol.,* 15, 235, 1952.
21. **Birren, J. E. and Wall, P. D.,** Age changes in conduction velocity, refractory period, number of fibers, connective tissue space and blood vessels in sciatic nerve of rats, *J. Comp. Neurol.,* 104, 1, 1956.
22. **LaFratta, C. W. and Smith, O. H.,** A study of the relationship of motor nerve conduction velocity in the adult to age, sex and handedness, *Arch. Phys. Med. Rehabil.,* 45, 407, 1964.
23. **Carlson, K. E., Alston, W., and Feldman, D. J.,** Electromyographic study of aging in skeletal muscle, *Am. J. Phys. Med.,* 43, 141, 1964.
24. **Fagg, G. E., Scheff, S. W., and Cotman, C. W.,** Axonal sprouting at the neuromuscular junction of adult and aged rats, *Exp. Neurol.,* 74, 847, 1981.
25. **Pestronk, A., Drachman, D. B., and Griffin, J. W.,** Effects of aging on nerve sprouting and regeneration, *Exp. Neurol.,* 70, 65, 1980.
26. **Rosenheimer, J. L. and Smith, D. O.,** Decreased sprouting and degeneration of nerve terminals of active muscles in aged rats, *Soc. Neurosci.,* 7, 184, 1981.
27. **Courtney, J. and Steinbach, J. H.,** Age changes in neuromuscular junction morphology and acetylcholine receptor distribution on rat skeletal muscle fibres, *J. Physiol. (London),* 320, 435, 1981.
28. **Gutmann, E. and Hanzlikova, V.,** Age changes of motor endplates in muscle fibres of the rat, *Gerontologia,* 11, 12, 1965.
29. **Gutmann, E., Hanzlikova, V., and Vyskocil, F.,** Age changes in cross striated muscle of the rat, *J. Physiol. (London),* 219, 331, 1971.
30. **Fujisawa, K.,** Some observations on the skeletal musculature of aged rats. III. Abnormalities of terminal axons found in motor endplates, *Exp. Gerontol.,* 11, 43, 1976.
31. **Gutmann, E. and Hanzlikova, V.,** The motor unit in old age, *Nature (London),* 209, 921, 1966.
32. **Tomonaga, M.,** Histochemical and ultrastructural changes in senile human skeletal muscle, *J. Am. Geriatr. Soc.,* 25, 125, 1977.
33. **Gutmann, E. and Hanzlikova, V.,** Fast and slow motor units in aging, *Gerontology,* 22, 280, 1976.
34. **Tůcek, S. and Gutmann, E.,** Choline acetyltransferase activity in muscles of old rats, *Exp. Neurol.,* 38, 349, 1973.
35. **Vyskocil, F. and Gutmann, E.,** Spontaneous transmitter release from nerve endings and contractile properties in the soleus and diaphragm muscles of senile rats, *Experientia,* 28, 280, 1972.
36. **Bass, A., Gutmann, E., and Hanzlikova, V.,** Biochemical and histochemical changes in energy supply enzyme pattern of muscles of the rat during old age, *Gerontologia,* 21, 31, 1975.
37. **Verkhratsky, N. S.,** Acetylcholine metabolism peculiarities in aging, *Exp. Gerontol.,* 5, 49, 1970.
38. **Gutmann, E., Jakoubek, B., Fischer, J., and Babicky, A.,** Autoradiographic study of protein metabolism in old and adolescent neurons, *Life Sci.,* 6, 2143, 1967.
39. **Gutmann, E., Hanzlikova, V., and Jakoubek, B.,** Changes in the neuromuscular system during old age, *Exp. Gerontol.,* 3, 141, 1968.
40. **Jakoubek, B., Gutmann, E., Fischer, J., and Babicky, A.,** Rate of protein renewal in spinal motoneurons of adolescent and old rats, *J. Neurochem.,* 15, 633, 1968.
41. **Gutmann, E.,** Nervous and hormonal mechanisms in the aging process, *Exp. Gerontol.,* 5, 357, 1970.
42. **McMartin, D. N. and O'Connor, J. A.,** Effect of age on axoplasmic transport of cholinesterase in rat sciatic nerves, *Mech. Ageing Dev.,* 10, 241, 1979.
43. **Brimijoin, S. and Dyck, P. J.,** Axonal transport of dopamine beta hydroxylase and acetylcholinesterase in human peripheral neuropathy, *Exp. Neurol.,* 66, 467, 1979.
44. **Tuffery, A. R.,** Growth and degeneration of motor endplates in normal cat hind limb muscles, *J. Anat.,* 110, 221, 1971.
45. **Gutmann, E.,** Considerations on neurotrophic relations in the central and peripheral nervous system, *Acta Neurobiol. Exp.,* 35, 341, 1975.
46. **Gutmann, E.,** Differentiation of metabolism in muscles of different function during ontogenesis, *Prog. Brain Res.,* 22, 566, 1968.
47. **Jennekens, F. G. I., Tomlinson, B. E., and Walton, J. N.,** Histochemical aspects of five limb muscles in old age, *J. Neurol. Sci.,* 14, 259, 1971.
48. **Gutmann, E.,** Maintenance and formation of neuromuscular synapses in senescent muscles, *Act. Nerv. Super.,* 18, 137, 1976.
49. **Larsson, L.,** Morphological and functional characteristics of the aging skeletal muscle in man. A cross sectional study, *Acta Physiol. Scand. Suppl.,* 457, 1, 1978.
50. **Barker, D. and Ip, M. C.,** Sprouting and degeneration of mammalian motor axons in normal and de-afferentiated skeletal muscle, *Proc. R. Soc. London,* 163, 538, 1966.
51. **Hooper, A. C.,** Length, diameter and number of aging skeletal muscle fibers, *Gerontology,* 27, 121, 1981.

52. **Rowe, R. W. D.,** The effects of senility on skeletal muscle in the mouse, *Exp. Gerontol.,* 4, 119, 1969.
53. **Berg, B. N.,** Muscular dystrophy in aging rats, *J. Gerontol.,* 11, 134, 1956.
54. **Karpati, G. and Engel, W. K.,** "Type grouping" in skeletal muscles after experimental reinnervation, *Neurology,* 18, 447, 1968.
55. **Mohan S. and Radha, E.,** Age related changes in muscle protein degradation, *Mech. Ageing Dev.,* 7, 81, 1978.
56. **Drahota, Z. and Gutmann, E.,** The effect of age on compensatory and "post functional hypertrophy" in cross striated muscle, *Gerontologia,* 6, 81, 1962.
57. **Srivastava, U. and Chaudhary, K. D.,** Effect of age on protein and ribonucleic acid metabolism in mouse skeletal muscle, *Can. J. Biochem.,* 47, 231, 1969.
58. **Syrovy, I. and Gutmann, E.,** Changes in speed of contraction and ATPase activity in striated muscle during old age, *Exp. Gerontol.,* 5, 31, 1970.
59. **Ermini, M.,** Ageing changes in mammalian skeletal muscle, *Gerontology,* 22, 301, 1976.
60. **Frolkis, V. V., Martynenko, O. A., and Zamostyan, V. P.,** Aging in the neuromuscular apparatus, *Gerontology,* 22, 244, 1976.
61. **Fudel-Osipova, S. I. and Rodionov, G. A.,** Relations between some physiological and histomorphological changes of neuromuscular system during aging, *Byull. Eksp. Biol. Med.,* 56, 50, 1963.
62. **Petersén, I. and Kurgelberg, E.,** Duration and form of action potential in the normal human muscle, *J. Neurol. Neurosurg. Psychiatry,* 12, 124, 1949.
63. **Fudel-Osipova, S. I. and Grishko, F. E.,** Features specific to electromyograms taken during voluntary muscle contraction in old age, *Byull. Eksp. Biol. Med.,* 3, 9, 1962.
64. **Sacco, G., Buchthal, F. and Resenfalck, P.,** Motor unit potential at different ages, *Arch. Neurol. (Chicago),* 6, 366, 1962.
65. **Grishko, F. I. and Litovchenko, S. V.,** Physiological characteristics of the neuromuscular apparatus in persons of advanced age, *Fiziol. Zh. (Kiev),* 10, 37, 1964.
66. **Vyskocil F. and Gutmann, E.,** Spontaneous transmitter release from motor nerve endings in muscle fibers of castrated and old animals, *Experientia,* 25, 945, 1969.
67. **Vyskocil, F.,** Action potentials of the rat diaphragm and the sensitivity to tetrodotoxin during postnatal development and old age, *Pfleugers Arch.,* 352, 155, 1974.
68. **Mitolo, M.,** Electromyography on aging, *Gerontologia,* 14, 54, 1968.
69. **Stålberg, E. and Thiele, B.,** Motor unit fibre density in the extensor digitorum communis muscle, *J. Neurol. Neurosurg. Psychiatry,* 38, 874, 1975.
70. **Tauchi, H., Yoshioka, T., and Kobayashi, H.,** Age changes of skeletal muscles, *Gerontologia,* 17, 219, 1971.
71. **Clarkson, P. M., Kroll, W., and Melchionda, A. M.,** Age, isometric strength, rate of tension development and fiber type composition, *J. Gerontol.,* 36, 648, 1981.
72. **Smith, D. O.,** Reduced capabilities of synaptic transmission in aged rats, *Exp. Neurol.,* 66, 650, 1979.
73. **Kalow, W.,** The distribution, destruction and elimination of muscle relaxants, *Anesthesiology,* 20, 505, 1959.
74. **Greene, N. M.,** Metabolism of drugs employed in anesthesia, *Anesthesiology,* 29, 327, 1968.
75. **Agoston, S., Vermeer, G. A., Kersten, V. W., and Scaf, A. H. J.,** A preliminary investigation of the renal and hepatic excretion of gallamine triethiodide in man, *Br. J. Anaesth.,* 50, 345, 1978.
76. **Paton, W. D. M. and Zaimis, E. J.,** Methonium compounds, *Pharm. Rev.,* 4, 219, 1952.
77. **Waser, P. G. and Luthi, U.,** Distribution and metabolism of curazizing and depolarizing drugs in cats, *J. Nucl. Biol. Med.,* 12, 4, 1968.
78. **Raaflaub, J. and Frey, P.,** Zur pharmadodinetic von diallyl-nor toxiferin beim menschen, *Arzneim. Forsch.,* 22, 73, 1972.
79. **Cohen, E. N., Brewer, H. W., and Smith, D.,** The metabolism and elimination of d-tubocurarine-H^3, *Anesthesiology,* 28, 309, 1967.
80. **Agoston, S., Vermeer, G. A., Kersten, U. W., and Meijer, D. K. F.,** The fate of pancuronium bromide in man, *Acta Anaesth. Scand.,* 17, 267, 1973.
81. **Somogyi, A. A., Shanks, C. A., and Triggs, E. J.,** Disposition kinetics of pancuronium bromide in patients with total biliary obstruction, *Br. J. Anaesth.,* 49, 1103, 1977.
82. **Friedman, S. M., Sreter, F. A., and Friedman, C. L.,** Distribution of water, sodium and potassium in the aged rat, *Gerontologia,* 7, 49, 1963.
83. **Yan, S. H. Y. and Franks, J. J.,** Albumin metabolism in elderly men and women, *J. Lab. Clin. Med.,* 72, 449, 1968.
84. **Misra, D. P., Loudon, J. M., and Staddon, G. E.,** Albumin metabolism in elderly patients, *J. Gerontol.,* 30, 304, 1975.
85. **Bender, A. D.,** The effect of increasing age on the distribution of peripheral blood flow in man, *J. Am. Geriatr. Soc.,* 13, 192, 1965.

86. **Rowe, J. W., Andres, R., Tobin, J. D., Norris, A. H., and Shock, N. W.,** The effect of age on creatinine clearance in men: a cross-section and longitudinal study, *J. Gerontol.,* 31, 155, 1976.

87. **Foldes, F. F. and Rhodes, D. H.,** The role of plasma cholinesterase in anesthesiology, *Curr. Res. Anesth. Analg.,* 32, 305, 1953.

88. **Oropollo, A. T.,** Abnormal peudocholinesterse levels in a surgical population, *Anesthesiology,* 48, 284, 1978.

89. **Somogyi, A. A., Shanks, C. A., and Triggs, E. J.,** Combined i.v. bolus and infusion of pancuronium bromide, *Br. J. Anaesth.,* 50, 575, 1978.

90. **Somogyi, A. A.,** Pancuronium plasma clearance and age, *Br. J. Anaesth.,* 52, 360, 1980.

91. **Duvaldestin, P., Saada, J., Berger, J. L., D'Hollander, A., and Desmonts, J. M.,** Pharmacokinetics, pharmacodynamics and dose-response relationships of pancuronium in control and elderly subjects, *Anesthesiology,* 56, 36, 1982.

92. **McLeod, K., Hull, C. J., and Watson, M. J.,** Effects of aging on the pharmacokinetics of pancuronium, *Br. J. Anaesth.,* 51, 436, 1979.

93. **Matteo, R. S., Brotherton, W. P., McDaniel, D. D., and Diaz, J.,** Pharmacokinetics of metocurine in the aged, *Anesthesiology,* 55, A215, 1981.

94. **Dripps, R. D.,** Abnormal respiratory response to various "curare" drugs during surgical anesthesia: incidence, etiology, treatment, *Ann. Surg.,* 137, 145, 1953.

95. **Miller, R., Marlar, K., and Silvay, G.,** Anesthesia for patients aged over ninety years, *N.Y. State J. Med.,* 77, 1421, 1977.

96. **Dundee, J. W.,** The relationship of the dosage of d-tubocurarine chloride and laudolissin to body weight, sex and age, *Br. J. Anaesth.,* 26, 174, 1954.

97. **Stovner, J., Theodorsen, L., and Bjelke, E.,** Sensitivity to tubocurarine and alcuronium with special reference to plasma protein pattern, *Br. J. Anaesth.,* 43, 385, 1971.

98. **Walts, L. F. and Dillon, J. B.,** durations of action of d-tubocurarine and gallamine, *Anesthesiology,* 29, 499, 1968.

99. **Vaughan, R. W. and Cobb, M. L.,** Pancuronium bromide as the sole muscle relaxant for major surgery, *Anesth. Analg. (Cleveland),* 53, 56, 1974.

100. **Lorhan, P. H. and Lippmann, M.,** Clinical apparaisal of pancuronium bromide for the aged patient, *Anesth. Analg. (Cleveland),* 51, 914, 1972.

101. **Durrans, S. F.,** Prolonged apnea, *Lancet,* 2, 539, 1952.

102. **Johnson, P. D.,** Prolonged apnoca following suxamethonium chloride, *Br. J. Anaesth.,* 26, 427, 1954.

103. **Foldes, F. F., Rendell-Baker, L., and Birch, J. H.,** Causes and prevention of prolonged apnea with succinylcholine, *Curr. Res. Anesth. Analg.,* 35, 609, 1956.

104. **Gray, T. C.,** The use of d-tubocurarine chloride in anaesthesia, *Ann. R. Coll. Surg. Eng.,* 1, 191, 1947.

105. **Foldes, F. F.,** *Muscle Relaxants in Anesthesiology,* Charles C Thomas, Springfield, Ill., 1947, 140.

106. **Foldes, F. F.,** Factors which alter the effect of muscle relaxants, *Anesthesiology,* 20, 464, 1959.

107. **Hunter, A. R.,** Neostigmine-resistant curarization, *Br. Med. J.,* ii, 919, 1956.

108. **Lippmann, M. and Rogoff, R. C.,** A clinical evaluation of pyridostigmine bromide in the reversal of pancuronium, *Anesth. Analg. (Cleveland),* 53, 20, 1974.

109. **Chmielewski, A. T., Pybus, D. A., Loach, A. B., and Goat, V. A.,** Recovery from neuromuscular blockade: a comparison between old and young patients, *Anaesthesia,* 33, 539, 1978.

110. **Owens, W. D., Waldbaum, L. S., and Stephen, C. R.,** Cardiac dysrhythmia following reversal of neuromuscular blocking agents in geriatric patients, *Anesth. Analg. (Cleveland),* 57, 186, 1978.

Miscellaneous Drugs

HISTAMINE AND ANTIHISTAMINES

G. Victor Rossi

HISTORY OF HISTAMINE

Histamine (β-imidazolylethylamine) was synthesized by Windaus and Vogt in 1907[1] and isolated from intestinal mucosa by Barger and Dale in 1911.[2] During the decade from 1910 to 1920, Dale et al.[3,4] revealed the diverse effects of histamine in several species. He speculated with remarkable prescience on the relationships of this amine to inflammatory and anaphylactic phenomena. Despite demonstration of a wide range of pharmacologic actions, the possibility of physiologic significance was clouded by the suspicion that histamine was not a product of normal tissue but was formed by the action of bacterial enzymes on the amino acid, histidine.[5] It was not until 1927 that Best et al.[6] succeeded in isolating crystalline histamine picrate from a variety of mammalian tissues by procedures that precluded histamine formation by bacterial action. Strong evidence for a role in allergy and anaphylaxis was provided in 1932 by identification of histamine in perfusates of sensitized tissues exposed to specific antigen.[7,8] The "histamine theory of anaphylaxis" provided major impetus in the search for selective antagonists of histamine activity. Compound 929F, described in 1937 by Bovet and Staub,[9] served as the prototype for a series of antihistaminic agents introduced into medical practice during the post-World War II period.

Yellin commented that the classical antihistamines proved useful as tools for delineating the pathophysiologic role of histamine but contributed relatively little to an understanding of the function of histamine in physiological processes, notably gastric secretion.[10] Black et al.[11] synthesized burimamide in 1972; it competitively blocks the stimulant effect of histamine on gastric secretion. Discovery of the linkage between histamine receptors and nucleotide cyclases reawakened interest in the possible biological regulatory role of histamine.

The first seven decades of histamine exploration have been reviewed comprehensively in two reference volumes edited by Eichler and Farah and by Rocha e Silva.[12,13] The renaissance of histaminology, catalyzed by development of the H_2-receptor antagonists, has been described masterfully in a monograph by Beaven.[14]

Storage and Synthesis of Histamine; Age-Related Changes

In man, as in most mammalian species, the mast cell is the chief repository of tissue histamine, whereas the basophil serves as the principle cytological depot for histamine in the blood. In certain structures, notably gastrointestinal mucosa and brain, a considerable fraction of tissue histamine is resistant to depletion by compound 48/80 and has been referred to as "nonmast cell histamine." The amine is associated with cells that have not been defined taxonomically. Nonmast cell histamine has a higher turnover rate than that stored in mast cells.[15]

Riley and West observed a correlation between mast cell concentration and histamine content in a variety of tissues in different species.[16] These investigators also reported an increase both in the number of mast cells and histamine levels in skin (cat), lungs and liver (ox, man) with progression from fetal to young to adult animals. Harvey noted that the histamine content of the heart was higher in old than in young rats.[17] Hardwick found that histamine levels in the skin remained fairly constant in rats from birth to 514 days, with transient high values occurring shortly after birth and at the time of weaning.[18] In contrast, Rocha e Silva reported a decrease in the histamine content of the skin in rabbits of increasing age, from newborns to adults.[19] Although weights of experimental animals were stated in most of these literature reports, ages usually were not specified. Based on these isolated observations, it is apparent that generalizations regarding the relationship between age and tissue content of histamine are not warranted.

Endogenous histamine originates in part by action of nonspecific L-amino-acid decarboxylase on the precursor amino acid, histidine; but principally by the enzymatic action of a selective L-histidine decarboxylase. This latter enzyme is inducible and is responsible for formation of induced or nascent histamine that is not stored, but exerts biological effects in proximity to sites of synthesis, and is rapidly inactivated by catabolic systems elucidated by Schayer et al.[20]

Håkanson et al.[21] and Aures and Håkanson[22] reported that, in rats, gastric histidine decarboxylase activity and gastric histamine concentration increase from birth until approximately 40 days of age, when the levels do not differ significantly from those observed in adults (age not specified). Isaac and Sapperstein found a linear increase in the histamine concentration in the glandular stomach from 25 to 179 days of age in the rat; histamine levels in the forestomach did not change with age.[23] The increase in histamine concentration associated with aging occurred in the muscular layer, not in the mucosal or serosal layers, of the rat glandular stomach. Lillehei and Wangensteen demonstrated increased susceptibility to histamine-induced gastroduodenal erosion in dogs progressing from those less than 1 year to over 10 years of age.[24]

Function

Although histamine was one of the first endogenous biologically active amines to be identified, its role in the natural economy remains to be established. Among the several proposed but unconfirmed roles for histamine in normal physiology are: (1) regulation of the microcirculation, (2) promotion of tissue growth and wound healing, (3) peripheral mediation of the sensory phenomena of pain and itch, (4) stimulation of gastric acid secretion, and (5) synaptic neurotransmission or neuromodulation in the central nervous system.[12-14,25] With the exception of possible involvement of histamine in gastric secretion and central neural processes, for which there is compelling evidence, the largely speculative functions of this amine will not be further considered.

Code,[26] and more recently Beaven[14] and Hirschowitz,[27] have summarized the multidimensional evidence supporting the role of histamine as a mediator of gastric secretion, notably:

1. The presence of this amine in relatively high concentrations in the gastric mucosa of all vertebrates, especially in the oxyntic gland area
2. The exquisite sensitivity of the gastric secretory apparatus to histamine and the exponential character of the relationship between the rate of histamine injection and the gastric secretory response
3. The decrease in gastric histamine levels and increase in gastric histidine decarboxylase activity which occur in response to a variety of stimuli (e.g., gastrin, cholinergic agents, insulin-induced hypoglycemia, food) that evoke acid secretion and, most critically
4. Inhibition of histamine activation of gastric mucosal adenylate cyclase and blockade of histamine-, pentagastrin- and food-induced gastric secretion by H_2-receptor antagonists

In 1956, Code stated that "no other chemostimulator is interposed between histamine and the parietal cells."[26] An alternative model, advanced more recently by Grossman and Konturek,[28] proposes three interdependent parietal cell receptors, i.e., for histamine, gastrin, and acetylcholine, with activation or blockade of any one reactive site altering the affinity of the remaining receptors for their specific agonist. Remarking on the diversity of natural processes and the evolutionary development of alternative mechanisms for regulating organ function, Code in 1977,[29] retreated somewhat from the absolutism of his earlier "final common pathway" hypothesis by stating "it is unlikely that histamine is the only route of stimulation to the parietal cells of all species." In this same publication, Code further remarked that histamine still appears to be the major route, if not the only route, to the parietal cell of many species, including man.

In comparison to the emphasis on catecholamines and 5-hydroxytryptamine, relatively little attention has been accorded to the possible involvement of histamine in central neural processes and psychotherapeutic drug action. Recent publications relating to (1) the selective distribution of histamine in the brain, (2) the identification in brain tissue of specific enzymatic systems for histamine synthesis and catabolism, (3) the ability of histamine to activate brain nucleotide cyclases, and (4) the demonstration of definitive electrophysiological and neuroendocrine responses upon intracerebroventricular injection or iontophoretic application of histamine have been offered as evidence that this amine may subserve a neurotransmitter or neuromodulatory function in the central nervous system.[30,31]

Inhibition of noradrenergic and serotonergic neuronal reuptake mechanisms by imipramine and related tricyclic derivatives has been advanced to account for the antidepressant activity of these drugs (see Dr. Horita's chapter in this handbook). That these molecular mechanisms are not generally applicable to all antidepressant compounds is indicated by the observation that the clinically effective antidepressants, iprindole and mianserin, have little or no influence on norepinephrine and serotonin reuptake. Several tricyclic antidepressants as well as iprindole and mianserin have been shown to block histamine activation of adenylate cyclase in homogenates of guinea pig cortex and hippocampus.[32,33] These studies suggest the possible involvement of a brain histamine-sensitive adenylate cyclase in antidepressant drug action. They indicate the need to consider further the possible contribution of histamine to the biogenic amine hypothesis of affective disorders.[34]

Age-related deficiencies in brain aminergic systems, assessed functionally and/or biochemically, have been observed in experimental animals and in man.[35-37] Histamine-stimulated adenylate cyclase activity in the hypothalamus, frontal cortex, and anterior limbic cortex was found to decline by approximately 50% in rabbits as they aged from less than 1 year to 5 years.[38] Although decreases in histamine-activated adenylate cyclases have not been linked to specific behavioral or functional deficits, it has been noted that these changes occurred in brain regions which, in man, are thought to be of importance in age-related decrements in central neuronal function.

Clinical Uses of Histamine

Pentagastrin, which has recently become available for diagnostic use, has largely displaced histamine phosphate in tests for the evaluation of gastric acid secretory function. Provocative tests, involving injection of histamine phosphate or methacholine chloride for the presumptive diagnosis of pheochromocytoma, have been superceded by quantitative determinations of urinary catecholamine metabolites. Histamine desensitization has been employed in allergic, vascular, and equilibrium disorders in which histamine is presumed to play an etiologic role; however, there is little objective evidence to support the efficacy of this therapeutic approach.[39] There are no documented specific precautions applicable to the diagnostic or therapeutic use of histamine in the elderly.

HISTORY OF ANTIHISTAMINES

A variety of synthetic compounds that function as competitive antagonists of histamine were developed subsequent to the pioneering work of Bovet and Staub in 1937.[9] Clinical experimentation established their usefulness in the palliation of local and systemic allergic disorders, in the prophylaxis and relief of motion sickness and other vestibular disturbances, and as adjuncts in the treatment of Parkinson's disease. Although the mechanistic classification "antihistamine" is convenient, it represents an oversimplification in that many compounds to which this term is applied possess, in addition to histamine-blocking activity, a variety of pharmacologic properties including anticholinergic, adrenolytic, local anesthetic, cardiac depressant, and central nervous system suppressant activity.

Systematic study revealed that antihistaminic agents antagonized most, but not all, effector organ responses to histamine; among those resistant to blockade were histamine-induced gastric acid secretion, stimulation of guinea pig atrial muscle, and inhibition of evoked contractions of rat uterine smooth muscle. Ash and Schild in 1966,[40] characterized the biological loci with which histamine interacts; they designated as H_1 receptors those reactive sites that are blocked by mepyramine and related antihistamines, and as non-H_1 receptors (later termed H_2 receptors) those which mediate responses to histamine that are refractory to mepyramine. Reevaluation of correlations between chemical structure and biological activity among a series of imidazole derivatives led, in 1972, to synthesis of the first H_2-receptor antagonist, burimamide, by Black and his co-workers.[11]

Burimamide, while of major experimental importance, exhibited relatively low potency and was not active orally. A molecular derivative, metiamide, was approximately ten times more potent than burimamide on a weight basis; it blocked histamine-stimulated gastric acid secretion selectively, following oral administration. Clinical trials of metiamide were suspended, however, after development of agranulocytosis in several patients undergoing therapy with this compound.[41] The thiourea moiety of metiamide, suspected of being responsible for the observed bone marrow depression, was replaced by a cyanoguanidine group forming cimetidine which, to date, is the only H_2-receptor antagonist approved for medical use in the U.S.[42]

H_1-Receptor Antagonists

The classical antihistamines (i.e., H_1-receptor antagonists) are associated with a very low incidence of serious adverse reactions. General acceptance of their considerable margin of safety underlies the availability of several antihistamines in nonprescription cough-cold, antiallergy, antimotion sickness, and sleep-aid formulations for patient self-medication.[43] Nevertheless, these drugs frequently cause untoward effects related largely to their central nervous system depressant and anticholinergic activities. The sedative effect is quite pronounced among antihistamines of the phenothiazine (e.g., promethazine) and ethanolamine (e.g., diphenhydramine, doxylamine) series but is usually less marked among those of the alkylamine (e.g., chlorpheniramine) group.[39] Although antihistamine-induced sedation may be advantageous in some clinical situations (e.g., insomnia associated with a distressful allergic disorder), drowsiness and somnolence represent potential hazards in ambulatory patients whose activities require mental alertness and motor coordination (e.g., operation of an automobile). The central nervous system effects of antihistamines may be manifested as dizziness, inability to concentrate, and ataxia.[44-46] While there is no firm evidence that impairment of mental and motor functions following administration of antihistamines of the H_1 type are age-related phenomena, the elderly would appear to be at substantial risk. Walson and Bressler have remarked that when the morbidity and mortality from falls resulting in broken bones are considered, side effects that are merely annoying in young adults may become life threatening in the elderly.[47] Special precautions and patient counseling are needed to minimize hazards that may arise from concomitant use of antihistamines and other central nervous system suppressants, notably alcohol, antianxiety agents, barbiturates, and nonbarbiturate sedative-hypnotics. Patients who have difficulty in reading fine print may be unaware that ethyl alcohol in concentrations as high as 25% v/v is incorporated in several over-the-counter antihistamine-containing cough-cold preparations.

Most drugs classified pharmacologically as antihistamines (i.e., H_1-antagonists) possess considerable anticholinergic activity which may account for such untoward reactions as (1) dryness of the mouth, throat, and respiratory passages, sometimes inducing cough; (2) urinary retention and dysuria, which are particularly distressful in elderly males with prostatic hypertrophy; (3) aggravation of constipation which is encountered frequently in older patients; (4) blurred vision and, in patients with narrow angle glaucoma, elevation of intraocular pressure; (5) palpitation and, occasionally, (6) postural hypotension. Atropine-like activity associated with large doses of antihistamines may be manifested as excitation, nervousness, incoordination, tremor, and may eventuate in convulsive seizures in patients who have focal lesions of the central nervous system.[39,44-46]

Although the pharmacokinetic profile and metabolic fate of relatively few of the 20 different H_1-receptor antagonists currently available for medical use have been determined in the elderly, nevertheless, certain generalizations appear valid. Following oral administration of liquid or solid preparations containing water-soluble salts of antihistaminic compounds, absorption is rapid and essentially complete. Although the available data are limited, there is little evidence to suggest any appreciable alteration in the absorption of most drugs from the gastrointestinal tract of elderly patients, especially weak bases (e.g., the antihistamines) that are absorbed by passive diffusion[48-50] (for additional discussion, see Dr. Richey's chapter in this handbook). Systemic effects are apparent within 15 to 30 min after oral administration of H_1-receptor antagonists. They are maximal in about 1 hour and usually persist for 3 to 6 hours, although some derivatives (e.g., chlorcyclizine) have an extended duration of action. As is characteristic of most lipid-soluble drugs, H_1-antagonists are metabolized extensively; only a relatively small fraction (5 to 15%) of unaltered drug is eliminated in the urine. Therefore, the decline in renal excretory capacity commonly associated with advancing age would not be expected to alter substantially the susceptibility of the elderly patient to the therapeutic or toxic effects of the conventional antihistamines.[51]

Metabolic reactions, identified primarily with the use of radiolabeled antihistaminic compounds, include ether cleavage, N-dealkylation, N-oxide formation, aromatic hydroxylation, and glucuronide and sulfate conjugation.[52] The liver is the major site of these synthetic and nonsynthetic biotransformations which, in the case of H_1-antagonists, lead almost invariably to inactive metabolites. Kato et al.[53] attributed the greater persistence of action of certain barbiturates and skeletal muscle relaxants in senescent rats to decreases in hepatic microsomal drug-metabolizing activity and in liver mass. Clinical pharmacokinetic studies have demonstrated either prolonged plasma half-life or reduced plasma clearance values, or both, for antipyrine and phenylbutazone in elderly subjects[49,54] (also see Dr. Baskin's chapter in this handbook). After single dose administration, the plasma levels of amobarbital, propranolol, and meperidine were significantly higher in elderly than in young patients; however, only in the case of amobarbital was there evidence to suggest that elevated plasma levels resulted from impaired drug metabolism. Gillette has cautioned that the findings obtained with one drug cannot be extrapolated to others although the same metabolic pathway may be presumably involved.[55] A literature search revealed no data on comparative plasma levels, or rates of metabolism of H_1-antagonists in young vs. elderly subjects.

H_2-Receptor Antagonists

In the relatively short time since its introduction into medical usage, numerous reports have attested to the effectiveness of the H_2-receptor antagonist, cimetidine, for the treatment of duodenal ulcer, benign gastric ulcer, pathological hypersecretory disorders (e.g., Zollinger-Ellison syndrome and systemic mastocytosis), erosive esophagitis, and upper gastrointestinal tract hemorrhage.[27,56-58] In several species, including man, cimetidine has been shown to suppress nocturnal and daytime basal gastric secretion, as well as acid secretion evoked by histamine, pentagastrin, stable choline esters, caffeine, insulin hypoglycemia, and food. As experimental tools, the H_2-receptor antagonists have firmly established the importance of endogenous histamine in the gastric secretory process. But whether histamine is the final common mediator of parietal cell secretion,[29] or one of the several interdependent gastric secretagogues,[28] continues to be debated.

Clinical experience has shown that while most duodenal ulcers will be healed after 6 to 8 weeks of cimetidine therapy, the rate of recurrence is high. Administration of maintenance doses of cimetidine, 400 mg nightly,[59] or twice daily,[60] for 6 to 12 months, has been reported to substantially reduce endoscopically verified recurrence of duodenal ulcer as compared to placebo-treated cases. Finkelstein and Isselbacher have suggested that such maintenance therapy should be considered for the elderly and poor-risk surgical patients with serious duodenal ulcer disease.[61] These investigators further noted that in patients with the Zollinger-Ellison syndrome, cimetidine therapy appears preferable to total gastrectomy, especially in elderly and malnourished patients in whom the surgical mortality may be high. Well-controlled comparative studies of cimetidine vs. intensive antacid therapy have demonstrated the fundamentally similar effectiveness of each of these medical approaches to the treatment of duodenal ulcer disease. Choice of treatment should be individualized and should take into account such factors as convenience and patient compliance[62] and, particularly in the case of elderly patients living on fixed incomes, medication costs.[63]

Cimetidine is largely ionized in a strongly acid environment, thus relatively little absorption occurs from the stomach; but the drug is absorbed rapidly from the small intestine. Compared to intravenous injection, the bioavailability of orally administered cimetidine is estimated to be approximately 75%; bioavailability of the drug does not appear to be grossly influenced by age.[64] Only 15 to 20% of the circulating drug is bound to plasma protein, thus there appears to be little risk of drug-drug interactions via the mechanism of competitive displacement from sites of plasma-protein binding. In contrast to the classical antihistamines, the H_2-receptor antagonist, cimetidine, is a hydrophilic molecule which is excreted in the urine largely in unchanged form; a relatively small fraction of the administered dose is eliminated in the form of inactive polar metabolites. In patients with renal failure, the elimination half-life is related inversely to creatinine clearance.[65]

Relatively minor side-effects associated with cimetidine therapy include headache, dizziness, fatigue, skin rash, diarrhea, constipation, and muscular pain. Gynecomastia has been observed in a small number of patients receiving cimetidine, several of whom had the Zollinger-Ellison syndrome and had been receiving the drug for more than 3 months. Serum creatinine levels tend to increase slightly in many patients on cimetidine therapy. Generally, the increase is within the normal range, but levels higher than 2 mg/dℓ have been found in about 3% of cimetidine-treated patients.[66,67] Dubb et al.[68] reported that single doses of cimetidine did not significantly alter the response to acid loading, maximal bicarbonate reabsorption, or urinary concentrating ability; it should be noted, however, that these observations were made in healthy young males.

Isolated or infrequent reports describe drug fever,[69] neutropenia,[70] leukopenia,[71,72] thrombocytopenia,[73] Stevens-Johnson syndrome,[74] severe diarrhea,[75] bradycardia and atrioventricular dissociation,[76,77] and hypotension (bolus intravenous injection)[78] in patients treated with cimetidine. In several of the cases cited in these clinical reports, a complicated medical history precludes establishment of cause-effect relationships; and there is no apparent association between these reported adverse reactions and patient age. Nevertheless, it would appear prudent to administer cimetidine with special caution in elderly patients with a history of allergic reactivity or heart disease.

Several cases of perforation of chronic peptic ulcers have been reported following abrupt cessation of cimetidine therapy.[79-81] Celestin and Spence remarked that perforation of chronic peptic ulcers is a potential complication of any inadequate therapy and that treatment must be continued until total healing is verified.[82] Particular vigilance is warranted in the use of cimetidine in the elderly patient where there is a history or suspicion of poor medication compliance.

There have been numerous reports of mental confusion with such symptoms as disorientation, restlessness, agitation, belligerence, and delirium associated with cimetidine administration; in most cases, the symptoms subsided upon cessation of cimetidine therapy.[83] Many of the patients in whom such confusional states have been observed were elderly, had serious underlying medical illness, were on multiple drug therapy, received higher than recommended doses of cimetidine, and had impaired renal function. The relative contribution of these factors to the development of neurological disturbances has not been ascertained, but it is apparent that cimetidine therapy should be carefully monitored in elderly, severely ill patients, particularly those with renal failure.

Based on assessments of mental status and serum cimetidine concentrations in 36 critically ill patients, Schentag et al.[84] suggested a relationship between mental status deterioration and blood levels of this H_2-receptor antagonist. These investigators further proposed that patients at high risk of cimetidine-induced confusional states are those with both severe renal and hepatic dysfunction. In their commentary on the study of Schentag et al.,[84] Flind and Rowley-Jones agree that dosage reduction is imperative in patients with renal failure.[85] However, they state that the evidence is not sufficient to recommend a reduction of cimetidine dosage in patients with isolated hepatic failure. Gugler and Somogyi observed a marked reduction in the plasma clearance of cimetidine in older patients and suggested that altered disposition of cimetidine, which occurs with age, may be a predisposing factor in the development of side effects such as mental confusion.[64]

Several case reports describe patients who had been treated with cimetidine for varying lengths of time and who were subsequently found to have carcinoma of the stomach.[86-88] In commentaries on these reports, the possibility of nitrosation of cimetidine, with formation of a potentially carcinogenic derivative is discussed, but no evidence is offered that such a reaction occurs in vivo.[86,89-91] Several clinicians emphasized the importance of a definitive diagnosis prior to treatment of gastric distress and warned that prescribing cimetidine for dyspeptic symptoms may confuse the diagnosis and delay identification of gastric malignancy.[89-92] Although the incidence has decreased sharply during the past several decades, carcinoma of the stomach remains a major cause of death in the U.S.; the neoplasm occurs in all age groups, but most commonly in patients over 50 years of age.[93]

REFERENCES

1. **Windaus, A. and Vogt, W.,** Synthese des imidazolylathylämins, *Ber. Dtsch. Chem. Ges.,* 40, 3691, 1907.
2. **Barger, G. and Dale, H. H.,** β-iminazolylethylamine, a depressor constituent of the intestinal mucosa, *J. Physiol. (London),* 41, 499, 1911.
3. **Dale H. H. and Laidlaw, P. P.,** The physiological action of β-iminazolylethylamine, *J. Physiol. (London),* 41, 318, 1910.
4. **Dale, H. H. and Richards, A. N.,** The vasodilator action of histamine and some other substances, *J. Physiol. (London),* 52, 110, 1918.
5. **Ackerman, D.,** Über den bacteriellen abbau des histidins, *Z. Physiol. Chem.,* 65, 504, 1910.
6. **Best, C. H., Dale, H. H., Dudley, H. W., and Thorpe, W. V.,** The nature of the vasodilator constituents of certain tissue extracts, *J. Physiol. (London),* 62, 397, 1927.
7. **Bartosch, R., Feldberg, W., and Nagel, E.,** Das freiwerden eines histaminähnlichen stoffes bei der anaphylaxie des meerschweinchens, *Arch. Gesante Physiol Pflugers,* 230, 120, 1932.
8. **Dragstedt, C. A. and Gebauer-Fuelnegg, E.,** Studies in anaphylaxis. I. The appearance of a physiologically active substance during anaphylactic shock, *Am. J. Physiol.,* 102, 512, 1932.
9. **Bovet, D. and Staub, A. M.,** Action pretectrice des ethers phenoliques au cours de l'intoxication histaminique, *C. R. Sceances Soc. Biol.,* 124, 547, 1937.
10. **Yellin, T. O., Ed.,** *Histamine Receptors,* Proceedings of the A. N. Richards Symposium, Spectrum Publications, New York 1979, 1.
11. **Black, J. W., Duncan, W. A., Durant, G. J., Ganellin, C. R., and Parsons, M. E.,** Definition and antagonism of histamine H_2-receptors, *Nature (London),* 236, 385, 1972.
12. *Handbook of Experimental Pharmacology, Histamine and Anti-Histamines, Part I,* Rocha e Silva, M., Ed., Springer-Verlag, New York, 1978, 18, 1.

13. *Handbook of Experimental Pharmacology, Histamine II and Anti-Histamines, Part II*, Rocha e Silva, M., Ed., Springer-Verlag, New York, 1978, 18, 2.
14. **Beaven, M.**, Histamine: its role in physiological and pathological processes, *Monogr. Allergy*, Karger, Basel, 1978, 13.
15. **Beaven, M. A., Horakova, Z., Severs, W. B., and Brodie, B. B.**, Selective labeling of histamine in rat gastric mucosa: application to measurement of turnover rate, *J. Pharmacol. Exp. Ther.*, 161, 320, 1968.
16. **Riley, J. F. and West, G. B.**, The occurrence of histamine in mast cells, in *Handbook of Experimental Pharmacology, Histamine and Antihistaminics, Part I*, Rocha e Silva, M., Ed., Springer-Verlag, New York, 1811, 1966, 116.
17. **Harvey, S. C.**, Comparative regional and subcellular distributions of histamine and norepinephrine in the hearts of rats, mice, guinea pigs, rabbits and dogs, *Jpn. Heart J.*, 19, 125, 1978.
18. **Hardwick, D. C.**, Changes in the histamine content of rat skin, *J. Physiol.*, 124, 157, 1954.
19. **Rocha e Silva, M.**, Histamine in the rabbit skin, *Proc. Soc. Exp. Biol. Med.*, 45, 586, 1940.
20. **Schayer, R. W.**, Catabolism of physiological quantities of histamine *in vivo*, *Physiol. Rev.*, 39, 116, 1959.
21. **Håkanson, R., Owman, C., and Sjöberg, N. O.**, Cellular stores of gastric histamine in the developing rat, *Life Sci.*, 6, 2535, 1967.
22. **Aures, D., and Håkanson, R.**, Histidine decarboxylase and DOPA decarboxylase in the stomach of the developing rat, *Experientia*, 15, 666, 1968.
23. **Isaac, L. and Sapperstein, R. L.**, Gastric histamine metabolism in the aging rat, *Biochem. Pharmacol.*, 26, 585, 1977.
24. **Lillehei, C. W. and Wangensteen, O. H.**, Effect of age on histamine-induced ulcer in dogs, *Proc. Soc. Exp. Biol. Med.*, 68, 129, 1948.
25. **Green, J. P.**, Histamine, in *Handbook of Neurochemistry, Control Mechanisms in the Nervous System*, Vol. 4, Lajtha, A., Ed., Plenum Press, New York, 1970, 221.
26. **Code, C. F.**, Histamine and gastric secretion, in *Ciba Foundation Symposium on Histamine*, Wolstenholme, G. E. W. and O'Connor, C. M., Eds., Little, Brown, Boston, 1956, 189.
27. **Hirschowitz, B. I.**, H_2-histamine receptors, *Ann. Rev. Pharmacol. Toxicol.*, 19, 203, 1979.
28. **Grossman, I., and Konturek, S. J.**, Inhibition of acid secretion in dog by metiamide, a histamine antagonist acting on H_2-receptors, in *International Symposium on Histamine H_2-Receptor Antagonists*, Wood, C. J. and Simkins, A. M., Eds., Research and Development Division, Smith, Kline and French Laboratories, Welwyn Garden City, 1973, 297.
29. **Code, C. F.**, Reflections on histamine, gastric secretion and the H_2-receptor, *N. Engl. J. Med.*, 296, 1459, 1977.
30. **Schwartz, J. C.**, Histaminergic mechanisms in brain, *Ann. Rev. Pharmacol. Toxicol.*, 17, 325, 1977.
31. **Green, J. P., Johnson, C. L., and Weinstein, H.**, Histamine as a neurotransmitter, in *Psychopharmacology: A Generation of Progress*, Lipton, M. A., DiMascio A., and Killam, K. F., Eds., Raven Press, New York, 1978, 319.
32. **Green, J. P. and Maayani, S.**, Tricyclic antidepressant drugs block histamine H_2 receptor in brain, *Nature (London)*, 269, 163, 1977.
33. **Kanof, P. D. and Greengard, P.**, Brain histamine receptors as targets for antidepressant drugs, *Nature (London)*, 272, 329, 1978.
34. **Editorial**, Antidepressants and histamine, *Lancet*, 1, 808, 1978.
35. **Finch, C. E.**, Neuroendocrine mechanisms and aging, *Fed. Proc., Fed. Am. Soc. Exp. Biol.*, 38, 178, 1979.
36. **McGeer, E. G. and McGeer, P. L.**, in *Neurobiology of Aging*, Terry, R. D. and Gershon, S., Eds., Raven Press, New York, 1976, 389.
37. **Weiss, B., Greenberg, L., and Cantor, E.**, Age-related alterations in the development of adrenergic denervation supersensitivity, *Fed. Proc., Fed. Am. Soc. Exp. Biol.*, 38, 1915, 1979.
38. **Makman, M. H. Ahn, H. S., Thal, L. J., Sharpless, N. S., Dvorkin, B., Horowitz, S. G., and Rosenfeld, M.**, Aging and monoamine receptors in brain, *Fed. Proc., Fed. Am. Soc. Exp. Biol.*, 38, 1922, 1979.
39. **Douglas, W. W.**, Histamine and antihistamines; 5-hydroxytryptamine and antagonists, in *The Pharmacological Basis of Therapeutics*, 5th ed., Goodman, L. S. and Gilman, A., Eds., Macmillan, New York, 1975, chap. 29.
40. **Ash, A. S. F. and Schild, H. O.**, Receptors mediating some actions of histamine, *Br. J. Pharmacol. Chemother*, 27, 427, 1966.
41. **Forrest, J. A., Shearman, D. J., Spence, R., and Celestin, L. R.**, Letter: neutropenia associated with metiamide, *Lancet*, 1, 392, 1975.
42. **Brimblecombe, R. W., Duncan, W. A., Durant, G. J., Emmett, J. C., Ganellin, C. R., and Parsons, M. E.**, Cimetidine — a non-thiourea H_2-receptor antagonist, *J. Int. Med. Res.*, 3, 86, 1975.
43. **Cormier, J. F. and Bryant, B. G.**, Cold and allergy products, in *Handbook of Non-prescription Drugs*, 6th ed., Goldberg, M. E., Ed., American Pharmaceutical Association, 1979, 73.

44. *AMA Drug Evaluations,* 3rd Ed., Publishing Sciences Group, Littleton, Maine, 1977, 672.
45. **Wyngaarden, J. B. and Seevers, M. H.,** The toxic effects of antihistaminic drugs, *J. Am. Med. Assoc.,* 145, 277, 1951.
46. **Bleumink, E.,** Antihistamines, in *Meyler's Side Effects of Drugs,* Vol. 8, Excerpta Medica, Amsterdam-Oxford, 1975, 406.
47. **Walson, P. D. and Bressler, R.,** Drugs and age, in *Drugs of Choice 1978-1979,* Modell, W., Ed., C. V. Mosby, St. Louis, 1978, 31.
48. **Triggs, E. J. and Nation, R. L.,** Pharmacokinetics in the aged: a review, *J. Pharmacokinet. Biopharm.,* 3, 387, 1975.
49. **Crooks, J., O'Malley, K., and Stevenson, I. H.,** Pharmacokinetics in the elderly, *Clin. Pharmacokinet.,* 1, 280, 1976.
50. **Vestal, R. E.,** Drug use in the elderly: a review of problems and special considerations, *Drugs,* 16, 358, 1978.
51. **Epstein, M.,** Effects of aging on the kidney, *Fed. Proc., Fed. Am. Soc. Exp. Biol.,* 38, 168, 1979.
52. **Witiak D. T. and Lewis, N. J.,** Absorption, distribution, metabolism and elimination of antihistamines, in *Handbook of Experimental Pharmacology; Histamine and Anti-Histaminics, Part I,* Eichler, O. and Farah, A., Eds., Springer-Verlag, New York, 1966, 18, 1, 513.
53. **Kato, R., Vassanelli, P., Frontini, G., and Chiessara, E.,** Variation in the activity of liver microsomal drug-metabolizing enzymes in rats in relation to the age, *Biochem. Pharmacol.,* 13, 1037, 1964.
54. **Richey, D. P. and Bender, A. D.,** Pharmacokinetic consequences of aging, *Ann. Rev. Pharmacol. Toxicol.,* 17, 49, 1977.
55. **Gillette, J. R.,** Biotransformation of drugs during aging, *Fed. Proc., Fed. Am. Soc. Exp. Biol .,* 38, 1900, 1979.
56. **Burland, W. L. and Simkins, M. A., Eds.,** *Cimetidine: 2nd Int. Symp.; Histamine H_2-Receptor Antagonists,* Excerpta Medica, Amsterdam, 1977, 392.
57. **Fordtran, J. S. and Grossman, M. I., Eds.,** 3rd Symp. Histamine H_2-Receptor Antagonists: Clinical Results with Cimetidine, *Gastroenterology,* 74, 338, 1978.
58. **Shearman, D J. C. and Hetzel, D.,** The medical management of peptic ulcer, *Ann. Rev. Med.,* 30, 61, 1979.
59. **Gray, G. R., Smith, I. S., Mackenzie, I., and Gillespie, G.,** Long term cimetidine in the management of severe duodenal ulcer dyspepsia, *Gastroenterology,* 74, 397, 1978.
60. **Bodemar, G. and Walan, A.,** Maintenance treatment of recurrent peptic ulcer by cimetidine, *Lancet,* 1, 403, 1978.
61. **Finkelstein, W. and Isselbacher, K. J.,** Drug therapy: cimetidine, *N. Engl. J. Med.,* 299, 992, 1978.
62. **Kenny, A. D.,** Designing therapy for the elderly, *Drug Therapy,* 9, 49, 1979.
63. **Bourinskie, J. E.,** Comparative costs of cimetidine and antacids, *N. Engl. J. Med.,* 300, 370, 1979.
64. **Gugler, R. and Somogyi, A.,** Reduced cimetidine clearance with age, *N. Engl. J. Med.,* 30, 435, 1979.
65. **Ma, K. W., Brown, D. C., Masler, D. S., and Silvis, S. E.,** Effects of renal failure on blood levels of cimetidine, *Gastroenterology,* 74, 473, 1978.
66. **Kruss, D. M. and Littman, A.,** Safety of cimetidine, *Gastroenterology,* 74, 478, 1978.
67. **Bleumink, E.,** Antihistamines, H_2-receptor antagonists, in *Meyler's Side Effects of Drugs,* Annual 3, Excerpta Medica, Amsterdam-Oxford, 1979, 138.
68. **Dubb, J. W., Stote, R. M., Familiar, R. G., Lee, K., and Alexander, F.,** Effect of cimetidine on renal function in normal man, *Clin. Pharmacol. Ther.,* 24, 76, 1978.
69. **Nistico, G., Rotiroti, D., De Sarro, A., and Naccari, F.,** Mechanism of cimetidine-induced fever, *Lancet,* 1, 265, 1978.
70. **Ufberg, M. M., Brooks, C. M., Bosanac, P. R., and Kintzel, J. E.,** Transient neutropenia in a patient receiving cimetidine, *Gastroenterology,* 73, 635, 1977.
71. **Johnson, N. McI., Black, A. E., Hughes, A. S. B and Clarke, S. W.,** Leucopenia with cimetidine, *Lancet,* 1, 1226, 1977.
72. **López-Luque, A., Rodriguez-Cuartero, A., Pérez-Galvez, N., Pomares-Mora, J., and Pena-Yañez, A.,** Cimetidine and bone-marrow toxicity, letter: *Lancet,* 1, 444, 1978.
73. **Idvall, J.,** Cimetidine-associated thrombocytopenia, *Lancet,* 2, 159, 1979.
74. **Ahmed, A. H., McLarty, D. G., Sharma, S. K., and Masawe, A. E. J.,** Stevens-Johnson syndrome during treatment with cimetidine, *Lancet,* 2, 433, 1978.
75. **Field, R. and Meyer, G. W.,** Diarrhea from cimetidine, *N. Engl. J. Med.,* 299, 262, 1978.
76. **Reding, P., Devroede, C., and Barbier, P.,** Bradycardia after cimetidine, *Lancet,* 2, 1227, 1977.
77. **Jeffreys, D. B. and Vale, J. A.,** Cimetidine and bradycardia, *Lancet,* 1, 828, 1978.
78. **Mahon, W. A. and Kolton, M.,** Hypotension after intravenous cimetidine, *Lancet,* 1, 828, 1978.
79. **Wallace, W. A., Orr, C. M. E., and Bearn, A. R.,** Perforation of chronic peptic ulcers after cimetidine, *Br. Med. J.,* 2, 865, 1977.

80. **Gill, M. J. and Saunders, J. B.,** Perforation of chronic peptic ulcers after cimetidine, *Br. Med. J.,* 2, 1149, 1977.
81. **Hoste, P., Ingels, J., Elewaut, A., and Barbier, F.,** Duodenal perforation after cimetidine, *Lancet,* 1, 666, 1978.
82. **Celestin, L. R. and Spence, R. W.,** Perforation of peptic ulcers after cimetidine, *Br. Med. J.,* 2, 1149, 1977.
83. **Wood, C A., Isaacson, M. I., and Hibbs, M. S.,** Cimetidine and mental confusion, *J. Am. Med. Assoc.,* 239, 2550, 1978.
84. **Schentag, J. J., Calleri, G., Rose, J. Q., Cerra, F. B., DeGlopper, E., and Bernhard, H.,** Pharmacokinetic and clinical studies in patients with cimetidine-associated confusion, *Lancet,* 1, 177, 1979.
85. **Flind, A. C. and Rowley-Jones, D.,** Mental confusion and cimetidine, *Lancet,* 1, 379, 1979.
86. **Elder, J. B., Ganguli, P. C., and Gillespie, I. E.,** Cimetidine and gastric cancer, *Lancet,* 1, 1005, 1979.
87. **Reed, P. I., Cassell, P. G., and Walters, C. L.,** Gastric cancer in patients who have taken cimetidine, *Lancet,* 1, 1234, 1979.
88. **Taylor, T. V., Lee, D., Howatson, A. G., Anderson, J., and MacLeod, I. B.,** Gastric cancer in patients who have taken cimetidine, *Lancet,* 1, 1235, 1979.
89. **Ruddell, W. S. J.,** Gastric cancer in patients who have taken cimetidine, *Lancet,* 1, 1234, 1979.
90. **Hill, M. J.,** Gastric cancer in patients who have taken cimetidine, *Lancet,* 1, 1235, 1979.
91. **Mullen, P. W.,** Gastric cancer in patients who have taken cimetidine, *Lancet,* 1, 1406, 1979.
92. **Guslandi, M.,** Gastric cancer in patients who have taken cimetidine, *Lancet,* 1, 1406, 1979.
93. **Brandborg, L. L.,** Malignant neoplasms of the stomach, in *Cecil-Loeb Textbook of Medicine,* Beeson, P. B. and McDermott, W., Eds., 14th ed., W. B. Saunders, Philadelphia, 1975, 1293.

PHARMACOLOGIC EFFECTS OF HEMATOPOIETIC DRUGS IN THE AGED

Barbara S. Beckman and James W. Fisher

INTRODUCTION

In spite of the fact that only 11% of the population in the U.S. is age 65 or older, the elderly use upwards of 25% of all medications.[1] Since anemias and coagulopathies are common in the elderly, the physician should have a good knowledge of the use of hematopoietic drugs. Although there are few published reports on the effects of hematopoietic drugs in the elderly, this chapter will attempt to organize the available information concerning the pharmacology of antianemia, anticoagulant, and plasma expander drugs, focusing on the characteristics of absorption, volume of distribution, protein binding, metabolism, renal excretion, and other pharmacokinetic differences in the disposition of hematopoietic drugs in young and old subjects.

In this handbook and elsewhere,[2] Richey has described physiologic changes which accompany aging and which can cause complex alterations in drug metabolism. There are greater individual disparities with aging which make it more difficult to propose rules for average geriatric dosages. The problems of drug metabolism in old age involve: (1) absorption, (2) transport and protein-binding in serum, (3) distribution and uptake at receptor sites, and (4) metabolic degradation and excretion. The absorption and transport of certain drugs are likely to occur at a slower rate although very little information exists concerning changes with age. A possible basis for decreased drug absorption is the decline in intestinal blood perfusion.[3,4] In a recent review of pharmacokinetics in the elderly,[5] the evidence suggested that drug absorption is not appreciably altered. The conjugation of drugs with body proteins may proceed at a slower rate because of reduced protein-binding capacities. The increased incidence of deleterious effects may be ascribed to the amount of drug that is nonprotein-bound or that has been displaced by competing drugs with an increase in toxicity which is proportional to the fraction in the free form. Local and systemic responses can be altered by a change in the number and properties of effector cells. Renal excretion is of considerable importance, and proper consideration should be given to primary renal senescence and the frequency of kidney infections.[6] Slower absorption, transport, and cell utilization may partially balance reduced renal excretion.

The liver is the primary site of drug metabolism; it is there that microsomal enzymes transform many drugs. As yet, no studies have been reported on age-related microsomal drug metabolism.[7] Specific studies of drug metabolism in geriatric patients have rarely been carried out, despite the fact that this segment of the population is the most highly medicated. Even data on aged animals is sparse.[8]

Important drug interactions may result from alterations in gastrointestinal motility and from the formation of insoluble and, therefore, nonabsorbable complexes within the lumen of the bowel. In a study of 137 female patients, the incidence of adverse reactions in those over 50 years of age was twice that in a corresponding group of younger females (38 vs. 19%).[9] The elderly, no doubt, have an increased sensitivity to drugs that may be related to a combination of existing pathology and altered physiological function.

ANTIANEMIA DRUGS

Anemias are common in the aged, although there are no specific anemias that are unique to the elderly population. Especially in the elderly, the complexities of pathologic states may be such that it is difficult for the physician to evaluate the underlying causes of the anemia. Complications, such as an occult malignant disorder, a chronic infection, or poor nutritional status[10-13] often may impair the capacity of the patient to respond to therapy.

Certain physiologic changes with aging affect the hematopoietic apparatus and thus set the stage for disease or reduce the capacity to deal with environmental stresses. Lymphoid tissue may atrophy, immunologic competence is occasionally decreased,[1] and the responsiveness of the bone marrow leukopoietic system is reduced.[14] Although the lifespan of red cells, as estimated by the technique of ^{51}Cr labeling, is unchanged in the elderly,[15] there may be a mild reduction in the circulating mass of red cells in older men. In women there is essentially no change, even after menopause. Any differences in hemoglobin between the sexes thus becomes smaller with advancing age.[16] The reduction in red cell mass observed in some older male subjects is postulated to be related to a decreased oxygen consumption secondary to loss of lean body mass, senile atrophy of body tissues in general, and to a decline in testosterone levels, which in turn, reduces circulating levels of erythropoietin. It has also been observed that older men have lower plasma levels of vitamin B_{12} than younger men.[17] Although an increase in iron stores in old age has been reported,[18,19] to our knowledge there are no published studies relating the possible changes in storage of iron in any animal species at age levels comparable to those of elderly men and women.

IRON DEFICIENCY ANEMIA

Data on the prevalence of anemia among the elderly have been obtained for each sex primarily from the following sources: healthy subjects living in their own homes or in homes for the aged; patients seen in clinics, doctors' offices, or hospitals.[20] In the latter group especially, as shown in Table 1,[22,29-34] there are considerable differences in the criteria for establishing anemia. Hemoglobin levels indicative of anemia, range from 10 g/100 mℓ to 13 g/100 mℓ. In addition, the criterion for age varies from a minimum of 60 years to 65 years. Irrespective of these differences, most studies conclude that iron deficiency anemia represents the majority of anemias. Many of these patients suffered blood loss from lesions of the gastrointestinal tract such as hiatal hernia, peptic ulcer, carcinoma of the stomach or colon, and diverticulitis.[21] According to Harant and Goldberger,[22] failure to obtain a good therapeutic effect with iron, which in their study occurred in more than half of the cases at a chronic disease hospital, may be due to the physician's failure to recognize the true underlying cause of the anemia.

Disposition of Iron

Iron absorption decreases with advancing age, even in healthy individuals,[23-25] consistent with the increasing incidence of atrophic gastritis and the consequent diminution of gastric secretion.[26-28] In the only study to compare absorption in healthy young and old subjects and young and old patients,[25] Marx found that iron absorption is modulated by the body's requirement for this mineral. Marx's criterion for iron deficiency was a lack of iron in the bone marrow. Much higher values for mucosal uptake (of ferrous sulfate), mucosal transfer, and retention of iron were found in the iron deficiency than in control groups. No difference in iron absorption was found between young and old patients with the same degree of iron deficiency, whereas healthy aged males had significantly higher mean values for mucosal uptake, transfer, and retention of iron than young males (no differences were observed in the healthy female groups.) However, uptake of Fe^{59} by red cells was significantly lower in aged persons than in young adults, suggesting progressively ineffective erythropoiesis in old age. This finding deserves further investigation, especially in relation to ferrokinetics and mean lifespan of red cells in old age.

Therapeutic Uses of Iron

A few reports are available which assess the therapeutic effects of iron preparations in the elderly.[35-41] Most of these reports are concerned with specific types of iron preparations.

Table 1
STUDIES OF ANEMIA IN THE ELDERLY

Criteria				Patients (%)				
Age	Sex	Hb/hmt[a]	Anemia	Iron def.	B_{12} and/or folate deficiency	Normochromic normocytic anemia	No. of patients	Ref.
>60	M/F	<11 /—	21	45	17	40	229	29
>60	M/F	<11.9/—	37	12	8	80	319	30
>65	M/F	<12/—	32	73	3	No data	400	31
>65	M/F	<10/—	6.4	67	51	6	2700	32
>60	F	<11.4/—	16	88	6	6	500	33
>65	M	<12/<40	32.6	[b]	[b]	[b]	1500	34
	F	<11.5/<37						
>60	M	<13/—	31	38	15	36	484	22
	F	<12/—						

[a] Hb = hemoglobin in grams per deciliter; Hmt = hematocrit in percent.
[b] Anemias were classified as due to (1) infection, 8.1%; (2) chronic renal disease, 7.5%; (3) carcinoma, 7.0%; (4) blood loss, 4.4%; (5) nutritional, 4.2%; (6) liver disease, 1.1%; (7) pernicious anemia, 0.3%.

For example, Pegel et al.[35] tested sustained-release capsules in 10 patients ranging in age from 64 to 97 years. Although iron therapy improved the hemoglobin levels of all patients, and produced minimal side effects, it is difficult to accept the conclusions of this study, since no other type of iron preparation was studied. Well-controlled studies of the therapeutic effects of iron preparations in the elderly seem not to be available.

Symptoms of gastrointestinal intolerance following orally administered iron frequently pose clinical problems in the treatment of iron-deficiency anemia; however, Kerr and Davidson reported no difference in the number of complaints with ferrous sulfate, other iron compounds, or with inert oral preparations containing only lactose.[41] A group of 20 elderly patients (65 to 95 years) with iron deficiency anemia, who had previously complained of gastrointestinal symptoms, were given a controlled-release compound of ferrous sulfate. Symptoms of gastrointestinal intolerance were more common with ferrous sulfate.[39]

MACROCYTIC ANEMIAS

Nutritional anemias occur more frequently in the elderly than in the young and may be the result of the patients' socioeconomic status. Folic acid and vitamin B_{12} (cyanocobalamin) are antianemia agents, deficiency of which leads to an alteration of normal bone marrow function with a resulting macrocytic megaloblastic anemia. Dietary deficiency of folic acid is particularly common among chronic alcoholics whose overall diets are often inadequate; dietary deficiency of vitamin B_{12} is not common.

Deficiencies in folic acid and vitamin B_{12} stem more commonly from malabsorption problems than from dietary deficiency. Absorption irregularities may be the result of several mechanisms: (1) insufficient secretion of the gastric intrinsic factor of Castle; or (2) organic or functional defects at the site of vitamin B_{12} absorption in the ileum. Regional ileitis and remedial surgical procedures for this disease are the most common abnormalities in the ileum that are likely to result in subnormal absorption of cyanocobalamin.[42] Deficiency of folic acid due to inadequate absorption is not as common as malabsorption of vitamin B_{12}, but may occur in alterations of the upper portion of the small bowel, as in sprue, celiac disease, or adult idiopathic steatorrhea.

Vitamin B₁₂ (Cyanocobalamin)

With regard to determining the effect of age on serum levels of vitamin B_{12}, Chow and Yeh suggest that studies meet several criteria:[17]

1. Surveys on the tissue level of vitamin B_{12} must include only those subjects who are known not to have received vitamin B_{12} parenterally prior to the test bleeding. The physiological, pathological, and medication profile of a subject or patient should be known, and test subjects or patients should be as uniform as possible with respect to this profile since.
2. Serum levels of vitamin B_{12} can be elevated or depressed by a number of physiological or pathological conditions and by medications. For example, patients with liver disease, myelogenous leukemia, or diabetes mellitus may have elevated levels, whereas patients with iron deficiency have lower vitamin B_{12} serum levels than do otherwise comparable subjects.
3. Statistical examinations must be critical in order to determine random distribution in the selection of samples and the uniformity of the subjects, in terms of environment and diets.
4. Great care must be practiced in the assay since the results will depend to a large extent on the precision of vitamin B_{12} serum level determinations

Few reports, according to Chow and Yeh,[17] on regression of vitamin B_{12} serum levels with age meet these criteria. However, studies from Chow's lab and from others,[43-46] show a convincing decrease of this vitamin with aging. The regression with increasing age of serum vitamin B_{12}, observed in prisoners consuming essentially the same diet, and in rats[17] raised on stock diet, is not likely due to altered dietary intake. The observation that injection of several different doses of vitamin B_{12} in young and old subjects results in the aged excreting less vitamin B_{12} in the urine than is excreted by the young[47] makes it unlikely that the age difference in serum levels is due to the inability of the elderly to retain absorbed vitamin B_{12}. Thus, the difference seems to be attributable to differences in absorption. Absorption depends on the presence of an adequate amount of intrinsic factor. The loss of intrinsic factor and subsequent failure to absorb vitamin B_{12} is the cause of pernicious anemia. The concentration of vitamin B_{12}-binding substance in gastric juice of older subjects is significantly lower than in younger ones.[48] Atrophy of the gastric mucosa and achlorhydria occur more frequently among the aged, leading to impairment of nutrient absorption. This, in turn, results in a loss of vitamin B_{12} and folic acid from the tissues; and thus a decrease in reserves.

Chow found that gastric secretion decreases with advancing age.[48] The composition of the gastric juice of old people often differs from that of the young; it is lower in hydrochloric acid, enzymes (e.g., pepsin), and vitamin B_{12} binding-substance. Since the absorption of vitamin B_{12} is dependent upon the intrinsic factor, this process is expected to be reduced with advancing age. However, experimentally this has not been demonstrated with any regularity.

Doscherholmen et al.[49] recently explored the relationship of age and serum vitamin B_{12} concentration, gastric acid production, vitamin B_{12} absorption, and intrinsic factor secretion. Vitamin B_{12} (as measured by ^{57}Co-cyanocobalamin) absorption showed no reduction with advancing age, but serum vitamin B_{12} and maximal acid output declined with advancing age. The authors suggested that patients with low maximum acid output had diminished or absent pepsin activity, resulting in decreased release of vitamin B_{12} from foods in the stomach, with consequent impaired assimilation of vitamin B_{12}. The role of gastric acid secretion and peptic activity in the absorption of vitamin B_{12} from foods and consequent maintenance of a normal serum concentration, remains to be determined.

A humoral role has been suggested for the thyroid and adrenal glands in vitamin B_{12} absorption. Although it is generally agreed that thyroid activity in older individuals is lower than in younger individuals, it is not known how important such a decline in thyroid function may be in the slight impairment of gastrointestinal absorption of large doses of vitamin B_{12} by older people. Additional studies are needed to support the hypothesis that the lower vitamin B_{12} serum levels in the aged, which are associated with reduced absorption, are the result of gastric atrophy or hormonal insufficiency.

Folic Acid

Deficiency of folic acid may arise from diminished intake of foodstuffs containing the conjugated vitamin, or from failure to break down or utilize the conjugate. A few studies have been published which specifically addressed the pharmacology of folic acid in geriatric patients.[50-55] Baker et al.[55] studied absorption of folates, vitamin B_6, pantothenate, and riboflavin from a natural food source (yeast) and from synthetic folylmonoglutamate in 24 elderly subjects (73 to 101 years of age) and in 12 healthy younger subjects (24 to 42 years of age). All subjects absorbed riboflavin, vitamin B_6, and pantothenate from yeast. Ingested folylmonoglutamate (the predominant folate in yeast) proved to be a very poor source of folate for the elderly, whereas synthetic folylmonoglutamate was a good source. It is suggested that the folate deficiencies, so common in the elderly, are caused by an impaired ability to obtain folate from ingested foods.

Multiple nutritional deficiencies occur more frequently in older than in younger individuals. These deficiencies can result in poor absorption and may gradually lead to a secondary deficiency of other vitamins caused by endocrine dysfunction. Experimental proof of such a complicated system in man is very difficult to obtain. For individuals with hormonal dysfunctions, additional problems are imposed. They may result in decreased absorption of iron and a defect in either the formation of hemoglobin or else erythropoiesis, both of which are influenced by hormones. In addition, anemia can result from deficiency or insufficiency of adrenal or thyroid functions, and even of certain pituitary hormones. Of the various known vitamins, folic acid, vitamin B_{12}, vitamin B_6, and vitamin C play important roles in hematopoiesis. Limited data are available from systemic, controlled studies on the subject of aging and marginal vitamin deficiencies.

NORMOCYTIC ANEMIAS

Normocytic-normochromic anemia, secondary to renal, hepatic, or other systemic disease, also represented a large proportion of the cases reported in the studies that comprise Table 1. In this variety, an attempt to diagnose the cause is essential. If the cause of the anemia is not identified and corrected, irreparable damage will be done. This type of anemia will respond only to blood transfusion and occasionally to androgenic steroids.[59,60]

Normocytic-normochromic anemia, frequently seen in chronic renal failure, is due to an inadequate production of erythropoietin needed to sustain erythropoiesis. In chronic renal failure, uremic toxins are increased in plasma and other biological fluids, exposing the blood-forming organs to high levels of these toxic substances, thus further aggravating the anemia. Uremic toxins may be responsible for the shortened lifespan of red cells seen in chronic renal failure.[56] Since erythropoietin deficiency is probably the major cause of the anemia of chronic renal failure, the therapeutic use of erythropoietin for the treatment of this disorder would obviously be a major advance in therapy. Indeed, some investigators have administered crude erythropoietin preparations to patients with the anemia of chronic renal failure, but without success.[57] Fever and other types of reaction were reported in patients treated with this crude urinary extract. Perhaps the purified erythropoietin prepared by Goldwasser et al.[58] would be more suitable to treat erythropoietic deficiency anemia.

Androgens also have been used widely for the treatment of anemia of renal diseases, with definite increases in red cell mass;[59,60] however, the deleterious side effects of androgens detract from their usefulness. Nonmasculinizing steroids such as the 5β-androstanes[61] or the 5β-pregnanes[62] hold some promise for the therapy of normocytic anemias, but much more clinical work is necessary to establish their usefulness as therapeutic agents. Prostaglandins, by triggering kidney production of erythropoietin,[63,64] as well as by acting directly on the erythroid progenitor cell compartment in bone marrow, may provide a useful means of treating normocytic-normochromic anemia in the future. Since no data are available regarding therapy of normocytic-normochromic anemias in elderly patients, controlled studies need to be made on their response to erythropoietin, androgenic steroids, 5β-androstanes and prostaglandins.

ANTICOAGULANT DRUG THERAPY IN THE ELDERLY

The not uncommon situation of the simultaneous existence of several pathological conditions in the elderly complicates use of anticoagulants in their therapy.[65] However, despite the risk, in certain conditions, anticoagulants are indicated. One of the major problems of therapy with oral anticoagulants is the marked interpatient variability in responsiveness to the drugs.[66,67] Nutritional state, vitamin K intake, age, sex, and rate of hepatic synthesis of clotting factors each plays a role. There are indications of a reduced hepatic synthesis of blood clotting factors in the elderly. This may, at least in part, contribute to a greater sensitivity in the elderly to the action of oral anticoagulants. Reports indicate that the risk of hemorrhagic episodes in the elderly on anticoagulant therapy is rather high.[68] Changes in gastrointestinal function, which bring about decreased absorption of vitamin K or of orally administered anticoagulant, can also alter the response to a given dose of anticoagulant. Although information is scarce relating incidence of thromboembolic complications to intensity of anticoagulant therapy, the available data are in support of more intensive therapy,[67] i.e., administration of drug sufficient to maintain prothrombin times at or above 10 to 20% as opposed to the more usual 30 to 49%.

Freeman states that there is controversy over appropriate therapy with anticoagulants in the aged patient.[65] Nevertheless, according to Quick,[69] more than 1/4 of the patients now on long-term therapy to depress prothrombin activity are over 60 years of age. The most common and important indications for anticoagulant therapy are deep venous thrombosis, pulmonary embolism, and prevention of coronary thrombosis;[21] arterial embolism constitutes a further indication for therapy, whenever complicated by a recent myocardial infarction or by rheumatic heart disease. The common practice of administering anticoagulants to prevent postoperative venous thrombosis in the elderly has been reported to produce favorable results. Anticoagulants have also been advocated in the treatment of senile dementia,[70-73] although the studies devised to demonstrate improvement were poorly controlled. Anticoagulant therapy for prevention of coronary thrombosis has failed to demonstrate any marked differences in response that can be attributed to age. In addition, it is uncertain whether long-term anticoagulant therapy will either delay or prevent the final episode. The advisability of anticoagulant therapy in cerebral thrombosis is seriously questioned;[74] furthermore, there is considerable hazard because of difficulties in distinguishing between symptoms due to cerebral hemorrhage or thrombosis. The diagnosis of venous thrombosis in the elderly is frequently difficult, and it is not rare for an elderly patient who has had no clinical evidence of venous thrombosis to die suddenly from massive pulmonary embolism.

Coumarin Derivatives

Warfarin sodium and dicumarol (bishydroxycoumarin) are the oral anticoagulants of choice for most thromboembolic disorders. Difficulties can arise because these drugs are long-acting and may gradually accumulate. If severe hemorrhage follows the use of warfarin, then blood transfusion is essential. The action of warfarin is potentiated in patients with liver disease; also by drugs such as phenylbutazone, salicylates, and broad spectrum antibiotics. In addition, Shepherd et al.[75] identified age differences in sensitivity to warfarin (in rats and humans) which may be related to increasing depression of hepatic clotting factor synthesis with increasing age.

Control of anticoagulants, particularly in long-term therapy, is complicated by some general features common to the older patient. Primarily, complications relate to considerations of: (1) reliability of the patient to take medication, (2) patient accessibility for examination, (3) patient mobility, (4) drug cost, (5) multiplicity of diseases, and (6) motivation of patient.

Older individuals may have clinical states that are not sufficiently characteristic to signal the need for tests. When a vascular crisis occurs, it may be impossible under these circumstances to institute routine investigations to identify all the elements involved. This increases the likelihood of bleeding during anticoagulant therapy in the elderly; and if bleeding occurs, it is likely to appear simultaneously at a number of sites. Contraindications to anticoagulant programs include the presence of gastrointestinal or genitourinary ulcers, diverticulitis of the colon, gastrointestinal malignancy, blood dyscrasias, impaired kidney or liver function, subacute bacterial endocarditis, or acute nephritis. When severe bleeding occurs in the elderly, it is more likely to precipitate cerebrovascular changes, myocardial infarction, irreversible shock, or renal shutdown.

The acute phase of myocardial infarction was one of the earliest disorders in which therapy with dicumarol was employed. While anticoagulants obviously do not reduce mortality due to massive infarction in the acute phase, if recovery occurs, they certainly have the potential for lessening the incidence of secondary thromboembolism. The earlier findings led to a number of large-scale clinical investigations, some of which indicated a marked decrease in mortality, while others reported no effect. Gifford and Feinstein evaluated 32 published studies on anticoagulant therapy and found that many of the favorable conclusions were not based on sound scientific and medical principles.[76] Often the prothrombin levels during anticoagulant therapy were not in a range which would have produced effective anticoagulation of blood. Those who were thought to benefit most were males under 60 years of age.[77] The finding was that the incidence of second occurrences of infarction during the 1st 6 months of therapy decreased. Patients with angina may benefit from anticoagulants if the condition is of recent origin. It has been claimed that old age per se is an indication for the use of anticoagulants in acute coronary occlusion. However, Russek has shown that there is no justification for the concept that age is an important factor in determining the prognosis in individual cases of coronary occlusion.[78] Russek concludes that the physician must judge the initial clinical appearance of the patient,[78] irrespective of age, and on that basis decide whether anticoagulants are indicated.

Pulmonary embolism is the most common cause of death in the injured elderly.[79] Foley and Wright indicated that mortality in pulmonary embolism,[80] secondary to thrombophlebitis, dropped from 18% to less than 1% by the introduction of anticoagulants. In a study of 1031 patients,[81] thromboembolic episodes occurred in 11% of 589 treated patients, compared with 26% of the 442 controls. Thromboembolic complications were higher in older patients. In the treated series of 589 persons 16% of the patients died (all causes) and 23.4% of the 442 controls died. Potential for death is naturally higher in those patients 60 years of age and over; indeed, death from a thromboembolic complication is almost doubled (23 to 42%) in this age group — partially due to impaired mobility. The reduction in deaths by proper anticoagulant treatment was "particularly dramatic in those 60 years and older."[81] Warfarin is probably the most effective drug for prophylactic therapy of thromboembolism.[79]

Heparin

The most common use for heparin in therapy is to provide immediate anticoagulation, while the coumarin drugs are chosen for long-term effects.[77] Jick et al.[82] studied 97 patients who received heparin therapy. Adverse reactions occurred in 18 out of 56 women (32%) and six out of 41 men (15%). The increased toxicity in women appeared to be limited to those over the age of 60. The authors suggest caution in the use of heparin in the elderly female population. Heparin is removed from the body predominantly by renal excretion of the unchanged drug; and to some extent by hepatic metabolism followed by urinary excretion of the inactive metabolites. This may account for the observed increased responsiveness in renal failure. Bleeding occurs more frequently with heparin than with oral anticoagulants, particularly in sick, elderly females.[84]

Vitamin K (Phytonadione)

Very little is known about the absorption, distribution, or excretion of this fat-soluble vitamin in the elderly.[85] The minimum daily requirement for normal persons has been estimated to be 0.03 μg/kg of body weight.[86,87]

Vitamin K is required for the synthesis of clotting factors II, VII, IX, and X. The oral anticoagulant drugs reduce the synthesis of these factors, probably by converting vitamin K to a less active form. Vitamin K therapy is indicated for (1) obstructive jaundice due to biliary cirrhosis, stone, or tumor; (2) in conditions of limited absorption as in sprue or ulcerative colitis; or (3) when anticoagulants have reduced the level of coagulation factors excessively.[88] Therapy is best controlled in most clinical settings by the original one-stage prothrombin test of Quick.[69] Both dietary deprivation and inhibition of intestinal synthesis of vitamin K are requisite to the development of deficiency symptoms in the adult, according to Frick et al.[89] These conditions may occur with greater frequency in the elderly, although further studies are needed to demonstrate this.

Plasma Expanders — Dextrans

Dextrans, the most commonly employed volume expanders, provide prophylactic antithrombotic therapy in surgical patients who are at high risk of thromboembolic complications. Comparative studies show dextrans to be as effective as warfarin for this purpose. However, anaphylaxis and other allergic reactions,[90,91] hypervolemia, renal failure, and a bleeding diasthesis make them less desirable as a drug of choice.[92] Although dextrans have been used widely to prevent thromboembolic disease in elderly individuals with a history of atherosclerotic or venous disease,[93,94] no studies have been published which assess the pharmacology of dextrans as they pertain specifically to the elderly patient.[95] Since dextrans produce more side effects than warfarin, their use in elderly patients is not recommended.[96]

CONCLUSIONS

Although a few generalized observations may be made concerning the manner whereby antianemic, anticoagulant, or plasma expander drugs affect the elderly patient, no consistent pattern of altered drug sensitivity in the aged has emerged. There is an increased sensitivity to drugs in general, which may be related to a combination of existing pathology and altered physiologic function. Absorption and transport of hematopoietic drugs probably occurs at a slower rate with advancing age, but this point has been investigated only with regard to iron, vitamin B_{12} and folic acid. Very little is known about changes in response at the receptor level, about changes in metabolic degradation or excretion of these drugs, except perhaps for vitamin B_{12}. Basic defects in experimental design abound and only one recent study compared pharmacologic effects of a drug in healthy elderly subjects and in those with recognized disease. This is a useful design which may allow a distinction between changes in physiologic function with aging, from changes due to disease. It is hoped that the sparse knowledge of the geriatric pharmacology of hematopoietic drugs will soon be corrected through well-designed studies and further support of research in this very important area of pharmacology.

REFERENCES

1. **Rabin, D. L.,** Use of Medicine: A Review of Prescribed and Non-Prescribed Medicine Use, U.S. Public Health Service, Department of Health, Education, and Welfare, Washington, D.C., 1972.
2. **Richey, D. P. and Bender, A. D.,** Pharmacokinetic consequences of aging, *Ann. Rev. Pharmacol. Toxicol.,* 17, 49, 1977.
3. **Bender, A. D.,** The effect of increasing age on the distribution of peripheral blood flow in man, *J. Am. Geriatr. Soc.,* 13, 192, 1965.
4. **Bender, A. D.,** Effect of age on intestinal absorption implications for drug absorption in the elderly, *J. Am. Geriatr. Soc.,* 16, 1331, 1968.
5. **Crooks, J., O'Malley, K., and Stevenson, I. H.,** Pharmacokinetics in the elderly, *Clin. Pharmacokinet.,* 1, 280, 1976.
6. **Friedman, S. A., Raizner, A. E., Rosen, H., Solomon, N. A., and Sy, W.,** Functional defects in the aging kidney, *Ann. Intern. Med.,* 76, 41, 1972.
7. **Gotz, B. E. and Gotz, V. P.,** Drugs and the elderly, *Am. J. Nurs.,* 78, 1347, 1978.
8. **Gorrod, J. W.,** Absorption, metabolism and excretion of drugs in geriatric subjects, *Gerontol. Clin.,* 16, 30, 1974.
9. **Seidl, L. G., Thornton, G. F., Smith, J. W., and Cluff, L. E.,** Studies on the epidemiology of adverse drug reactions. III. Reactions in patients on a general medical service, *Bull. Johns Hopkins Hosp.,* 119, 299, 1966.
10. **Clifford, G. O.,** Hematologic problems in the elderly, in *Clinical Geriatrics,* Rossman, I., Ed., Lippincott, Philadelphia, 1971, 253.
11. **Gillum, H. L. and Morgan, A. F.,** Nutritional status of the aging. I. Hemoglobin levels, packed cell volumes and sedimentation rates of 577 normal men and women over 50 years of age, *J. Nutr.,* 55, 265, 1955.
12. **Hobson, W. and Blackburn, E. K.,** Haemoglobin levels in a group of elderly persons living at home alone or with spouse, *Br. Med. J.,* 1, 647, 1953.
13. **Hallberg, L. and Hogdahl, A M.,** Anaemia and old age. Observations in a population sample of women in Goteborg, *Gerontol. Clin., (Basel),* 13, 31, 1971.
14. **Timaffy, M.,** A comparative study of bone marrow function in young and old individuals, *Gerontol. Clin.,* 4, 13, 1962.
15. **Woodford-Williams, E., Webster, D., Dixon, M. P., and MacKenzie, W.,** Red cell longevity in old age, *Gerontol. Clin.,* 4, 183, 1962.
16. **Williamson, C. S.,** Influence of age and sex on hemoglobin, *Arch. Intern. Med.,* 18, 505, 1916.
17. **Chow, B. F. and Yeh, S. D. J.,** Vitamins and mineral supplements in the diet of the elderly, in *Clinical Principles and Drugs in the Aging,* Freeman, J. T., Ed. Charles C Thomas, Springfield, Ill., 1963, 219.
18. **Benzie, R. M.,** The influence of age upon the iron content of bone marrow, *Lancet,* 1, 1074, 1963.
19. **Cape, R. D. T. and Zirk, M. H.,** Assessment of iron stores in old people, *Gerontol. Clin.,* 17, 101, 1975.
20. **Elwood, P. C.,** Epidemological aspects of iron deficiency in the elderly, *Gerontol. Clin.,* 13, 2, 1971.
21. **Judge, T. G. and Caird, F. I.,** Drug treatment of the elderly patient, Pitman Medical Publishing Co., Ltd., London, 1978, 101.
22. **Harant, Z. and Goldberger, J. V.,** Treatment of anemia in the aged: a common problem and challenge, *J. Am. Geriatr. Soc.,* 23, 127, 1975.
23. **Freiman, H. D., Tauber, S. A., and Tulsky, E. G.,** Iron absorption in the healthy aged, *Geriatrics,* 18, 716, 1963.
24. **Jacobs, A. M. and Owen, G. M.,** The effect of age on iron absorption, *J. Gerontol.,* 24, 95, 1969.
25. **Marx, J. J. M.,** Normal iron absorption and decreased red cell iron uptake in the aged, *Blood,* 53, 204, 1979.
26. **Jacobs, A. and Owen, G. M.,** Gastric secretion and iron absorption, *Br. J. Haematol.,* 15, 324, 1968.

27. **Jacobs, A., Rhodes, J., Peters, D. K., Campbell, H., and Eakins, J. D.,** Gastric acidity and iron absorption, *Br. J. Haematol.,* 12, 728, 1966.
28. **Edwards, F. C. and Coghill, N. F.,** Aetiological factors in chronic atrophic gastritis, *Br. Med. J.,* 2, 1409, 1966.
29. **Bose, S. K., Andrews, J., and Roberts, P. D.,** Haematological problems in a geriatric unit with special reference to anaemia, *Gerontol. Clin.,* 12, 339, 1970.
30. **Lawson, I. R.,** Anaemia in a group of elderly patients, *Gerontol. Clin.,* 2, 87, 1960.
31. **Davison, W.,** Anaemia in the elderly with special reference to iron deficiency, *Gerontol. Clin.,* 9, 393, 1967.
32. **Evans, D. M. D., Pathy, M. S., Sanerkin, N. G., and Deeble, T. J.,** Anaemia in geriatric patients, *Gerontol. Clin.,* 10, 228, 1968.
33. **Griffiths, H. J. L., Nicholson, W. J., and O'Gorman, P.,** A haematological study of 500 elderly females, *Gerontol. Clin.,* 12, 18, 1970.
34. **Cooper, W. M., Hieber, R. D., and Chapman, W. L.,** Anemia in the aged, *J. Am. Geriatr. Soc.,* 15, 568, 1967.
35. **Pegel, L. A.,** Iron therapy for aged patients, *J. Am. Geriatr. Soc.,* 6, 621, 1958.
36. **Gershoff, S. N., Brusis, O. A., Nino, H. V., and Huber, A. M.,** Studies of the elderly in Boston. I. The effects of iron fortification on moderately anemic people, *Am. J. Clin. Nutr.,* 30, 226, 1977.
37. **Migden, J.,** The treatment of iron deficiency in the aged: a controlled study, *J. Am. Geriatr. Soc.,* 7, 928, 1959.
38. **Wright, W. B.,** Iron deficiency anaemia of the elderly treated by total dose infusion, *Gerontol. Clin.,* 9, 107, 1967.
39. **Morrison, B. O.,** Tolerance to oral hematinic therapy: controlled release versus conventional ferrous sulfate, *J. Am. Geriatr. Soc.,* 14, 757, 1966.
40. **Geill, T.,** On the treatment of the nephrogenic anaemias with a combined cobalt-iron preparation, *Gerontol. Clin.,* 11, 48, 1969.
41. **Kerr, D. N. S. and Davidson, S.,** Gastrointestinal tolerance to oral iron preparations, *Lancet,* 2, 489, 1958.
42. **Freeman, G. T.,** Some principles of medication in geriatrics, *J. Am. Geriatr. Soc.,* 22, 289, 1974.
43. **Boger, W. P., Wright, L. D. Strickland, S. C., Gylfe, J. S., and Ciminera, J. C.,** Vitamin B_{12}: correlation of serum concentration and age, *Proc. Soc. Exp. Biol. Med.,* 89, 375, 1955.
44. **Cape, R. D. T. and Shinton, N. K.,** Serum-vitamin B_{12} concentration in the elderly, *Gerontol. Clin.,* 3, 163, 1961.
45. **Gaffney, G. W., Horonick, A., Okuda, K., Meier, P., Chow, B. F., and Shock, N. W.,** Vitamin B_{12} serum concentrations in 528 apparently healthy human subjects of ages 12-94, *J. Gerontol.,* 12, 32, 1957.
46. **Kilpatrick, G. S. and Withey, J. L.,** The serum vitamin B_{12} concentration in the general population, *Scand. J. Haematol.,* 2, 220, 1965.
47. **Watkin, D. M., Lang, C. A. Chow, B. F., and Shock, N. W.,** Agewise differences in the urinary excretion of vitamin B_{12} following intramuscular administration, *J. Nutr.,* 50, 341, 1953.
48. **Chow, B. F.,** Vitamin B_{12} and aging, *Fed. Proc., Fed. Am. Soc. Exp. Biol.,* 13, 453, 1954.
49. **Doscherholmen, A., Ripley, D., Chang, S., and Silvis, S. E.,** Influence of age and stomach function on serum vitamin B_{12} concentration, *Scand. J. Gastroenterol.,* 12, 313, 1977.
50. **Hansen, H. A. and Nystrom, B.,** Blood folic acid levels and folic acid clearance in geriatric cases, *Gerontol. Clin.,* 3, 173, 1961.
51. **MacLennan, W. J.,** Xylose absorption and serum carotene levels in the elderly, *Gerontol. Clin.,* 13, 370, 1971.
52. **Sheridan, D. J., Temperley, I. J., and Gatenby, P. B. B.,** Blood indices, serum folate and vitamin B_{12} levels in the elderly, *J. Irish Coll. Phys. Surg.,* 4, 39, 1974.
53. **Girdwood, R. H.,** Folate depletion in old age, *Am. J. Clin. Nutr.,* 22, 234, 1969.
54. **Markkanen, T. and Ruikka, I.,** Folic acid excretion in the urine of elderly women, *Gerontol. Clin.,* 4, 304, 1962.
55. **Baker, H., Jaslow, S. P., and Frank, O.,** Severe impairment of dietary folate utilization in the elderly, *J. Am. Geriatr. Soc.,* 26, 218, 1978.
56. **Fisher, J. W.,** Mechanism of the anemia of chronic renal failure, *Nephron,* 25(3), 106, 1980.
57. **Van Dyke, D. C., Keighley, G., and Lawrence, J. H.,** Decreased responsiveness to erythropoietin in a patient with anemia secondary to chronic uremia, *Blood,* 22, 838, 1963.
58. **Miyake, T., Kung, C. K. H., and Goldwasser, E.,** Purification of human erythropoietin, *J. Biol. Chem.,* 252, 5558, 1977.
59. **Hendler, D., Coffinet, J. A., Ross, S., Longnecker, R., and Bakovic, E.,** Controlled study of androgen therapy in anemia of patients on maintenance hemodialysis, *N. Engl. J. Med.,* 291, 1046, 1974.
60. **Williams, J. S., Stein, J. H., and Ferris, J. F.,** Nandrolone decanoate therapy for patients receiving hemodialysis, *Arch. Int. Med.,* 134, 289, 1974.

61. **Modder, B., Foley, J. E., and Fisher, J. W.,** The *in vitro* and *in vivo* effects of testosterone and steroid metabolites on erythroid colony forming cells (CFU-E), *J. Pharm. Exp. Ther.,* 207, 1004, 1978.
62. **Besa, E. C., Dale, D. C., Wolff, S. M. and Gardner, F. H.,** Treatment of refractory anemia with etiocholanolone and prednisolone (etio-pred), Initial clinical experience in 8 patients, 8th Annual Meeting of the American Society of Hematology, Dallas, Texas, December 6-9, 1975, (Abstr.), 47.
63. **Fisher, J. W., Gross, D. M., Foley, J. E., Nelson, P. K., Rodgers, G. M., George, W. J., and Jubiz W.,** A concept for the control of kidney production of erythropoietin involving prostaglandins and cyclic nucleotides, Symposium Monograph on Kidney Hormones, Hanover, West Germany, *Contr. Nephrol.,* 13, 37, 1978.
64. **Ortega, J. A., Malekzadeh, M., Dukes, P. P., Fine, R. N., and Shore, N. A.,** Potential role of erythropoietin and prostaglandins in the treatment of anemia of chronic renal disease, 16th Inter. Cong. of Hematology, Kyoto, Japan, September 5-11, 1976, (Abstr.) 15.
65. **Freeman, J. T., Ed.,** *Clinical Principles and Drugs in the Aging,* Charles C Thomas, Springfield, Ill., 1963, 485.
66. **Greppi, E.,** Use of anticoagulants in the old, *Geront. Clin.,* 1, 13, 1959.
67. **Coon, W. W. and Willis, P. W.,** Some aspects of the pharmacology of oral anticoagulants, *Clin. Pharmacol. Ther.,* 11, 312, 1970.
68. **Bochner, F., Carruthers, G., Campmann, J., and Steiner, J.,** in *Handbook of Clinical Pharmacology,* Little, Brown, Boston, 1978, 65.
69. **Quick, A. J.,** Anticoagulants in the aging, in *Clinical Principles and Drugs in the Aging,* Charles C Thomas, Springfield, Ill., 1963, 411.
70. **Walsh, A. C.,** Prevention of senile and pre-senile dementia by bishydroxycoumarin (Dicumarol) therapy, *J. Am. Geriatr. Soc.,* 17, 477, 1969.
71. **Walsh, A. C.,** Anticoagulant therapy as a potentially effective method for the prevention of pre-senile dementia: two case reports, *J. Am. Geriatr. Soc.,* 16, 472, 1968.
72. **Walsh, A. C.,** Senile and presenile dementia: further observations on the benefits of a dicumarol-psychotherapy regimen, *J. Am. Geriatr. Soc.,* 20, 127, 1972.
73. **Ratner, J., Rosenberg, G., Krae, V. A., and Englesmann, F.,** Anticoagulant therapy for senile dementia, *J. Am. Geriatr. Soc.,* 20, 556, 1972.
74. **Editorial,** Possible risks in anticoagulation. Treatment of cerebral vascular disease, *J. Am. Med. Assoc.,* 176, 223, 1961.
75. **Shepherd, A. M., Hewick, D. S., Moreland, T. A., and Stevenson, I. H.,** Age as a determinant of sensitivity to warfarin, *Br. J. Clin. Pharmacol.,* 4, 315, 1977.
76. **Gifford, R. H. and Feinstein, A. R.,** A critique of methodology in studies of anticoagulant therapy for acute myocardial infarction, *N. Engl. J. Med.,* 280, 351, 1976.
77. **Meyers, F. H., Jaewtz, E., and Goldfien, A.,** in *Review of Medical Pharmacology,* 6th ed., Lange Medical Publications, Los Altos, Calif., 1978, 174.
78. **Russek, H. I.,** The place of anticoagulant therapy in acute myocardial infarction, *J. Am. Geriat. Soc.,* 5, 255, 1957.
79. **Clagett, G. P. and Salzman, E. W.,** Prevention of venous thromboembolism in surgical patients, *N. Engl. J. Med.,* 290, 93, 1974.
80. **Foley, W. T. and Wright, I. S.,** The use of anticoagulants, *Med. Clin. N. Am.,* 40, 1339, 1956.
81. **Wright, I. S., Beck, D. F., and Marple, C. D.,** Myocardial infarction and its treatment with anticoagulant, *Mod. Concepts Cardiovas. Dis.,* 23, 208, 1954.
82. **Jick, H., Slone, D., Borda, I. T., and Shapiro, S.,** Efficacy and toxicity of heparin in relation to age and sex, *N. Engl. J. Med.,* 279, 284, 1968.
83. **Teien, A. N.,** Heparin elimination in patients with liver cirrhosis, *Thromb. Haemostas.,* 38, 701, 1977.
84. **O'Reilly, R. A.,** Therapy with anticoagulant drugs, *Ration. Drug. Ther.,* 8, 1, 1974.
85. **Koch-Weser, J. and Sellers, E. M.,** Drug interactions with coumarin anticoagulants, *N. Engl. J. Med.,* 285, 487, 1971.
86. Response of human beings to vitamin K, *Nutr. Rev.,* 27, 287, 1969.
87. Vitamin K deficiency in adults, *Nutr. Rev.,* 26, 165, 1968.
88. **Melmon, K. L. and Morrelli, H. F.,** in *Clinical Pharmacology — Basic Principles in Therapeutics,* Macmillan, New York, 1972, 376.
89. **Frick, P. G., Riedler, G., and Brogli, H.,** Dose response and minimal daily requirement for Vitamin K in man, *J. Appl. Physiol.,* 23, 387, 1967.
90. **Michelson, E.,** Anaphylactoid reactions to dextrans, *N. Engl. J. Med.,* 278, 552, 1968.
91. **Furhoff, A. K.,** Anaphylactoid reaction to dextran . . . a report of 133 cases, *Acta Anaesthesiol. Scand.,* 21, 161, 1977.
92. **Harris, W. H., Salzman, E. W., DeSanctis, R. W., and Coutts, R. D.,** Prevention of venous thromboembolism following total hip replacement: warfarin vs. dextran *J. Am Med. Assoc.,* 40, 220, 1319, 1972.

93. **Bryant, M. F., Bloom, W. L., and Brewer, S. S.,** Experimental study of the antithrombotic properties of dextrans of low molecular weight, *Am. Surg.,* 29, 256, 1963.
94. **Borchgrevink, C. F.,** Low molecular weight dextran in acute myocardial infarction, *Geriatrics,* 24, 138, 1969.
95. **Data, J. L. and Nies, A. S.,** Dextran 40, *Ann. Intern. Med.,* 81, 500, 1974.
96. **Atik, M.,** Dextran 40 and dextran 70: a review, *Arch. Surg.,* 94, 664, 1967.

ANTIMICROBIAL AND ANTIFUNGAL AGENTS

Jerome Santoro and Donald Kaye

INTRODUCTION

The success or failure of antimicrobial therapy of any infection is determined by (1) the susceptibility of the infecting organism to the antimicrobial agent, (2) the integrity of host defense mechanisms against the infecting agent, and (3) the ability to deliver adequate quantities of the antimicrobial agent to the site of infection without undue toxicity to the host. It is in the latter two categories that the elderly patient may differ from other hosts. In what follows, differences in the susceptibility and response to infection in the elderly will be discussed briefly and problems likely to be encountered with the use of various antimicrobial agents in the geriatric population will be delineated.

HOST FACTORS

T cell function has been shown to be decreased in the elderly.[1-3] In one study,[2] T cells from older individuals were shown to have a diminished response to various antigens. Others,[3] have found decreased delayed skin test reactivity, response to phytohemagglutinin, and T cell dependent IgG response to certain antigens, in people over 60 years as compared to a group of younger (less than 25 years) individuals. B cell function, as measured by the level of antibody response to influenza vaccine, is also diminished in the elderly.[4] Antibody levels were lower in older individuals compared to a younger control population.

The elderly are more likely to develop disease processes, which can compromise host defense. Diabetes mellitus has been shown to be associated with diminished neutrophil function.[5,6] Chronic lymphocytic leukemia and multiple myeloma are disease entities in which there is decreased immunoglobulin production following antigenic challenge.[7] In advanced Hodgkin's Disease, T cell function is severely depressed.[7] A variety of chemotherapeutic agents, such as corticosteroids and immunosuppressive drugs which are likely to be used in older people, are capable of depressing normal defense mechanisms.[3] Arteriosclerotic cardiovascular disease makes older individuals more susceptible to a variety of infections. Breakdown of the skin barrier of the lower extremities, especially in diabetics, predisposes to severe infections of the lower limbs. Cerebrovascular disease and cardiac arrhythmias, which can result in loss of consciousness, may lead to aspiration pneumonia. Periods of immobility may predispose to decubitus ulcers. Prostatic hypertrophy and carcinoma in aging males and the resultant instrumentation lead to more frequent urinary tract infections. Foley catheterization, often utilized in the elderly, is an obvious cause of infectious morbidity. Bacteremia caused by gram negative bacilli from intravenous catheters, urinary catheters, and other invasive procedures is also commonly encountered in geriatric patients.

It would appear that elderly patients are more prone to infection and are less likely to be able to defend adequately against infection than their younger counterparts. Thus, the delivery of adequate concentrations of antimicrobial agents to sites of infection in these individuals is imperative. However, this is often made difficult by the impaired physiologic processes of the elderly. These impaired processes may also predispose patients to unexpected drug toxicity. Further difficulties are encountered when the patient is receiving other drugs which may interact adversely with a given antimicrobial agent, or when the aging process itself causes unpredictable adverse drug effects.[8]

DECLINE IN PHYSIOLOGIC PROCESSES RELATED TO AGE

The aging process is associated with a decline in a number of physiologic processes which do not result in clinically overt disease.[8] Several reviews on the subjects of absorption, distribution, metabolism, and excretion of drugs in the elderly have recently appeared.[9-11] These, along with many other pharmacokinetic data as they relate to the elderly, are put into perspective by Dr. Richey in this handbook. For the most part, studies have shown that drug absorption and distribution are essentially unaltered in old age. However, achlorhydria is common in the elderly, and with achlorhydria certain antibiotics such as the penicillins may have enhanced absorption.[12] The plasma half-life of drugs that are presumably metabolized by the liver seems to be prolonged in geriatric populations. However, these differences are generally not of great clinical significance. In contrast, the rate of elimination of drugs excreted by the kidneys is often markedly decreased in the elderly. This occurs because there is an age-related ''physiologic'' decline in renal function, as reviewed by Dr. Richey in this handbook.

Davies and Shock showed that in a group of males between 20 and 90 years of age[13] there was an age-dependent fall in the glomerular filtration rate (GFR).

$$\text{GFR} = \text{Inulin clearance (m}\ell\text{/min/1.73m}^2) = 153.2 - 0.96 \text{ age}$$

Thus, by age 70, a normal individual would have a fall in GFR of about 70 mℓ/min or 45%. Siersbaek-Nielsen et al.[14] have pointed out that although creatinine clearance decreases considerably with advancing years, serum creatinine values were about the same regardless of age. Based on a study measuring urinary creatinine per kilogram body weight per 24 hr in different age groups, they developed a nomogram for the rapid evaluation of creatinine clearance (Figure 1). This demonstrates that the serum creatinine should *fall* as patients age and lose muscle mass. In the elderly, maintenance of serum creatinine levels at adult values is, therefore, an indication of diminishing renal function. Similarly, a moderate elevation of serum creatinine (e.g., to 2 to 3 mg/dℓ) may represent a severely depressed GFR in elderly individuals. For instance, if a 75 year old man who weighs 70 kg has a serum creatinine of 2.0 mg/dℓ, the nomogram (Figure 1) estimates his creatinine clearance to be only about 32 mℓ/min.

For discussion of the evidence that tubular function also diminishes with advancing age, the reader is referred to the work of Schock et al., begun several decades ago,[15] and to Dr. Richey's review of excretion in the elderly, in this handbook.

Many antimicrobial agents are primarily eliminated by the kidneys. For the reason just stated (normal decline in renal function), alterations in dose of many of these drugs may not be required. However, in addition to the ''physiologic'' decrease in renal function in the elderly, clinically significant renal failure may be found because of renal disease from concomitant hypertension, arteriosclerotic cardiovascular disease, gout, or diabetes mellitus. These often change renal function to a degree which does necessitate dose modification.

Guidelines for administration of antimicrobial agents in the face of renal insufficiency are outlined in Table 1. Antimicrobial agents that require substantial dose reductions in the presence of renal failure include the aminoglycosides, polymyxins' tetracyclines (except doxycycline and minocycline), flucytosine, and vancomycin. Agents such as the penicillins, cephalosporins, minocycline, and trimethoprim-sulfamethoxazole require only a moderate decrease in dose. The loading dose is unchanged in the presence of renal insufficiency. Dose reduction is applied only to the maintenance doses.[16] It should be noted that the incidence of nephrotoxicity is increased when cephalosporins are administered simultaneously with aminoglycosides.[17]

The aminoglycoside antibiotics represent a very special group of antimicrobial agents with

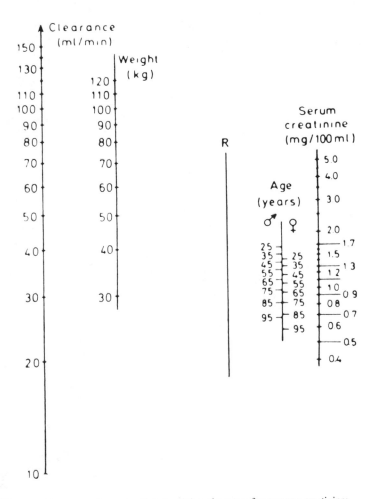

FIGURE 1.   Nomogram for estimating creatinine clearance from serum creatinine:

1.   Connect the patient's age, sex, and weight with a straight edge and determine the intercept with line R.
2.   Connect intercept on line R with patient's serum creatinine level using a straight edge. This plane then intercepts the estimated creatinine clearance.

(From Siersback-Nielsen, K., Hansen, J. M., Kampman, J., and Kristensen, M., *Lancet*, 1, 1133, 1971. With permission.)

regard to renal function and toxicity. These drugs are eliminated primarily by glomerular filtration,[18,19] and possibly to a small extent by tubular secretion.[19,20] The drugs are reabsorbed in the renal cortex; this may be an important mechanism in their toxicity.[19,21] The amino-glycosides have a very low therapeutic index, that is, therapeutic serum levels of these drugs are very close to toxic levels. Thus, in elderly individuals with "normal" serum creatinines, overdosage and, therefore, toxicity (renal and auditory) will be commonly encountered if consideration is not given to the physiologic reduction in renal function. Furthermore, a vicious cycle is frequently encountered clinically; namely, overdose of an aminoglycoside leads to a decrease in GFR which leads to toxic levels of the drug, further reduction in renal function, and possibly ototoxicity.

Of the available aminoglycosides, only gentamicin, tobramycin, and amikacin are commonly administered by the parenteral route, in the treatment of serious gram negative bacillary infections. Kanamycin is generally avoided because of its severe ototoxicity and current

Table 1
ANTIBIOTIC DOSAGE ADJUSTMENTS FOR RENAL FAILURE[16]

Drug	Pharmacology Half-life (hr) GFR normal	GFR <10mℓ/ min	Usual dose interval (hr)	Method[a]	Adjustment for renal failure GFR (mℓ/min) >50	10—50	<10
Antifungal Agents							
Amphotericin B	24	40	24	Int	24	24	36
5-Fluorocytosine[b]	3—6	70	6	Int	6	12—24	24—48
Antituberculous Agents							
Aminosalicylic acid	0.75	23	8	Int	8	12	c
Ethambutol	4	8	24	Int	24	24—36	48
Isoniazid	2—4	4	24		None	None	None
Rifampin	2—5	2—5	24		None	None	None
Aminoglycosides[b]							
Amikacin	2—3	27—36	12	Dose	≥90	50—90	15—35
Kanamycin							
Gentamicin	2	24—48	8	Dose	≥70	35—70	10—25
Tobramycin							
Cephalosporins							
Cephalexin	0.9	5—30	6	Int	6	6	6—12
Cephalothin	0.6	3—18	4—6	Int	4—6	4—6	6—12
Cefamandole	0.9	9	4—6	Int	4—6	6—9	9
Cefazolin	1.4—2.2	18—36	6—8	Int	8	12	24—48
Cephapirin	0.6	—	4—6	Int	4—6	4—6	6—12
Cephradine	0.9	8—15	6	Int	6	6	6—12
Cefoxitin	0.9	17.5	4—6	Int	4—6	6—9	9
Cefotaxime	1.1	2.5	4—8	Dose	None	50—80	50
Cefoperazone	1.9	2.5	8—12	Dose	None	None	None
Moxalactam	2.3	19	8—12	Dose	75	50	10—20
Chloramphenicol	2.5	3—7	6		None	None	None
Chloroquine	48	?	24	Dose	None	None	50
Clindamycin	2—2.5	1.5—3.5	6—8		None	None	None
Colistimethate[b]	3—8	10—20	12	Dose	75—100	c	d
Erythromycin	1.2—2.6	4—6	6		None	None	None
Lincoymcin	4—5	10	6	Int	6	6—12	12—24
Methenamine Mandelate	3—6	?	6		None	c	d
Metronidazole	6—14	?	8		8	?	?
Nalidoxic Acid	1.5	21	6		None	None	d
Nitrofurantoin	0.3	1	8	Dose	None	c	d
Penicillins							
Amoxicillin	1	7	8	Int	8	12	16
Ampicillin	1.5	8—20	6	Int	6	9	12—15
Carbenicillin	1.5	10—20	4	Dose	100	50—75	15—25
Cloxacillin or Dicloxacillin	0.5	0.8	6		None	None	None
Methicillin	0.5	4	4	Int	4	4	6—12
Nafcillin-Oxacillin	0.5	1	6		None	None	None
Penicillin G	0.5	6—20	Varied	Dose	100	20—50	10—20
Ticarcillin	1—1.5	15	4	Dose	100	50—75	15—25
Azlocillin	1/0	5.0	4—6	Dose	None	30—80	30
Mezlocillin	1.0	3—4	4—6	Dose	None	60—70	40—80
Piperacillin	1.0	3—4	4—6	Dose	None	60—70	40—50
Pyrimethamine	1.5—5	?	24		None	None	None
Sulfamethoxazole-	S(9—11)	20—50	12	Int	12	18	24
trimethoprim	T(10—15)	24					
Sulfisoxazole	3—7	6—12	6	Int	6	8—12	12—24

Table 1 (continued)
ANTIBIOTIC DOSAGE ADJUSTMENTS FOR RENAL FAILURE[16]

Drug	Pharmacology Half-life (hr) GFR normal	GFR <10mmℓ/min	Usual dose interval (hr)	Method[a]	Adjustment for renal failure GFR (mℓ/min) >50	10—50	<10
Tetracyclines							
Tetracycline	6—12	36—80	6	Int	6—12	c	c
Doxycycline	15—24	15—36	12		None	None	None
Minocycline	12	30	12		12	18—24	24—36
Vancomycin[b]	6—8	240	6—12		12—24	24—240	240

Note: GFR = glomerular filtration rate; None = no adjustment necessary.

a Int = interval method expressed as hours between repeated loading dose; dose = reduction method as percent loading dose given at usual interval.
b Important to measure blood levels in renal insufficiency.
c Avoid if possible in renal failure.
d Should never be used in renal failure.

Modified from Bennett, W. M., Singer, I., Golper, T., Feig, P., and Coggens, C. J., *Ann. Intern. Med.*, 86, 754, 1977; and other sources.

lack of antibacterial spectrum. Streptomycin is used mainly in the therapy of tuberculosis and bacterial endocarditis. Neomycin is reserved for oral use to decrease the normal bowel flora in patients with hepatic failure or in pre-operative bowel preparation.

Dosage schedules and adjustments take into account a loading dose based on age, lean body weight, and the desired serum concentration. Factors beside GFR and weight which might alter aminoglycoside levels include: anemia (hematocrit <25%), obesity, high fever, and burns. Aminoglycosides are bound to red blood cells; therefore, anemia tends to increase serum levels. Since aminoglycosides do not enter adipose tissue, obesity may result in overdose if these agents are given on a total body weight rather than a lean body weight basis.[22] High fever causes more rapid clearance of aminoglycosides, thereby lowering serum levels.[23] Aminoglycoside levels are also underestimated in burn victims because of an apparent increase in GFR.[24] The therapeutic peak serum concentration for gentamicin and tobramycin, using 8-hr dosing intervals, is between 4 and 10μg/mℓ, with a concentration of less than 2.0 μg/mℓ being desirable just before the next dose (trough or valley).[22] Kanamycin, amikacin, and streptomycin are given every 12 hr, and peak levels of 15 to 35 μg/mℓ and troughs of less than 5.0 μg/mℓ are sought.[22]

The loading dose of these drugs, based on lean body weight, is the same in all age groups regardless of renal function. For gentamicin and tobramycin, a loading dose of 1.7 to 2.0 mg/kg is used, and for kanamycin, streptomycin, and amikacin, 7.5 mg/kg are administered.[22] In patients under age 50 without renal failure, the same dose of gentamicin or tobramycin given at 8-hr intervals (or of kanamycin, streptomycin, or amikacin every 12 hr) will generally reproduce the desired peak and valley levels or show some slight accumulation of the antibiotic.[22] If peak levels of gentamicin or tobramycin are less than 4 μg/mℓ on day 2 of therapy, the daily dose can be increased by 2 mg/kg (0.67 mg/kg every 8 hr), which will generally result in a therapeutic peak level. Similarly, downward adjustments can be made for levels that are too high.[22] Kanamycin, streptomycin, and amikacin are managed by modifying the dose in a similar, proportional fashion for peak levels below 15 μg/mℓ or levels that are too high. In patients with renal failure or patients over 50, establishment of the maintenance dose is more complicated. Tables,[25] nomograms,[26] and computer programs[27,28] have been advocated to aid proper dose selection in the presence of renal dysfunction. The needed adjustment in maintenance dose can be accomplished by changing the dosage interval or the dose given at the usual interval. We prefer the latter method so that prolonged periods with subtherapeutic levels of antibiotic are avoided. Table 1 can be used to select a reasonable maintenance dose based on the patients' lean body weight and creatinine clearance (calculated from Figure 1).

Example: a 70 year old, nonobese man, weighing 70 kg, has chronic renal failure due to obstructive uropathy and a stable serum creatinine of 3.0 mg/dℓ for several months. The patient develops high fever and chills, and pyuria and bacteria are noted in a urinalysis. The patient is given a loading dose of 120 mg of gentamicin (70 kg × 1.7 mg/kg). What would be the maintenance dose of gentamicin in this patient provided stable renal dysfunction continued?

Estimated Ccr (Figure 1) = 20 mg/min

Maintenance dose (Table 1) = about 45% of loading dose

0.45 × 120 mg = 54 mg every 8 hr

Note that these guidelines can only be used in the presence of stable renal function. On the other hand, in the face of acute renal failure, a serum creatinine rise from 1.0 to 3.0 mg/dℓ in 24 hr indicates almost no GFR. It is obvious that with a serum creatinine of 3.0 mg/dℓ reached in this fashion, the above guidelines are not applicable. Several studies have emphasized that nomograms and tables are to be used only as guidelines and that individual differences make levels relatively unpredictable.[29-31] Thus in the elderly, especially if renal failure is present, frequent measurement of serum aminoglycoside levels is imperative. Several methods for measurement are available.[32,33] In patients requiring frequent hemodialysis, approximately half of the loading dose should be given after dialysis provided the predialysis levels were in the proper range.[34]

ADVERSE DRUG EFFECTS RELATED TO AGING PER SE

It seems clear that adverse effects of drugs are more common in the elderly. This is, in part, due to a decline in physiologic processes and to use of other pharmacologic agents (for underlying disease) resulting in adverse interactions. However, certain agents seem to cause problems in older individuals without any specific factor, other than age itself being identified as the cause.

Perhaps the most notorious adverse drug reaction that seem to be in large part related to age is isoniazed (INH)-induced hepatitis. Serum transaminase elevations (> 100 mU/mℓ) occur in 10 to 20% of patients receiving the drug.[35-37] However, most of these patients are asymptomatic and the drug can be continued without difficulty.[36,37] In contrast, only 1% of patients develop overt hepatitis (characterized by malaise, anorexia, nausea, and abdominal distress) with transaminase values above 250 mU/mℓ, alkaline phosphatase elevations, and clinically detectable icterus.[36,37] Fever, rash, and eosinophilia are uncommon but may be encountered. INH hepatitis rarely occurs before age 20, but in individuals over 50 the incidence climbs to 2.3%.[36,37] Hepatitis begins during the first 2 months of therapy in about 1/2 of the patients but cases beginning as late as 11 months after initiation of therapy have been described. Late onset tends to be associated with more severe disease. The histologic appearance of the liver is indistinguishable from that of viral hepatitis.[35] Death occurs in 8 to 12% of patients with clinical hepatitis.[35]

INH hepatic necrosis appears to be caused by the acetylhydrazine metabolite of the drug.[37] Rapid acetylators have higher concentrations of this metabolite, thus they seem to be more prone to hepatic injury.[37] Since transaminase elevation occurs in at least 10% of patients receiving INH, the American Thoracic Society does not recommend routine measurements of serum transaminase but suggests monthly patient evaluations and biochemical studies if symptoms compatible with hepatitis become manifest.[38] Others have advocated routine screening and discontinuance of INH when transaminase levels exceed 200 mU/mℓ.[39] In any event, the "prophylactic" use of INH in elderly individuals should be undertaken with extreme caution and only in special clinical situations.[38]

Hypersensitivity reactions to antimicrobial agents are said to be more common in older individuals.[40] Some authors have postulated that this may be due to a greater likelihood of exposure and thus sensitization to these drugs.[8] Accordingly it has been shown that the frequency of positive skin tests to major and minor penicillin determinants increases with age.[40]

Nephrotoxicity and ototoxicity with chemotherapeutic agents is more likely to occur and have more serious consequences in the elderly than in the young, since both nephrons and neural tissue are lost with aging. An age-related increase in prevalence of nephrotoxicity with aminoglycosides and polymixins and perhaps other antibiotics has been demonstrated in clinical studies.[21,41]

Ototoxicity caused by the aminoglycosides is thought to be more common among elderly individuals. An estimate of the incidence of overt toxicity in the average patient, regardless of age, is 1, 2, and 3% for tobramycin, gentamicin, and amikacin, respectively,[22] but toxicity is undoubtedly higher in the elderly. When sensitive methods are used to detect eighth nerve dysfunction (e.g., audiograms or nystagmagrams), toxicity may be three to five times greater.[22,42,43] Risk factors for ototoxicity include prior aminoglycoside administration, other ototoxic drugs (e.g., ethacrynic acid), initial abnormal audiograms, and diminished renal function.[22] The latter two risk factors are more common in the elderly and would make then more susceptible to eighth nerve damage.

Several reports have emphasized that lincomycin- and clindamycin-related pseudomembranous colitis occurs with greater frequency among elderly patients and age may be the most important risk factor.[44-47] Acute penumonitis produced by nitrofurantoin is more likely to occur in the elderly.[48]

DRUG INTERACTIONS

Because simultaneous disease states are commonly encountered in the elderly, necessitating the use of drugs other than antimicrobial agents, it is important to be vigilant about possible drug interactions when administering antimicrobials. For example, geriatric patients are often receiving digitalis preparations. It is known that carbenicillin and ticarcillin act as nonabsorbable anions in the urine and can produce severe hypokalemic metabolic alkalosis,[49] or worsen existing hypokalmia due to diuretic therapy. Therefore, the use of these agents can produce digitalis intoxication. The antifungal agent, amphotericin B, also produces hypokalemia by a toxic effect on the renal tubule and thus may also potentiate cardiac glycoside toxicity. Certain oral antimicrobial preparations, particularly neomycin, have been shown to diminish digitalis absorption when administered for prolonged periods.[50]

Patients with congestive heart failure are unable to handle large loads of sodium because of impaired renal excretion. Carbenicillin and ticarcillin contain large amounts of sodium (approximately 5.0 mEq/g).[51] For serious infection, a dose of 30 to 40 g in 24 hr is often administered. Thus, if about 150 to 200 mEq of sodium (equal to 1ℓ of normal saline solution) is given daily, congestive heart failure may be exacerbated.

As another example, diuretics are frequently used agents in older patients with heart

Table 2
ADVERSE INTERACTION OF ANTIMICROBIALS WITH DRUGS LIKELY TO BE USED IN ELDERLY PATIENTS[59-64]

Interacting drugs	Adverse effect	Probable mechanism (where known)
Amantadine (Symmetrel®) with anticholingergics and anti-Parkinson agents	Confusion and hallucinations	
Aminoglycoside antibiotics with		
Cephaloridine	Increased nephrotoxicity	
Cephalothin	Increased nephrotoxicity	
Curare-like drugs	Neuromuscular blockade	Additive
Digoxin	Possible decreased digoxin effect with oral neomycin	Decreased absorption
Ethacrynic acid (Edecrin®)	Increased ototoxicity	Additive
Polymyxins (Aerosporin® Coly-Mycin®)	Increased nephrotoxicity	Additive
Anticoagulants	Increased anticoagulant effect	Decreased Vitamin K production
Amphotericin B (Fungizone®) with		
Curare-like drugs	Increased curare effect	Hypokalemia
Digitalis drugs	Increased digatalis toxicity	Hypokalemia
Carbenicillin (Geopen,® Pyopen®) or Ticarcillin (Ticar®) with		
Aminoglycoside antibiotics	Decreased aminoglycoside activity	Inactivation of aminoglycoside
Digitalis drugs	Increased digitalis toxicity	Hypokalemia
Cephaloridine (Loridine®) with		
Aminoglycoside antibiotics	Increased nephrotoxicity	
Ethacrynic acid (Edecrin®)	Increased nephrotoxicity	Additive
Furosemide (Lasix®)	Increased nephrotoxicity	Additive
Cephalothin (Keflin®), with		
Aminoglycoside antibiotics	Increased nephrotoxicity	Not established
Chloramphenicol (Chloromycetin® and others) with		
Anticoagulants	Increased anticoagulant effect	Microsomal enzyme inhibition
Oral hypoglycemics	Increased sulfonylurea effect	Microsomal enzyme inhibition
Phenytoin (Dilantin® and others)	Increased phenytoin toxicity	Microsomal enzyme inhibition
Griseofulvin (Fulvicin-U/F® and others) with		
Anticoagulants, oral	Decreased anticoagulant effect	Microsomal enzyme induction
Alcohol	Disulfiram (Antabuse®)-like reaction	
Isoniazid with		
Alcohol	Decreased isoniazid effect in some patients with chronic alcohol abuse	Increased metabolism
Aluminum antacids	Decreased isoniazid effect	Decreased isoniazid absorption
Disulfiram (Antabuse®)	Psychotic episodes, ataxia	Alteration of dopamine metabolism
Phenytoin (Dilantin® and others)	Increased phenytoin toxicity	Microsomal enzyme inhibition
Rifampin (Rifadin® Rimactane®)	Increased chance of hepatotoxicity	
Lincomycin (Lincocin®) with		
Kaolin-pectin (Kaopectate®)	Decreased lincomycin effect	Decreased lincomycin absorption

Table 2 (continued)
ADVERSE INTERACTION OF ANTIMICROBIALS WITH DRUGS LIKELY TO BE USED IN ELDERLY PATIENTS[59-64]

Interacting drugs	Adverse effect	Probable mechanism (where known)
Metronidazole		
Alcohol	Antabuse®-like reaction	
Disulfiram (Antabuse®)	Psychotic episodes	
Nalidixic acid (NegGram®) with		
Anticoagulants, oral	Increased anticoagulant effect	Displacement from albumin
Neomycin (oral) with		
Digitalis drugs	Decreased digitalis effect	Decreased absorption
Nitrofurantoin		
Antacids	Decreased effect of Nitrofurantoin	Decreased absorption
Para-aminosalicylic Acid		
Anticoagulants Oral	Increased anticoagulant effect	
Phenytoin (Dilantin®)	Increased Toxicity	
Isoniazid	Increased blood levels	Decreased acetylation of Isoniazid
L-dopa	Decreased effectiveness of L-dopa	
Probenecid (Benemid®)	Increased PAS toxicity	Decreased renal excretion
Polymyxins (Aerosporin®, Coly-Mycin®) with		
Aminoglycoside antibiotics	Increased nephrotoxicity	Additive
Cephalothin	Increased nephrotoxicity	
Curare-like drugs	Neuromuscular blockade	Additive
Rifampin (Rifadin®, Rimactane®) with		
Anticoagulants, oral	Decreased anticoagulant effect	Microsomal enzyme induction
Contraceptives, oral	Decreased contraceptive effect	Increased estrogen metabolism
Corticosteroids	Decreased corticosteroid effect	Microsomal enzyme induction
Hypoglycemics	Possible decreased tolbutamide (Orinase®) effect	Microsomal enzyme induction
Methadone and other narcotics	Narcotic withdrawal symptoms	Microsomal enzyme induction
Sulfonamides with		
Anticoagulants, oral	Increased anticoagulant effect	Displacement from binding sites
Oral hypoglycemics	Increased sulfonylurea hypoglycemia	Structural similarity
Methotrexate	Increased antifolate effect	Additive
Phenytoin	Increased phenytoin toxicity	Structural similarity
Tetracyclines with		
Antacids, oral	Decreased effect of tetracyclines	Decreased tetracycline absorption
Barbiturates	Decreased doxycycline (Vibramycin® and others) effect	Microsomal enzyme induction
Carbamazepine (Tegretol®)	Decreased doxycycline (Vibramycin® and others) effect	Microsomal enzyme induction
Iron, oral	Decreased effect of tetracyclines	Decreased tetracycline absorption
Methoxyflurane (Penthrane®)	Increased nephrotoxicity	
Oral anticoagulants	Increased anticoagulant effect	
Zinc sulfate	Decreased effect of tetracyclines	Decreased absorption

disease or hypertension. Ethacrynic acid and perhaps furosemide can potentiate the ototoxicity of the aminoglycosides.[52] Another commonly prescribed group of drug is the coumarin anticoagulants. Rifampin and griseofulvin, by inducing microsomal enzymes in the liver, diminish the effectiveness of anticoagulants.[53] However, antimicrobials more commonly potentiate the action of dicumerol derivates by interfering with the gut flora that produce vitamin K (broad spectrum antibiotics), by displacing the anticoagulant from protein binding sites in serum (nalidixic acid, sulfonamides), or by inhibiting microsomal enzyme activity (chloramphenicol).[54]

Two other important drugs whose effects are altered by antimicrobial agents are the sulfonylureas and the phenytoin derivatives. The hypoglycemic activity of agents such as tolbutamide and chlorpropamide is enhanced by the sulfonamides and their structural analogues and by chloramphenicol, through the mechanism of enzyme inhibition.[55,56] Chloramphenicol, by the same mechanism, can increase the activity of phenytoin, thus predisposing to toxicity.[57] Isoniazid apparently has a similar effect upon phenytoin metabolism and toxicity.[58]

There are many other potential interactions to consider in addition to those outlined above. Some of the additional ones are listed in Table 2, along with those already discussed.

REFERENCES

1. **Gladstone, J. L. and Recco, R.,** Host factors and infectious diseases in the elderly, *Med. Clin. North Am.,* 60, 1225, 1976.
2. **Weksler, M. E., and Hütteroth, T. H.,** Impaired lymphocyte function in aged humans, *J. Clin. Invest.,* 53, 99, 1974.
3. **Roberts-Thomson, I. C., Whittingham, S., Youngchaiyud, U., and Mackay, I. R.,** Ageing, immune response, and mortality, *Lancet,* 2, 368, 1974.
4. **Howells, C. H., Vesselinova-Jenkins, C. K., Evans, A. D., and James, J.,** Influenza vaccination and mortality from bronchopneumonia in the elderly, *Lancet,* 1, 381, 1975.
5. **Drachman, R. H., Root, R. K., and Wood, W. B., Jr.,** Studies on the effect of experimental non-ketotic diabetes on antibacterial defense. I. Demonstration of a defect in phagocytosis, *J. Exp. Med.,* 124, 227, 1966.
6. **Mowat, A. and Baum, J.,** Chemotaxis of polymorphonuclear leukocytes from patients with diabetes mellitus, *N. Engl J. Med.,* 284, 621, 1971.
7. **Remington, J. S.,** The compromised host, *Hosp. Pract.,* 7, 59, 1972.
8. **Moellering, R. C.,** Factors influencing the clinical use of antimicrobial agents in elderly patients, *Geriatrics,* 33, 83, 1978.
9. **Gorrod, J. W.,** Absorption, metabolism and excretion of drugs in geriatric subjects, *Gerontol. Clin.,* 16, 30, 1974.
10. **Triggs, E. J. and Nation, R. L.,** Pharmacokinetics in the aged, a review, *J. Pharmacokinet. Biopharm.,* 3, 387, 1975.
11. **Crooks, J., O'Malley, K., and Stevenson, I. H.,** Pharmacokinetics in the elderly, *Clin. Pharmacokinet.,* 1, 280, 1976.
12. **Weinstein, L. and Dalton, C. A.,** Host determinants of response to antimicrobial agents, *N. Engl. J. Med.,* 279, 467, 1968.
13. **Davies, D. F. and Shock, N. W.,** Age changes in glomerular filtration rate, effective renal plasma flow, and tubular excretory capacity in adult males, *J. Clin. Invest.,* 29, 496, 1950.
14. **Siersback-Nielsen, K., Hansen, J. M., Kampmann, J., and Kristensen, M.,** Rapid evaluation of creatinine clearance, *Lancet,* 1, 1133, 1971.
15. **Miller, J. H., McDonald, R. K., and Shock, N. W.,** Age changes in the maximal rate of tubular reabsorption of glucose, *J. Gerontol.,* 7, 196, 1952.

16. **Bennett, W. M., Singer, I., Golper, T., Feig, P., and Coggens, C. J.,** Guidelines for drug therapy in renal failure, *Ann. Intern. Med.,* 86, 754, 1977.
17. **EORTC International Antimicrobial Therapy Project,** Three antibiotic regimens in the treatment of infection in febrile granulocytopenic patients with cancer, *J. Infect. Dis.,* 137, 14, 1978.
18. **Ritt, L. J. and Jackson, G. G.,** Pharmacology of gentamicin in man, *J. Infect. Dis.,* 124, 98, 1971.
19. **Appel, G. B. and Neu, H. C.,** The nephrotoxicity of antimicrobial agents, *N. Engl. J. Med.,* 296, 663, 1977.
20. **Gyselynck, A. M., Forrey, A., and Cutler, R.,** Pharmacokinetics of gentamicin, distribution and plasma and renal clearance, *J. Infect. Dis.,* 124, 70, 1971.
21. **Chiu, P. J. S., Brown, A., Miller, G., and Long, J. F.,** Renal excretion of gentamicin in anesthetized dogs, *Antimicrob. Agents Chemother.,* 10, 277, 1976.
22. **Jackson, G. G.,** Present status of aminoglycoside antibiotics and their safe, effective use, *Clin. Therapeut.,* 1, 200, 1977.
23. **Pennington, J. E., Dale, D. C., Reynolds, H. Y., and MacLowry, J. D.,** Gentamicin sulfate pharmacokinetics, lower levels of gentamicin in blood during fever, *J. Infect. Dis.,* 132, 270, 1975.
24. **Zaske, D., Sawchuck, R. J., Gerding, D. N., and Strate, R. G.,** Increased dosage requirements of gentamicin in burn patients, *J. Trauma,* 16, 824, 1976.
25. **McHenry, M. C., Gavan, T. L., Gifford, R. W., Jr., Geurkink, N. A., Van Ommen, R. A., Town, M. A., and Wagner, J. G.,** Gentamicin dosages for renal insufficiency, adjustments based on endogenous creatinine clearance and serum creatinine concentration, *Ann. Intern. Med.,* 74, 192, 1971.
26. **Chan, R. A., Benner, E. J., and Hoeprich, P. D.,** Gentamicin therapy in renal failure, a nomogram for dosage, *Ann. Intern. Med.,* 76, 773, 1972.
27. **Jelliffe, R. W., Knight, R., Buell, J. et al.,** Computer assistance for gentamicin therapy, *Clin. Res.,* 18, 441, 1970.
28. **Hull, J. H. and Sarubbi, F. A., Jr.,** Gentamicin serum concentrations, pharmacokinetic predictions, *Ann. Intern. Med.,* 85, 183, 1976.
29. **Kaye, D., Levison, M. E., and Labovitz, E. D.,** The unpredictability of serum concentrations of gentamicin, pharmacokinetics of gentamicin in patients with normal and abnormal renal function, *J. Infect. Dis.,* 130, 150, 1974.
30. **Barza, M., Brown, R. B., Shen, D., Gibaldi, M., and Weinstein, L.,** Predictability of blood levels of gentamicin in man, *J. Infect. Dis.,* 132, 165, 1975.
31. **Schumacher, G. E.,** Pharmacokinetic analysis of gentamicin dosage regimens recommended for renal impairment, *J. Clin. Pharmacol.,* 15, 656, 1975.
32. **Finegold, S. M., Martin, W. J., and Scott, E. G.,** *Diagnostic Microbiology,* ed. C. V. Mosby, St. Louis, Mo., 1978, 402.
33. **Broughton, A. and Strong, J. E.,** Radioimmunoassay of antibiotics and chemotherapeutic agents, *Clin. Chem.,* 22, 726, 1976.
34. **Christopher, T. G., Korn, D., Blair, A. D., Forrey, A W., O'Neill, M. A., and Cutler, R. E.,** Gentamicin pharmacokinetics during hemodialysis, *Kidney Int.,* 6, 38, 1974.
35. **Black, M., Mitchell, J. R., Zimmerman, H. J., Ishak, K. G., and Epler, G. R.,** Isoniazid-associated hepatitis in 114 patients, *Gastroenterology,* 69, 289, 1975.
36. **Mitchell, J. R., Zimmerman, H. J., Ishak, K. G., Thorgiersson, U. P., Timbrell, J. A., Snodgrass, W. R., and Nelson, S. D.,** Isoniazid liver injury, clinical spectrum, pathology, and probable pathogenesis, *Ann. Intern. Med.,* 84, 181, 1976.
37. **Rahal, J. J. and Simberkoff, M. S.,** Adverse reactions to anti-infective agents, *Disease-A-Month,* 25, 1, 1978.
38. **American Thoracic Society,** Preventive therapy of tuberculosis infection, *Am. Rev. Resp. Dis.,* 110, 371, 1974.
39. **Lefrak, S. S., Byrd, R., Senior, R. M. et al.,** Chemoprophylaxis of tuberculosis, *Arch. Intern. Med.,* 135, 606, 1975.
40. **Stember, R. H. and Levine, B. B.,** Prevalence of allergic diseases, penicillin hypersensitivity, and aeroallergin hypersensitivity in various populations, *J. Allergy Clin. Immunol.,* 51, 100, 1973.
41. **Koch-Weser, J., Sidel, V. W., Federman, E. B., Konarek, P., Finer, D. C., and Eaton, A. E.,** Adverse effects of sodium colistimethate, manifestations and specific reaction rates during 317 courses of therapy, *Ann. Intern. Med.,* 72, 857, 1970.
42. **Lerner, S. A., Seligsohn, R., and Matz, G. J.,** Comparative clinical studies of ototoxicity and nephrotoxicity of amikacin and gentamicin, *Am. J. Med.,* 62, 919, 1977.
43. **Black, R. E., Lau, W. K., Weinstein, R. J., Young, L. S., and Hewitt, W. L.,** Ototoxicity of amikacin, *Antimicrob. Agents Chemother.,* 9, 956, 1976.
44. **Smart, R. E., Ramsden, M. W., Gear, M. W., Nicol, A., and Lennox, W. M.,** Severe pseudomembranous colitis after lincomycin and clindamycin, *Br. J. Surg.,* 63, 25, 1976.

45. **Schwartzberg, J. E., Maresca, R. M., and Remington, J. S.,** Clinical study of gastrointestinal complications associated with clindamycin therapy, *J. Infect. Dis.,* 135, 599, 1977.
46. **Gurwith, M. J., Rabin, H. R., and Love, K.,** Diarrhea associated with clindamycin and ampicillin therapy, preliminary results of a cooperative study, *J. Infect. Dis.,* 137, S104, 1977.
47. **Neu, H. C., Prince, A., Neu, O. C., and Garvey, J.,** Incidence of diarrhea and colitis associated with clindamycin therapy, *J. Infect. Dis.,* 137, S120, 1977.
48. **Dawson, R. B.,** Pulmonary reactions to nitrofurantoin, *N. Engl. J. Med.,* 274, 522, 1966.
49. **Lipner, H. I., Ruzany, F., Dasgupta, M., Lief, P. D., and Bank, N.,** The behavior of carbenicillin as a nonreabsorbed anion, *J. Lab. Clin. Med.,* 86, 183, 1975.
50. **Lindenbaum, J., Maultiz, R. M., Saha, J. R., Shea, N., and Butler, V. P., Jr.,** Impairment of digoxin absorption by neomycin, *Clin. Res.,* 20, 410, 1972.
51. **Weinstein, L.,** The penicillins, in *The Pharmacologic Basis for Therapeutics,* 5th ed., Goodman, L. S. and Gilman, A., Eds., Macmillan, New York, 1975, 1130.
52. **Schwartz, G. H., David, D. S., Riggio, R. R., Stengel, K. H., and Rubin, A. L.,** Ototoxicity induced by furosemide, *N. Engl. J. Med.,* 282, 1413, 1970.
53. **Cullin, S. I. and Catalano, P. M.,** Griseofulvin-warfarin antagonism, *J. Am. Med. Assoc.,* 199, 582, 1967.
54. **O'Reilly, R. A. and Aggeler, P. M.,** Determinants of the response to oral anticoagulant drugs in man, *Pharmacol. Rev.,* 22, 35, 1970.
55. **Dall, J. L. C., Conway, H., and McAlpine, S. G.,** Hypoglycemia due to chlorpropamide, *Scot. Med. J.,* 12, 403, 1967.
56. **Petitpiere, B. and Fabre, J.,** Chlorpropamide and chloramphenicol, *Lancet,* 1, 789, 1970.
57. **Ballek, R. E., Reidenberg, M. M., and Orr, L.,** Inhibition of diphenylhydantoin metabolism by chloramphenicol (letter), *Lancet,* 1, 150, 1973.
58. **Kutt, H., Brennan, R., Dehejia, H., and Verbely, K.,** Diphenylhydantoin intoxication, A complication of isoniazid therapy, *Am. Rev. Resp. Dis.,* 101, 377, 1970.
59. Adverse interactions of drugs, *Med. Lett. Drugs Ther.,* 21, 5, 1979.
60. **Kabins, S. A.,** Interactions among antibiotics and other drugs, *J. Am. Med. Assoc.,* 219, 206, 1972.
61. **Sanford, J.,** *Guide to Antimicrobial Therapy,* Sanford, J. (publisher), Bethesda, 1978.
62. **Hansten, P. D.,** *Drug Interactions,* Lea & Febiger, Philadelphia, 1979.
63. **American Pharmaceutical Association,** *Evaluation of Drug Interactions,* 2nd ed., Washington, D. C., 1976.
64. **James, J. D. et al.,** *A Guide To Drug Interactions,* McGraw-Hill, New York, 1978.

THE INFLUENCE OF AGING ON ANTINEOPLASTIC THERAPY

Rosaline R. Joseph

INTRODUCTION

The incidence of malignant neoplastic disease increases with age, with the majority of cases occurring in individuals over 50 years old.[1] Proper medical therapy of malignancies is thus vitally concerned with the problems of response to antineoplastic agents peculiar to the older age group.

The recognized decreases in organ function[2] and immune reactivity[3] accompanying aging play significant roles in modifying response to cancer chemotherapy in the elderly. The slower rate of tumor growth occurring with advancing age also undoubtedly influences response to drugs. This phenomenon has been demonstrated experimentally in mice,[4] and empirically in humans, as evidenced by the often prolonged survival of older cancer patients.[5]

Available information concerning the properties of the major antineoplastic agents in current clinical use is summarized in Table 1,[6-16] which will serve as a reference for the discussion that follows of age-related problems in cancer chemotherapy.

AGE-RELATED TOXICITY

Disposition of antineoplastic agents by elderly patients is dependent on the level of those functions important in the biotransformation and/or excretion of the particular drug in question. Absorption by the gastrointestinal tract is unaffected by age, and body distribution of drugs remains essentially unchanged.[17] Although hepatic size declines with age, liver function usually remains within normal limits,[18] so that the disposition of antineoplastic drugs chiefly metabolized by the liver such as adriamycin, is not significantly impaired.[19] The progressive decrease in renal function which occurs with aging,[18] however, has important clinical effects on the fate of drugs such as methotrexate and platinum which are excreted in active form almost entirely by the kidneys.

For example, in a group of 49 patients with advanced cancer and normal serum creatinine and/or blood urea nitrogen levels, the only factor which predicted methotrexate toxicity was the patient's age.[20] Glomerular filtration rate decreases 46% from age 20 to 90. At the same time, the renal blood flow decreases 53%. Tubular functions are also diminished.[21] Caution must thus be observed in administering these drugs to elderly patients. Creatinine clearances should be performed prior to institution of treatment with methotrexate or platinum and appropriate dose de-escalations made for borderline values.

The decline in immune response associated with aging decreases the margin of safety of the antineoplastic agents, almost all of which produce at least a temporary immunosuppression. The elderly patient who is taking immunosuppressive agents should be followed especially closely and advised of the necessity for immediate contact with his physician at the first sign of possible infection.

The increased risks of toxicity from antineoplastic drugs in the elderly are not related only to the usual consequences of aging. There are several toxic reactions to these agents which are intensified in the older age group with no correlation to any factor other than age itself. Adriamycin, one of the most useful of the antineoplastic compounds because of its broad spectrum of activity, is associated with the development of dose-related cardiomyopathy at any age. Since adriamycin-associated congestive heart failure carries a mortality rate of about 50%,[22] it is imperative to keep within the dose limits generally considered to be below those known to induce clinically significant cardiac damage. A recent study demonstrated that evidence of myocardial degeneration precedes functional abnormalities,[22] and that overt heart failure occurs only after a critical degree of morphologic damage. In

Table 1
COMMONLY USED ANTINEOPLASTIC AGENTS

Drug	Mode of Action	Principle routes of biotransformation and/or disposition	Toxicity	Ref.
Antimetabolites				
Methotrexate	Inhibition of dihydro-folate reductase blocking nucleotide synthesis	90% excreted as intact compound in urine	Myelosuppression, mucositis, cirrhosis, interstitial pneumonitis	6, 7
5 Fluoro Uracil	Inhibition of thymi-dylate synthetase and nucleotide synthesis	Activation to 5-Fluo-rouridine monophos-phate and 5-Fluorodeoxyuridylate Hepatic degradation	Oral and gastrointes-tinal ulceration, diar-rhea, myelosuppress-ion	6, 7
Cytosine arabino-side	Inhibition of DNA-dependent DNA polymerase	Conversion to active nucleotide arabinoside cytidine triphosphate Hepatic degradation to uracil arabinoside	Nausea and vomiting, myelosuppression	6, 7, 8
6-Mercaptopurine	Purine nucleotide inhibition	Rapid, extensive bio-transformation, uri-nary excretion of urates	Myelosuppression	6, 13
Alkylating Agents				
Cyclophosphamide	Transfer of alkyl groups resulting in crosslinked DNA strands	Activation of hepatic microsomal enzymes Urinary excretion of metabolites	Myelosuppression, hemorrhage, cystitis, alopecia	6, 7
Melphalan	Transfer of alkyl groups resulting in cross-linked DNA strands	Rapid biotransformation Urinary excretion of metabolites	Myelosuppression	6, 13
Natural Products **Antibiotics**				
Adriamycin™	Intercalation between adjacent base pairs on DNA strand Inhibition of RNA synthesis by tem-plate disordering	Hepatic and tissue biotransformation Biliary excretion	Myelosuppression, nausea, alopecia, cardiotoxicity	7, 9
Bleomycin	Fragmentation of DNA	High tissue concentra-tion and degradation Urinary excretion	Pulmonary fibrosis, skin toxicity, pyrexia	
Mitomycin	Inhibition of DNA-dependent RNA synthesis	Enzymatic activation and deactivation — exact mechanism unknown	Myelosuppression, alo-pecia, hypocalcemia	11
Vinca Alkaloids				
Vincristine	Mitotic inhibition by metaphase arrest	Rapid local uptake or destruction Hepatic Excretion	Neurotoxicity	12
Vinblastine	Mitotic inhibition by metaphase arrest	Rapi local uptake or destruction Hepatic excretion	Myelosuppression, alopecia	13
Carmustine (BCNU)	Alkylation Inhibition of DNA replication	Rapid tissue uptake and biotransforma-tion. Specific metabo-lites unknown	Myelosuppression	6, 7

Table 1 (continued)
COMMONLY USED ANTINEOPLASTIC AGENTS

Drug	Mode of Action	Principle routes of biotransformation and/or disposition	Toxicity	Ref.
Lomustine (CCNU)	Alkylation, Inhibition of DNA replication	Rapid uptake and biotransformation	Myelosuppression	6, 7
Cis Platinum	Crosslinkage of DNA	Urinary excretion of unchanged compound and metabolites	Myelosuppression, Nephrotoxicity, Ototoxicity	14
Procarbazine	Uncertain, ? inhibition of RNA and DNA synthesis	Rapid biotransformation Urinary excretion	Myelosuppression, CNS Suppression	6, 15
1-Asparaginase	Hydrolysis of asparagine	? Phagocytosis by reticuloendothelial system ? Extravascular sequestration ? Cellular penetration into liver	Hepatotoxicity, Pancreatitis, CNS depression	6, 16

this report, patients older than 70 years of age appeared to be predisposed to the development of heart failure even though their degree of myocardial degeneration did not exceed that anticipated at their particular adriamycin dose levels. It is suggested, therefore, that anyone age 70 or more should have a substantial reduction in the total cumulative dose of adriamycin below the usual limit of 550 mg/m². A total dose of 450 mg/m² is recommended. The question of safety in using adriamycin in patients with pre-existing cardiac disease, a situation frequently encountered in older patients, has never been satisfactorily resolved. There is no evidence that preexisting cardiac disease predisposes to early development of adriamycin myocardiopathy and/or congestive failure.[23] Most authors state that, given the proper indications, the drug may be used in patients with cardiac disease, perhaps with a dosage limitation of 450 mg/m², regardless of age. Cyclophosphamide and mediastinal irradiation potentiate the cardiotoxicity of adriamycin and extreme caution should be used in administering the drug to patients over 70 who are also receiving one or both of these treatment modalities.

A major concern in the use of bleomycin has been the unpredictable development of pulmonary fibrosis, sometimes with a fatal outcome, in 5 to 10% of treated patients.[24,25] Clinically, pulmonary toxicity is first manifested by dyspnea, cough, and occasionally low grade fever. Physical examination reveals bibasilar rales. A bilateral interstitial infiltrate is seen on chest X-ray. Patients over age 70 have a significantly greater risk of pulmonary toxicity,[25] with 14.5 % of these patients being affected, as opposed to 6 to 8% in the younger age groups. Special precautions, such as regular monitoring of chest X-rays and frequent performance of pulmonary function tests, are indicated in this age group. The drug should be discontinued in the face of any new abnormality in these studies or with the appearance of bibasilar rales.

The use of intrathecal methotrexate is associated with greater toxicity in adults than in children.[26] This phenomenon may be related to the common practice of calculating cancer chemotherapy dosages in terms of body surface area. Since the central nervous system reaches its full volume before the rest of the body has completed its growth, dose calculation on the basis of body surface area results in the delivery of a relatively greater dose to adults than to children. It is suggested that a standard total dose, rather than one dependent on body surface area, be given to adults. In addition, patients over 60 years old may require lower doses since the volume of the brain begins to decrease after this age and because cerebrospinal fluid turnover may also be diminished in patients of advanced age.[17]

Table 2
DISSEMINATED NEOPLASMS CURABLE BY ANTINEOPLASTIC DRUGS (1979)

Acute lymphocytic leukemia	Embryonal rhabdomyosarcoma
Burkitt's lymphoma	Ewing's tumor
Advanced hodgkins disease	Choriocarcinoma
Wilm's tumor	Embryonal testicular carcinoma

Neurotoxicity from asparaginase, an agent used to treat acute lymphocytic leukemia, is also more frequent in the adult.[27] Although the mechanism for this neurotoxicity is unclear, it is suggested[28] that, at least in older animals, it may be due to an impaired ability to eliminate asparaginase through the reticuloendothelial system or to a failure to counterbalance the depletion of asparagine through asparagine synthetase. No increase in the common neurotoxicity produced by the more widely used compound, vincristine, has been reported in the elderly.

AGE-RELATED DIMINISHED RESPONSES

At the present time, several disseminated malignant neoplasms are curable by treatment with antineoplastic drugs. These are listed in Table 2. It is noteworthy that with the exception of Hodgkin's disease, the list is composed of tumors occurring primarily in children and young adults. A possible explanation of the success of antineoplastic agents in this group of tumors is that selective toxicity of antitumor drugs has been demonstrated for those tumors with rapid growth fractions, allowing curative schedules to be achieved by application of animal data relative to cellular and drug kinetics.[29] The majority of the common malignant neoplasms of the elderly are of the slow-growth-fraction variety, where the slowly proliferating tumor cells are less drug sensitive. Doses of cytotoxic agents sufficient to kill these tumor cells often impose an unacceptable toxicity on normal cells.

There are some situations in which even *within* the same tumor type, treated by the same agents, the response to therapy is poorer in the older population than in the younger. Perhaps the most striking of these tumors are the acute leukemias. In acute lymphocytic leukemia, several large studies[30-32] have found that patients over 15 years of age have a poorer response to therapy and a shorter survival time than those under 15, with survival appearing to be a decreasing function of age. In one report of combination chemotherapy in leukemia,[31] adult patients showed 18 complete remissions out of 23 cases (78%), where the children had 74 remissions out of 75 cases (98%). This difference was highly significant. Of 5 adult nonresponders, 2 were over 60 years old.

In the adult population, about 80% of cases of acute leukemia are of the nonlymphocytic variety. In the past, it has been emphatically stated that, when acute nonlymphocytic leukemia occurs in patients over age 50, chemotherapy only very rarely produces remissions.[33] The reasons for this lack of responsiveness remain unclear, but it has been postulated that in the older age group rather than drug resistance, increased risk of infection and hemorrhage is responsible for therapeutic failure.[34] Since approximately 45 to 50% of patients with this disease fall into the over-50 age category,[35] their poor response represents a major problem in the management of this disorder. Recent reports are more optimistic, reporting nearly the same response rate and survival in the over-50 age group as in younger patients with acute nonlymphocytic leukemia when using newer combination chemotherapy regimens.[36,37] The agents most effective in this situation at the present time are cytosine arabinoside, daunomycin (or adriamycin), and thioguanine. It is probable that improved supportive care with antibiotics and replacement of blood components, particularly platelets and white blood cells, has also contributed to the greater remission rate now obtainable in elderly individuals.

Poor response to treatment in the older patient is noted in other hematologic neoplasms. Multiple myeloma patients more than 60 years old have a significantly worse prognosis than younger patients given the same chemotherapeutic regimen.[38] In persons with Hodgkin's disease treated with multiple drug chemotherapy, the probability of surviving for 5 years was found to be significantly higher in patients under 40 years of age than in patients over that age.[39]

With adjuvant chemotherapy of breast carcinoma, where treatment is aimed at the prevention of tumor recurrence following removal of all known tumor burden, a marked difference in result between pre- and postmenopausal women has been noted in two large studies.[40,41] Whereas adjuvant chemotherapy significantly diminished the rate of recurrence in premenopausal women with positive axillary nodes at the time of surgery, no such benefit resulted from the same treatment of postmenopausal women. This finding seems to be independent of the effect of chemotherapy on menstrual function, since the benefit occurred whether or not the premenopausal women were rendered amenorrheic by chemotherapy. No adequate explanation has yet come forth for this observation.

DRUG INTERACTIONS

Since the elderly often receive multiple medications, an additional concern in devising antineoplastic treatment regimens for these patients is the possibility of interaction of these agents with other drugs prescribed for coexisting disorders. Table 3 lists significant interactions between antineoplastic agents and other drugs the elderly are likely to use.

Although the possibility of all of the listed interactions should be kept in mind when prescribing any of the listed combinations, it is usually not necessary to diminish the initial dosage. If a clinical problem develops, appropriate adjustments can then be made. There are a few situations, however, in which the interactions are critical. In these cases, the offending combinations should be avoided or an initial dose adjustment made. The concomitant use of salicylates with methotrexate may lead to increased and prolonged serum levels of free methotrexate and thus increase its toxicity. This interaction does not occur with acetaminophen,[43] which may, therefore, be substituted for salicylates in patients receiving methotrexate.

Of utmost clinical importance is the interaction between allopurinol and 6-mercaptopurine or its closely related compound, azathioprine. Allopurinol, a xanthine oxidase inhibitor, delays the catabolism of the latter substances, causing greatly increased levels of the parent compounds. Since allopurinol is often prescribed to prevent urate deposition in the kidneys during cytoxic therapy, the combination of allopurinol and antipurine metabolites is a frequent one. At the start of such combination therapy, the dose of mercaptopurine or azathioprine should be reduced to one third or one fourth of the usual level.

Procarbazine has weak monoamine oxidase inhibitor properties which have been implicated in several adverse interactions. There is an apparent synergism between procarbazine and central nervous system depressants such as antihistamines, barbiturates, and phenothiazines. Caution should be used when administering procarbazine in combination with such drugs, and a reduced dosage of the central nervous system depressant may be indicated. The combination of monoamine oxidase inhibitors with sympathomimetic drugs such as are found in cold and allergy preparations has produced hypertensive reactions. If possible, the concomitant use of these drugs and procarbazine should be avoided. Finally, procarbazine should not be given with tricyclic antidepressants which themselves are monoamine oxidase inhibitors.

Table 3
DRUG INTERACTIONS INVOLVING ANTINEOPLASTIC AGENTS

Interacting drugs	Adverse effect	Probable mechanism
Methotrexate with		
Salicylates	Increased cytotoxicity	Displacement of methotrexate
Sulfonamides		from plasma binding sites
Diphenylhydantoin		
Chloramphenicol		
Tetracycline		
Penicillin G		
Cyclophosphamide with		
Succinylcholine	Prolonged apnea	Decrease in plasma cholinesterase
Chloramphenicol	Decreased cytotoxicity	Inhibition of activation by micro-somal enzymes
Phenobarbital	Increased cytotoxicity	Increased microsomal activation of drug
Allopurinol	Increased cytotoxicity	Unknown
6-Mercaptopurine with		
Allopurinol	Increased cytotoxicity	Inhibition of degradation to thiouric acid
Procarbazine with		
Alcohol	Disulfiram-like reaction	Monoamine oxidase inhibiting properties of procarbazine
Central nervous system	Increased central nervous system	Monoamine oxidase inhibiting
Depressants	depression	properties of procarbazine
Sympathomimetics	Hypertensive reaction	
Tricyclic antidepressants	Hypertensive reaction	

REFERENCES

1. **Cutler, S. J. and Eisenberg, H.,** Cancer in the aged, *Ann. N.Y. Acad. Sci.,* 771, 1964.
2. **Richey, D. P. and Bender, A. D.,** Pharmacokinetic consequences of aging, *Ann. Rev. Pharmacol. Toxicol.,* 17, 49, 1977.
3. **Teller, M. N.,** Age changes and immune resistance to cancer, *Adv. Gerontol. Res.,* 4, 25, 1972.
4. **Teller, M. N., Bowie, M., and Mountain, I. M.,** Influence of age of host on the chemotherapy of murine myeloma LCP-1, *J. Gerontol.,* 29, 360, 1974.
5. **Cowdry, E. V.,** Influence of aging on the skin, *Natl. Cancer Inst. Monograph,* 10, 335, 1963.
6. **Carter, S. K. and Slavik, M.,** Chemotherapy of cancer, *Ann. Rev. Pharmacol.,* 157, 1974.
7. **Chabner, B. A., Myers, C. E., Coleman, C. N., and Johns, D. G.,** The clinical pharmacology of antineoplastic agents, *N. Engl. J. Med.,* 292, 107, 1975.
8. **Kremer, W. B.,** Cytarabine, *Ann. Intern. Med.,* 82, 684, 1975.
9. **Blum, R. H. and Carter, S. K.,** Adriamycin, a new anticancer drug with significant clinical activity, *Ann. Intern. Med.,* 80, 249, 1974.
10. **Blum, R. H., Carter, S. K., and Agre, K.,** A clinical review of bleomycin — a new antineoplastic agent, *Cancer,* 31, 903, 1973.
11. **Crooke, S. T. and Bradner, W. T.,** Mitomycin C: a review, *Cancer Treatment Rev.,* 3, 121, 1976.
12. **Bennett, W. M., Singer, I., Golper, T., Feig, P. and Coggins, C. T.,** Guidelines for drug therapy in renal failure, *Ann. Intern. Med.,* 86, 754, 1977.
13. **Mihich, E.,** Pharmacologic principles and the basis for selectivity of drug action, in *Cancer Medicine,* Holland, J. F. and Frei, E., Eds., Lea & Febiger, Philadelphia, 1973, 650.
14. **Rozencweig, M., Von Hoff, D. D., Slavik, M., and Muggia F. M.,** Cisdiamminedichloroplatinum (II). A new anticancer drug *Ann. Intern. Med.,* 86, 803, 1977.
15. **Spivack, S. D.,** Procarbazine, *Ann. Intern. Med.,* 81, 795, 1974.

16. **Capizzi, R. L. and Handschumacher, R. E.,** Asparaginase, in *Cancer Medicine,* Holland, J. F. and Frei, E., Eds., Lea & Febiger, Philadelphia, 1973, 850.

17. **Gorrod, J. W.,** Absorption, metabolism and excretion of drugs in geriatric subjects, *Gerontol. Clin.,* 16, 30, 1974.

18. **Goldman, R.,** Decline in organ function with aging, in *Clinical Geriatrics,* Rossman, I., Ed., J. B. Lippincott, Philadelphia, 1971, 19.

19. **Exton-Smith, A. N. and Windsor, A. C. M.,** Principles of drug treatment in the aged, in *Clinical Geriatrics,* Rossman, I., Ed., Lippincott, Philadelphia, 1971, 369.

20. **Hansen, H. H., Selawry, O. S., Holland, J. F., and McCall, C. B.,** The variability of individual tolerance to methotrexate in cancer patients, *Br. J. Cancer,* 25, 298, 1971.

21. **Davies, D. F. and Shock, N. W.,** Age changes in glomerular filtration rate, effective renal plasma flow and tubular excretory capacity in adult males, *J. Clin. Invest.,* 29, 496, 1950.

22. **Bristow, M. R., Mason, J. W., Billingham, M. E., and Daniels, J. R.,** Doxorubicin cardiomyopathy: evaluation by phonocardiography, endomyocardial biopsy and cardiac catheterization, *Ann. Intern. Med.,* 88, 168, 1978.

23. **Blum, R. H. and Carter, S. K.,** Adriamycin — a new anticancer drug with significant clinical activity, *Ann. Inter Med.,* 80, 249, 1974.

24. **Blum, R. H., Carter, S. K., and Agre, R.,** A clinical review of bleomycin — a new antineoplastic agent, *Cancer,* 31, 903, 1973.

25. **Gottlieb, J. A.,** *New Drugs and Clinical Trials in Cancer Chemotherapy,* Fundamental Concepts and Recent Advances, Yearbook Medical Publishers, Chicago, 1975, 79.

26. **Bleyer, W. A.,** Clinical pharmacology of intrathecal methotrexate II — an improved dosage regimen derived from age-related pharmacokinetics, Cancer Treatment Rep., 61, 1419, 1977.

27. **Weiss, H. D., Walker, M. D., and Wernic P.,** Neurotoxicity of commonly used antineoplastic agents, *N. Engl. J. Med.,* 291, 75, 1974.

28. **Khan, A.,** Age and asparginase side effects, *Lancet,* 1, 206, 1972.

29. **Zubrod, C. G.,** Selective toxicity of anticancer drugs: presidential address, *Cancer Res.,* 38, 4377, 1978.

30. **Henderson, E. S.,** Treatment of acute leukemia, *Sem. Hematol.,* 6, 271, 1969.

31. **Gee, T. S., Hoghbin, M., Dowling, M., Cunningham, I., Middleman, M. P., and Clarkson, B. D.,** Acute lymphoblastic leukemia in adults. Difference in response with similar therapeutic regimens, *Cancer,* 37, 1256, 1976.

32. **Gehan, E. A., Smith T. L., Freireich, E. J., Bodey, G., Rodriguez, V., Speer, J., and McCredie, K.,** Prognostic factors in acute leukemia, *Semin. Oncol.,* 3, 271, 1976.

33. **Crosby, W. H.,** To treat or not to treat acute granulocytic leukemia, *Arch. Int. Med.,* 122, 79, 1968.

34. **Ellison, R. R., Glidewell, O. J., and Holland, J. F.,** Prognostication of survival of adults with acute myelocytic leukemia (Abstract) *Proc. Am. Assoc. Cancer Res.,* 10, 22, 1969.

35. **Gunz, F. W. and Hough, R. F.,** Acute leukemia over the age of fifty, a study of its incidence and natural history, *Blood,* 11, 882, 1956.

36. **Grann, V., Erickson, R., Flannery, J., Finch, S., and Clarkson, B.,** The therapy of acute granulocytic leukemia in patients more than 50 years old, *Ann. Int. Med.,* 80, 15, 1974.

37. **Crowell, E. B., Jr., MacKinney, A. A., Pisciotta, A. V., Schloesser, L. L., and Keimovitz, R. M.,** Age and treatment response in acute non-lymphoblastic leukemia, *J. Gerontol.,* 33, 52, 1978.

38. **Matzner, Y., Benbassat, J., and Polliack, A.,** Prognostic factors and the effect of alkylating agents on survival in multiple myeloma. A review of 80 patients, *Israel J. Med. Sci.,* 13, 797, 1977.

39. **Sutcliffe, S. B., Wrigley, P. F., Peto, J., Lister, T. A., Stansfeld, A. G., Whitehouse, J. M., Crowther, D., and Malpas, J. S.,** MVPP Chemotherapy regimen for advanced Hodgkin's disease, *Br. Med. J.,* 1, 679, 1978.

40. **Bonadonna, G., Brusamolino, E., Valagussa, P., Rossi, A., Brugnatelli, L., Brambilla, C., Dehena, M., Toncini, G., Bajella, E., Musumeci, R., and Veronesi, U.,** Combination chemotherapy as an adjuvant treatment in operable breast cancer, *N. Engl. J. Med.,* 294, 405, 1976.

41. **Fisher, B., Carbone, P. Economou, S. G., Freleck, R., Glass, A., Herner, H., Redmond, C., Zelen, M., Band, P., Kabrych, D. L., Wolmark, N., and Fisher, E. R.,** L-phenylalanine mustard (L-PAM) in the management of primary breast cancer, *N. Engl. J. Med.,* 292, 117, 1975.

42. **Buckingham, R. B.,** Interactions involving cytotoxic drugs, *Bull. Rheumatic Dis.,* 28, 962, 1977.

43. **Rosenberg, J. M.,** Antineoplastic agents, interactions that really matter, *Current Prescribing,* April, 74, 1978.

Index

INDEX

A

Metoprolol, 46
  pharmacokinetics of, 7
  treatment of hypertension and, 162
Metronidazole
  adverse interactions with drugs of, 235
  renal failure and, 230
Meyer-Overton theory, of mechanisms of anesthetic
    block, 146
Miniature endplate potentials (mepp), measurement
    of, 191—192
Minoxidil, in antihypertension therapy, 57—58
Mitomycin, pharmacokinetics of, 240
Monoamine oxidase (MAO), 84
  aging and, 157
  heart and, 159
Monoamine oxidase inhibitors (MAOI), 81
Morphine, 109—110
  oral vs. parenteral administration, 110
  pharmacokinetics of, 8
Multiple myeloma, and host defense, 227
Muscle
  degeneration with age of, 187
  effects of autonomic drugs on, 176
Muscle contraction
  age-related changes in, 191
  effects of age on, 193
  measurement of, 197
Myasthenia gravis, 195
Myocardial infarction, and atherosclerosis, 67
Myocardium, in angina pectoris, 43

N

Nalidixic acid
  adverse interaction with drugs of, 235
  renal failure and, 230
Narcotic analgesics
  adverse interaction with antimicrobials of, 235
  codeine, 109
  fentanyl, 111
  meperidine, 110
  morphine, 109—110
  pentazocine, 111
National Health Examination Survey, 51
Nausea, in antiatherosclerotic therapy, 68—70
Neomycin, 231
  adverse effects of, 233
  adverse interaction with drugs of, 235
Neoplastic disease, see also Antineoplastic agents,
    239
Neostigmine, 197, 198
Nephrectomies, and antihypertension therapy, 58
Nephrotoxicity, of antimicrobial agents, 233
Netilmicin, pharmacokinetics of, 7
Neuroleptic drugs
  butyrophenones, 83
  phenothiazines, 83
  reserpine, 82—83
Neuromuscular blocking drugs

changes in effector organ sensitivity and, 194—
    195
  pharmacokinetics of, 195—198
Neuromuscular junction
  age-related changes in, 187—189
  microphysiology of, 191
Neuromuscular system, aging
  anatomy of, 187—191
  physiology of, 187—191
Neurotransmitters
  drug effects in aging brain and, 84—85
  effect of autonomic drugs on, 155—159
Niacin, double-blind trial of, 95
Nicotine
  metabolism of, 159
  transmitter content and, 168, 169
Nicotinic acid
  double-blind trial of, 94, 95
  pharmacokinetics of, 68
Nitrates, 44
  antianginal effects of, 45
  concomitant use of β-blockers with, 46
Nitrazepam, pharmacokinetics of, 7, 10
Nitrofurantoin
  adverse interaction with drugs of, 235
  renal failure and, 230
Nitroglycerin, see also Antianginal agents, 44
  antianginal effects of, 45
  side effects of, 45
Nondepolarizing compounds
  cardiotoxicity of, 197
  effectiveness of, 195
Noradrenaline, chronotropic response to, 168
Noradrenergic synapse, 79, 80
Norepinephrine (NE), 79
  aging and, 162—163, 168, 170
  blood pressure changes in aging and, 160—161
  cardiovascular sensitivity to, 161
  heart rate and, 167
  heart rate after exercise and, 165
Norepinephrine concentration, hindbrain, 158
Norepinephrine uptake, effect of nicotine on, 169
Normocytic-normochromic anemia, 219—220
Nortriptyline, double-blind trial of, 90
Nutritional anemias, 217
Nutritional deficiencies, 219

O

Opiate therapy, side effects related to, 109
Ototoxicity
  antimicrobial agents, 233
  salicylate, 118
Ouabain
  distribution of, 17
  inotropic response, 16
Oxazepam, pharmacokinetics of, 7
Oxyphenbutazone, 121
Oxyprenolol, cardiovascular sensitivity to, 162

P

Pacemaker activity, effects of lidocaine on, 25
Pain, see also Analgesics
  chronic, 118
  narcotic analgesics for, 109
Pancuronium
  elimination kinetics of, 196
  neostigmine and, 198
Papaverine, double-blind trial of, 95
Papillary muscle, digoxin concentrations in plasma
    and, 18
Para-aminosalicylic acid, adverse interaction with
    drugs of, 235
Paracetamol
  pharmacokinetics of, 8
  potential fatality of, 119
Parasympthetic agonists, actions on heart of, 171—
    173
Parasympathetic antagonists, actions on heart of,
    171—173
Parkinsonism, and process of aging, 84
Penicillin
  interaction with antineoplastic agents of, 244
  pharmacokinetics of, 7
  protein binding of, 9
  renal failure and, 230
Pentaerythritol tetranitrate, 45
Pentazocine, 111
Pentylenetetrazol
  double-blind trial of, 94, 95
  early studies of, 93
Pepsin-alcohol elixir, double-blind trial of, 94
Peptic ulcers
  aspirin in, 119
  nicotinic acid therapy and, 68
Peripheral nerves, aged, 187
Perphenazine, 89
  double-blind trial of, 87, 90, 96
  efficacy of, 86
pH, and local anesthetic block, 138—140
Pharmacogerontology, 3—4
Pharmacokinetics, equations for, 9—11
Phenacetin, 121
Phenobarbital
  interaction with antineoplastic agents of, 244
  pharmacokinetics of, 8
Phenobarbituric acid, protein binding of, 9
Phenothiazines, 83
  antihistamines of, 208
  commonly prescribed, 89
  sedative effects of, 86
Phenylbutazone
  absorption of, 121
  pharmacokinetics of, 8, 114, 117
  plasma half-life of, 122
  protein binding of, 6, 9
  volume of distribution of, 121
Phenylephrine
  cardiovascular sensitivity to, 161

dilation of pupils and, 175, 176
  effect on left ventricular performance, 166
Phenylethanolamine-*N*-methyltransferase (PNMT),
    and aging, 156—159
Phenytoin
  adverse interaction with antimicrobials of, 234—
    236
  adverse reactions to, 30
  pharmacokinetics of, 29—30
  protein binding of, 9
Phytonadione, in anticoagulant therapy, 222
Piperacetazine
  double-blind trial of, 87
  efficacy of, 86
Pipradrol, 93
Placebo
  anginal pain and, 44
  codeine vs., 109
  double-blind trials of, 87, 90, 94—96, 279
Plaques, athersclerotic, 63
Plasma concentration, peak, 7—8
Plasma expanders, in anticoagulant therapy, 222
Plasma renin activity (PRA), 52
Polymyxins, adverse interaction with drugs of, 235
Polythiazide, 53
Practolol, pharmacokinetics of, 7
Prazosin, in hypertension therapy, 52, 57
Probenecid, adverse interaction with antimicrobials
    of, 235
Probucol, in antiatherosclerotic therapy, 70
Procainamide
  adverse reactions to, 29
  pharmacokinetics of, 28—29
Procaine
  calcium action and, 140—141
  pH and local block, 139
Procarbazine
  drug interactions with, 244
  pharmacokinetics of, 241
Progeria, 120
Propicillin, pharmacokinetics of, 7
Propranolol
  adverse reactions to, 32
  antiarrhythmic effects of, 30—31
  cardiovascular sensitivity to, 161, 162
  hypertension therapy and, 52
  metabolism of, 159
  pharmacokinetics of, 7, 31
  sudden withdrawal of, 32
Prostaglandins (PGs), biosynthetic pathway of, 114
Protein, see Lipoproteins
Protein binding, 9
  aging and, 6, 215
  phenytoin, 30
  procainamide, 28
  propranolol, 31
  quinidine, 27
  verapamil, 33
Protriptyline, double-blind trial of, 96
Pruritis, in antiatherosclerotic therapy, 68